With compliments

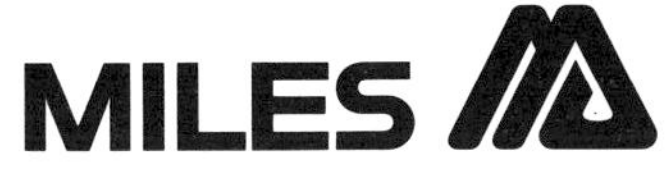

M. Bergener B. Reisberg (Eds.)

Diagnosis and Treatment of Senile Dementia

With 91 Figures and 54 Tables

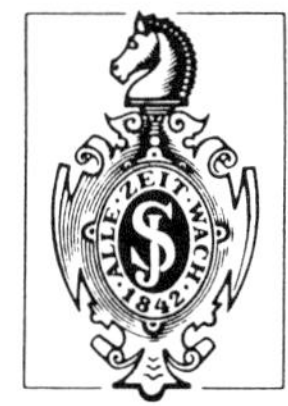

Springer-Verlag
Berlin Heidelberg New York
London Paris Tokyo

Professor Dr. med. Manfred Bergener
Rheinische Landesklinik Köln
Wilhelm-Griesinger-Straße 23
D-5000 Köln 91

Professor Barry Reisberg, M. D.
NYU Medical Center
550 First Avenue
New York, NY 10016
USA

ISBN 3-540-50800-7 Springer-Verlag Berlin Heidelberg New York
ISBN 0-387-50800-7 Springer-Verlag New York Berlin Heidelberg

Library of Congress Cataloging-in-Publication Data
Diagnosis and treatment of senile dementia / M. Bergener, B. Reisberg (eds.)
   p. cm.
  Includes index.
  ISBN 0-387-50800-7 (U.S. : alk. paper)
  1. Senile dementia. 2. Senile dementia – Chemotherapy.
3. Nimodipine – Therapeutic use. I. Bergener, Manfred.
II. Reisberg, Barry.
  [DNLM: 1. Dementia, Senile – diagnosis. 2. Dementia, Senile – drug
therapy. 3. Nimodipine – therapeutic use. WT 150 D536]
RC524.D53 1989
616.89'83 – dc20
DNLM/DLC
for Library of Congress   89-6145
                                              CIP

The use of general descriptive names, trade names, trade marks, etc. in this publication,
even if the former are not especially identified, is not to be taken as a sign that such names,
as understood by the Trade Marks and Merchandise Marks Act, may accordingly be used
freely by anyone.

Product Liability: The publisher can give no guarantee for information about drug dosage
and application thereof contained in this book. In every individual case the respective user
must chock its accuracy by consulting other pharmaceutical literature.

Printed and bookbinding: Zechnersche Buchdruckerei, 6720 Speyer
2127/3140/54321 – Printed on acid-free paper

Preface

Senile dementia is one of the major health problems confronting mankind in this century. To some extent the problem has, of course, always existed. The condition was sufficiently troubling to classical philosophers and jurists to have apparently provoked comments by Solon in approximately 500 B.C. and Plato in the fourth century B.C. (Plutarch 1967 translation; Plato 1921 translation). Medical recognition can be traced at least as far back as the second century A.D. (Adams 1861). However, several factors have converged in this century to extend the absolute dimensions of the problem of senile dementia and to increase societal, medical, and scientific recognition of the magnitude of the condition.

Perhaps the most important factor relating to the present importance of senile dementia is demographic. Although the human population has been increasing since the mid-eighteenth century, it has only been since the advent of the twentieth century that a decrease in mortality has been noted for those over the age of 45 (McKeown 1976). Consequently, the absolute number of aged persons and the proportion of increasingly aged persons in the populations of the world's industrial nations have been steadily increasing. For example, in the United States, 4% of the population was over the age of 65 in 1900. In the 1970 census, this proportion had grown to 10%. More generally, the World Health Organization notes that from 1900 to 1980 "the life expectancy in industrialized countries increased by 50%, resulting in a 20–40% increase in the number of individuals over age 65" (World Health Organization 1981). These trends are continuing and are now projected to be of increasing relevance for developing countries as well as industrialized nations (Andrews and Davidson 1984).

Epidemiologic aspects of senile dementia are discussed in this volume. Eastwood notes, however, that a review by Ineichen (1987) of 20 studies resulted in the "conservative estimate that DAT (dementia of the Alzheimer type) afflicts 1% of the population 65–74 years of age and 10% of those over age 75." Hasegawa and Imai, also in this volume, report that in Japan the prevalence rate of dementia in the community is approximately 5% of the population over age 65. This prevalence rate for senile dementia of varying etiology is similar to that which has been noted in a recent U.S. NIMH Epidemiologic Catchment Area study which indicated a prevalence of approximately 6% for senile dementia in an American community sample over age 65 (Folstein et al. 1985).

It should be noted that the true prevalence of dementia and any calculation of the burden of the disorder must incorporate information regarding the many persons with dementia in old-age institutions. The proportions of institutionalized elderly with dementia vary by nation. However, in the United States it is clear that the majority of the well over a million persons in nursing homes suffer from dementia. The best current numerical estimate of the number of persons with dementia in U. S. nursing homes would be approximately 900 000 individuals (68% of 1.3 million U. S. nursing home residents). Consequently, the incidence figures cited by Hasegawa and Imai of the NIMH Epidemiologic Catchment Area Program, revealing a prevalence rate for dementia of approximately 6% of the over 65 population in the U. S., should be adjusted to incorporate these additional 900 000 institutionalized persons with dementia for a comprehensive view of the dimensions of the problem. Such adjustments raise the true prevalence of dementia in the U. S. to perhaps 9% of the over 65 population. All community surveys of dementia prevalence should be similarly adjusted to include the enormous institutional burden of the disorder on a nation-by-nation basis. Regardless of the final numbers, it is clear that dementia is an enormous problem which afflicts a significant proportion of the world's elderly.

Dementia is also a major cause of institutionalization in the world today. For example, in the U. S., dementia afflicts the great majority of persons in long-term care facilities and approximately 40% of all persons in hospitals and other institutional settings at any given time. Dementia is also a major cause of death. The average life expectancy following the diagnosis of dementia of the Alzheimer type has been estimated to be approximately 5 years (American Psychiatric Association DSM-III 1987). Most studies show an even more rapid demise for individuals with dementia associated with cerebral infarction and/or ischemia (Molsa et al. 1986). Calculations based upon the incidence and prevalence of dementia and the time course of the disorder indicate that it is one of the leading causes of death in developed nations today. Clearly, the above statistics indicate that dementia is today a major health problem in terms of morbidity and mortality. The dimensions of the problem have been increasing as life expectancy has increased and the proportion of the elderly population has grown. Other somewhat related factors have resulted in increased societal recognition of the enormity of the problem. Perhaps the most important of these factors has been the recognition that senile dementia is the result of pathologic processes rather than "natural causes" associated with old age.

The pathogenesis of senile dementia has been a subject of continuing debate. Confounding the debate at all stages has been a tendency to confuse association with causality. More specifically, senile dementia, an age-associated disorder, has often been thought of as an entity "caused by the aging process." There have been two reasons for this continued confusion until recently. One reason is that senile dementia by definition affects mental processes, and mankind has always had great difficulty understanding mental disorders in general. Since senile dementia is an age-associated mental disorder, primarily afflicting the elderly, understanding appears to have been particularly difficult to achieve. Secondly, senile dementia is the result of pathologic processes which are most strikingly revealed upon postmortem examination. Postmortem clinical-pathologic correlation is a very difficult process which is accomplished successfully only rarely.

Consequently, it has only been in the course of this decade that the medical and scientific communities, and with them the wider lay community, have concluded that senile dementias are clearly the result of pathology associated with, but distinct from, more general aging phenomena. These pathologic processes are now widely investigated. These investigations have resulted in improved understanding of many basic aspects of dementia. In particular, there has been in this decade an explosive increase in knowledge regarding the behavioral characteristics and clinical evolution of senile dementia.

Aging patients can no longer be seen purely as a collection of symptoms and diseases nor as individuals in whom dementia or other forms of psychopathology are simply an expected part of normal aging. Accurate differentiation between behaviors that are to be expected in normal aging and maladaptive aspects of behavior amenable to modification or even change by treatment is an important goal for further inquiry. Not the isolated assessment by one specialty, but the comprehensive evaluation from the vantage point of an interdisciplinary approach, will lead, ultimately, to proper understanding.

It is essential that we recognize the importance of international activity and collaboration in psychogeriatrics. There is no one country or single school of psychiatry, neurology, psychology, genetics, biochemistry, or morphology that has developed all of the possible answers.

In dementia, all efforts are directed toward further progress in basic research. Morphology, genetics, and biochemistry together might point towards a new approach or reveal the heterogeneous etiology and pathogenesis of the disorder. In fact, it remains unsettled whether one basic disease process, at different localizations and in different stages of progression, is involved in senile as well as in presenile forms of dementia, or whether different disease processes are involved simultaneously or consecutively, leading to a steady decline in cerebral function.

While the essential role of the cholinergic system appears to be fairly well established, it remains an open question to what extent other neurotransmitter systems are also involved. More extensive clinical and also clinically based genetic investigations are necessary, and of great importance, as a basic condition for further progress.

More recently, the significance of vascular processes has been discussed with increasing intensity. Congophilic angiopathy seems to play an important role here. Assuming amyloid and congophilic substances are present, a specific dispersion pattern has been suggested. This pattern appears to affect only arterioles from the pia mater entering the cerebral cortex and terminates without exception at the cortica-medullar line.

One assumption is that the vascular complications evident in congophilic angiopathy might be attributed to perivascular atypical nuclear plaque, in the sense that permeability disturbances in arterioles and capillaries lead to an influx of a serum component, thus inducing amyloid precipitation into the nervous parenchym. Assuming that, morphologically, the central nervous system has only limited possibilities of reaction that can be made visible, a formation of vascular as well as neuronal and glial-side plaque could be a possible explanation for the observed findings.

The varying clinical progressive forms correspond to certain histomorphological dispersion patterns. So one can show that plaque dispersion and intensity in the cerebral cortex are correlated with symptoms of dementia that can be clinically differentiated. These advances are summarized in many of the contributions in this volume. Perhaps the most significant result of the improved recognition of the dimensions and importance of senile dementia and its recognition as a pathologic condition, is the widespread current belief that senile dementia is potentially amenable to treatment. Consequently, it is of note that in this decade, when promising compounds with potential central nervous system effects are introduced. These compounds are routinely investigated for efficacy in the treatment of senile dementia. This volume documents one such approach. Naturally, mankind will be well served if this approach is effective. The important message, of course, is that these and similar attempts must be repeated with disparate strategies until the devastating scourge of the senile dementias – the widespread age-associated, generalized cognitive impairments literally destroying the minds of so great a proportion of humanity – are alleviated and, ultimately, eradicated.

This volume contains papers presented by eminent scientists on the occasion of the Workshop "Diagnosis and Treatment of Senile Dementia" held in Seefeld, Austria. We would like to express our gratitude to all the contributors for their efforts not only during the symposium, but also for their helpful collaboration during the preparation of this volume.

We are also very much obliged to all those responsible at Bayer AG, Leverkusen. Without their support, it would have been impossible to bring together clinicians and scientists from around the world for this symposium.

This volume, with in its international scope, provides a comprehensive overview of current knowledge in diagnostics, prevention, and treatment of senile dementia, as well as of present research activities that are taking place across the world to illuminate the dementing processes, one of the greatest challenges of our time.

References

Adams F (ed) (1861) The extant works of Aretaens, the Cappadocian. Syndenham Society, London

American Psychiatric Association (1987) Diagnostic and statistical manual of mental disorders (3rd edn revised). American Psychiatric Association, Washington (DC), p 120

Andrews GR, Davidson AH (1984) Aging and dementia in the developing world – a challenge for the future. In: Wertheimer J and Marois M (eds) Dementia: outlook for the future. Liss, New York, pp 479–490

Folstein M, Anthony JC, Parhad I, Duffy B, Gruenberg EM (1985) The meaning of cognitive impairment in the elderly. J Am Geriatr Soc 33: 228–235

Ineichen B (1987) Measuring the rising tide: how many dementia cases will there be by 2001? Br J Psychiatry 150: 193–200

McKeown T (1976) The modern rise of population. Academic, New York

Molsa PK, Martilla RJ, Rinne UK (1986) Survival and cause of death in Alzheimer's disease and multi-infarct dementia. Acta Neurol Scand 74: 103–107

Plato (1921) The laws (ed trans.) Book IX. Manchester University Press, Manchester

Plutarch (1967) Lives (T. North, trans.). AMS, New York

World Health Organization (1981) Neuronal aging and its implications in human neuronal pathology. In: World Health Organization Technical Report Series 665, World Health Organization, Geneva

Manfred Bergener, M.D. and Barry Reisberg, M.D.

Manfred Bergener, M.D. and Barry Reisberg, M.D.

Contents

Differential Diagnosis of Dementia

Psychological Assessment of Aging and Dementia

Basic Clinical and Diagnostic Characteristics of Senile Dementia

An Approach to the Treatment of Senile Dementia: Calcium Channel Modulation

Pharmacology

Clinical Results with Nimodipine

List of Contributors

ADEM, A.
Department of Geriatric Medicine, Karolinska Institute, Huddinge Hospital B 56,
S-141 86 Huddinge

ADOLFSSON, R.
Department of Psychiatry, Umeå University, Umeå, Sweden

ALAFUZOFF, I.
Department of Pathology, Karolinska Institute, Stockholm, Sweden

ALBA, R.
Department of Psychiatry, NYU Medical Center, 550 First Avenue, New York,
NY 10016, USA

APECECHEA, M.
KFM Klinische Forschung GmbH, München, Elsenheimerstraße 41–43,
D-8000 München 21

BAUMEL, B.
Baumel-Eisner Neuromedical Institute, 1135 Kane Concourse,
Bay Harbor Islands, Miami Beach, FL 33154-2025, USA

BERGENER, M.
Rheinische Landesklinik Köln, Wilhelm-Griesinger-Straße 23,
D-5000 Köln 91

BIGORRA, J.
Qumica-Farmacéutica Bayer S.A. Calabria 268, E-08029 Barcelona

BOEHME, K.
BAYER AG, Institut für Biometrie, Aprather Weg, D-5600 Wuppertal 1

BONO, G.
Departments of Neurology and Neuroradiology, IRCCS C. Mondino,
University of Pavia, Via Palestro 3, I-27100 Pavia

BORENSTEIN, J.
Department of Psychiatry, NYU Medical Center, 550 First Avenue, New York,
NY 10016, USA

VAN BUSKIRK, R.
Department of Biology, State University of New York, Binghamton, NY 13901,
USA

COPELAND, J. R. M.
Department of Psychiatry, Royal Liverpool Hospital, P.O. Box 147,
Liverpool L69 3BX, UK

CROOK, TH. H.
Memory Assessment Clinics, Inc., 8311 Wisconsin Avenue, Bethesda, MD 20814,
USA

DANKS, A. M.
Department of Psychology, State University of New York, Binghamton,
NY 13901, USA

DAVIDSON, I. A.
Royal Liverpool Hospital, P.O. Box 147, Liverpool L69 3BX, UK

DEWEY, M. E.
Department of Psychiatry, Liverpool University, Liverpool, UK

DREWES, L. R.
Department of Biochemistry, University of Minnesota, Duluth, MN 55812, USA

DYCKA, J.
BAYER AG, Institut für Biometrie, Aprather Weg, D-5600 Wuppertal 1

EASTWOOD, M. R.
Clarke Institute of Psychiatry, 250 College Street, Toronto, Ontario M5T 1R8,
Canada

EISDORFER, C.
Department of Psychiatry, Mental Health Building, Jackson Memorial Hospital,
P.O. Box 016960, Miami, FL 33101, USA

EISNER, L. S.
Baumel-Eisner Neuromedical Institute, 1135 Kane Concourse,
Bay Harbor Islands, Miami Beach, FL 33154–2025, USA

ERZIGKEIT, H.
Psychiatrische Klinik mit Poliklinik der Universität Erlangen,
Schwabachanlage 6 und 10, D-8520 Erlangen

FAHEY, J.M.
Department of Psychology, State University of New York, Binghamton,
NY 13901, USA

FERRIS, S.H.
Department of Psychiatry, NYU Medical Center, 550 First Avenue, New York,
NY 10016, USA

FISCHHOF, P.
Psychiatrische Klinik Wien, Baumgartner Höhe, A-1090 Wien

FLICKER, C.
Department of Psychiatry, NYU Medical Center, 550 First Avenue, New York,
NY 10016, USA

FRAUSSEN, E.
Department of Psychiatry, NYU Medical Center, 550 First Avenue, New York,
NY 10016, USA

GERRITSEN VAN DER HOOP, R.
RMI, Institute of Molecular Biology, University of Utrecht, Vondellaan 6,
NL-3521 GL Utrecht

GISPEN, W.H.
RMI, Institute of Molecular Biology, University of Utrecht, Vondellaan 6,
NL-3521 GL Utrecht

GLOSSMANN, H.
Institut für Biochemische Pharmakologie der Universität Innsbruck,
Peter-Mayr-Straße 1, A-6020 Innsbruck

GOTTFRIES, C.G.
Department of Psychiatry and Neurochemistry, Gothenburg University
St. Jörgen's Hospital, S-42203 Hisings Backa

GRASSEGGER, A.
Institut für Biochemische Pharmakologie der Universität Innsbruck,
Peter-Mayr-Straße 1, A-6020 Innsbruck

GUTERMAN, A.
Department of Psychiatry, Mental Health Building, Jackson Memorial Hospital,
P.O. Box 016960, Miami, FL 33101, USA

HASEGAWA, K.
Department of Psychiatry, St. Marianna University, School of Medicine,
2–16–1 Sugao Miyamae-ku, Kawasaki 213, Japan

Hiersemenzel, R.
KFB, Klinische Forschung GmbH, Berlin, Kurfürstendamm 217,
D-1000 Berlin 15

Hoffmeister, F.
BAYER AG, PH Forschung und Entwicklung, Aprather Weg,
D-5600 Wuppertal 1

Hüppe, M.
Psychologisches Institut der Universität Würzburg, Domerschulstraße 13,
D-8700 Würzburg

Imai, Y.
Department of Psychiatry, St. Marianna University, School of Medicine,
2–16–1 Sugao Miyamae-ku, Kawasaki 213, Japan

Isaacson, R. L.
Department of Psychology, State University of New York, Binghamton,
NY 13901, USA

Janke, W.
Psychologisches Institut der Universität Würzburg, Domerschulstraße 13,
D-8700 Würzburg

Jenike, M. A.
Harvard Medical School, Massachusetts General Hospital, Bulfinch 3,
Fruit Street, Boston, MA 02114, USA

Kanowski, S.
Freie Universität Berlin, Universitätsklinikum Charlottenburg,
Abteilung für Gerontopsychiatrie, Reichsstraße 15, D-1000 Berlin 19

Karukin, M.
Baumel-Eisner Neuromedical Institute, 1135 Kane Concourse,
Bay Harbor Islands, Miami Beach, FL 33154-2025 USA

van den Kerckhoff, W.
BAYER AG, Institut für Pharmakologie, Postfach 101709,
D-5600 Wuppertal 1

Kern, U.
KFB, Klinische Forschung GmbH, Berlin, Kurfürstendamm 217,
D-1000 Berlin 15

Kluger, A.
Department of Psychiatry, NYU Medical Center, 550 First Avenue, New York,
NY 10016, USA

KNAUS, H.-G.
Institut für Biochemische Pharmakologie der Universität Innsbruck,
Peter-Mayr-Straße 1, A-6020 Innsbruck

KRANZHOFF, E. U.
Rheinische Landesklinik Köln, Wilhelm-Griesinger-Straße 23, D-5000 Köln 91

LANDFIELD, PH.
The Bowman Gray, School of Medicine, Wake Forest University, Department
of Physiology and Pharmacology, 300 South Howthorne Road, Winston-Salem,
NC 27103, USA

LÅNGSTRÖM, N.
Department of Geriatric Medicine, Karolinska Institute, Huddinge Hospital B 56,
S-14186 Huddinge

LANSKA, D. J.
Alzheimer Centes, University Hospitals of Cleveland, 2047 Abington Road,
Cleveland, Ohio 44106, USA

DE LEON, M. J.
Department of Psychiatry, NYU Medical Center, 550 First Avenue, New York,
NY 10016, USA

LITTSCHAUER, L.
Psychiatrische Klinik Wien, Baumgartner Höhe, A-1090 Wien

MacNAMARA, R.
Baumel-Eisner Neuromedical Institute, 1135 Kane Concourse,
Bay Harbor Islands, Miami Beach, FL 33541-2025, USA

MAIER, D. L.
Department of Psychology, State University of New York, Binghamton,
NY 13901, USA

MANDEL, A. H.
Department of Psychology, State University of New York, Binghamton,
NY 13901, USA

MARTELLI, A.
Departments of Neurology and Neuroradiology, IRCCS C. Mondino,
University of Pavia, Via Palestro 3, I-27100 Pavia

MAURI, M.
Departments of Neurology and Neuroradiology, IRCCS C. Mondino,
University of Pavia, Via Palestro 3, I-27100 Pavia

MCWILLIAM, C.
Leighton Hospital, Crewe, Cheshire, UK

MERLO, P.
Departments of Neurology and Neuroradiology, IRCCS C. Mondino,
University of Pavia, Via Palestro 3, I-27100 Pavia

MEYER, E.
McConnell Brain Imaging Unit, Montreal Neurological Institute,
3801 University Street, Montreal, Quebec H3A 2B4, Canada

MITTELMANN, M.
Department of Psychiatry, NYU Medical Center, 550 First Avenue, New York,
NY 10016, USA

NAPPI, G.
Departments of Neurology and Neuroradiology, IRCCS C. Mondino,
University of Pavia, Via Palestro 3, I-27100 Pavia

NEAL, C.D.
Leighton Hospital, Crewe, Cheshire, UK

NILSSON-HÅKANSSON, L.
Department of Pharmacology, Uppsala University, Uppsala, Sweden

NORDBERG, A.
Department of Geriatric Medicine, Karolinska Institute, Huddinge Hospital B 56,
S-141 86 Huddinge

PEDROMINGO, A.
Department of Biometrics, Bayer Spain, E-Barcelona

POON, L. W.
Gerontology Center, The University of Georgia, 100 Cantler Hall, Athens,
GA 30602, USA

RAMESHWAR, K.
Department of Psychiatry, NYU Medical Center, 550 First Avenue, New York,
NY 10016, USA

RAPHAN, H.
MILES Pharmaceuticals, 400 Morgan Lane, West Haven, CT 06516, USA

REISBERG, B.
Department of Psychiatry, NYU Medical Center, 550 First Avenue, New York,
NY 10016, USA

RIFAT, S. L.
Clarke Institute of Psychiatry, 250 College Street. Toronto. Ontario M5T 1R8.
Canada

RÖHMEL, J.
AFB, Arzneiforschung GmbH Berlin, Kurfürstendamm 217,
D-1000 Berlin 15

RÜTHER, E.
Zentrum Psychologische Medizin, Abteilung Psychiatrie,
Georg-August-Universität Göttingen, von-Siebold-Straße 5, D-3400 Göttingen

SCHMAGE, N.
BAYER AG, Institut für Klinische Forschung,
Aprather Weg, D-5600 Wuppertal 1

SCHMITZ, H.
BAYER AG, Institut für Biometrie, Aprather Weg, D-5600 Wuppertal 1

SCHUURMAN, T.
Troponwerke GmbH, Neurobiologische Forschung, Berliner Straße 156,
D-5000 Köln 80

SHAMOIAN, C. A.
New York Hospital-Cornell Medical Center, Westchester Division,
21 Bloomingdale Road, White Plains, NY 10605, USA

SINFORIANI, E.
Departments of Neurology and Neuroradiology, IRCCS C. Mondino,
University of Pavia, Via Palestro 3, I-27100 Pavia

STRIESSNIG, J.
Institut für Biochemische Pharmakologie der Universität Innsbruck,
Peter-Mayr-Straße 1, A-6020 Innsbruck

TABATON, M.
Department of Neurology, University of Genoa, I-16100 Genoa

TOBARES, N.
Hospital F. Primo de Rivera, c/Gabriela Mistral 6, 6-B, E-27935 Madrid

TRABER, J.
Troponwerke GmbH, Neurobiologische Forschung, Berliner Straße 156,
D-5000 Köln 80

UNNERSTALL, J. R.
Alzheimer Center Basic Research Laboratories, Case Western Reserve
University, 2074 Abington Road, Cleveland, Ohio 44106, USA

WAGNER, G.
  Psychiatrische Klinik Wien, Baumgartner Höhe, A-1090 Wien

WALLACE, B.
  Department of Psychiatry and Arthur M. Fishberg Center of Neurobiology,
  Mount Sinai School of Medicine, New York, NY, USA

WHITEHOUSE, P. J.
  Alzheimer Center, Division of Behavioral Neurology, Case Western Reserve
  University, 2047 Abington Road, Cleveland, Ohio 44106, USA

WINBLAD, B.
  Department of Geriatric Medicine, Karolinska Institute, Huddinge Hospital B 56,
  S-141 86 Huddinge

ZECH, C.
  Institut für Biochemische Pharmakologie der Universität Innsbruck,
  Peter-Mayr-Straße 1, A-6020 Innsbruck

ZERNIG, G.
  Institut für Biochemische Pharmakologie der Universität Innsbruck,
  Peter-Mayr-Straße 1, A-6020 Innsbruck

VAN DER ZEE, C. E. E. M.
  RMI, Institute of Molecular Biology, University of Utrecht, Vondellaan 6,
  NL-3521 GL Utrecht

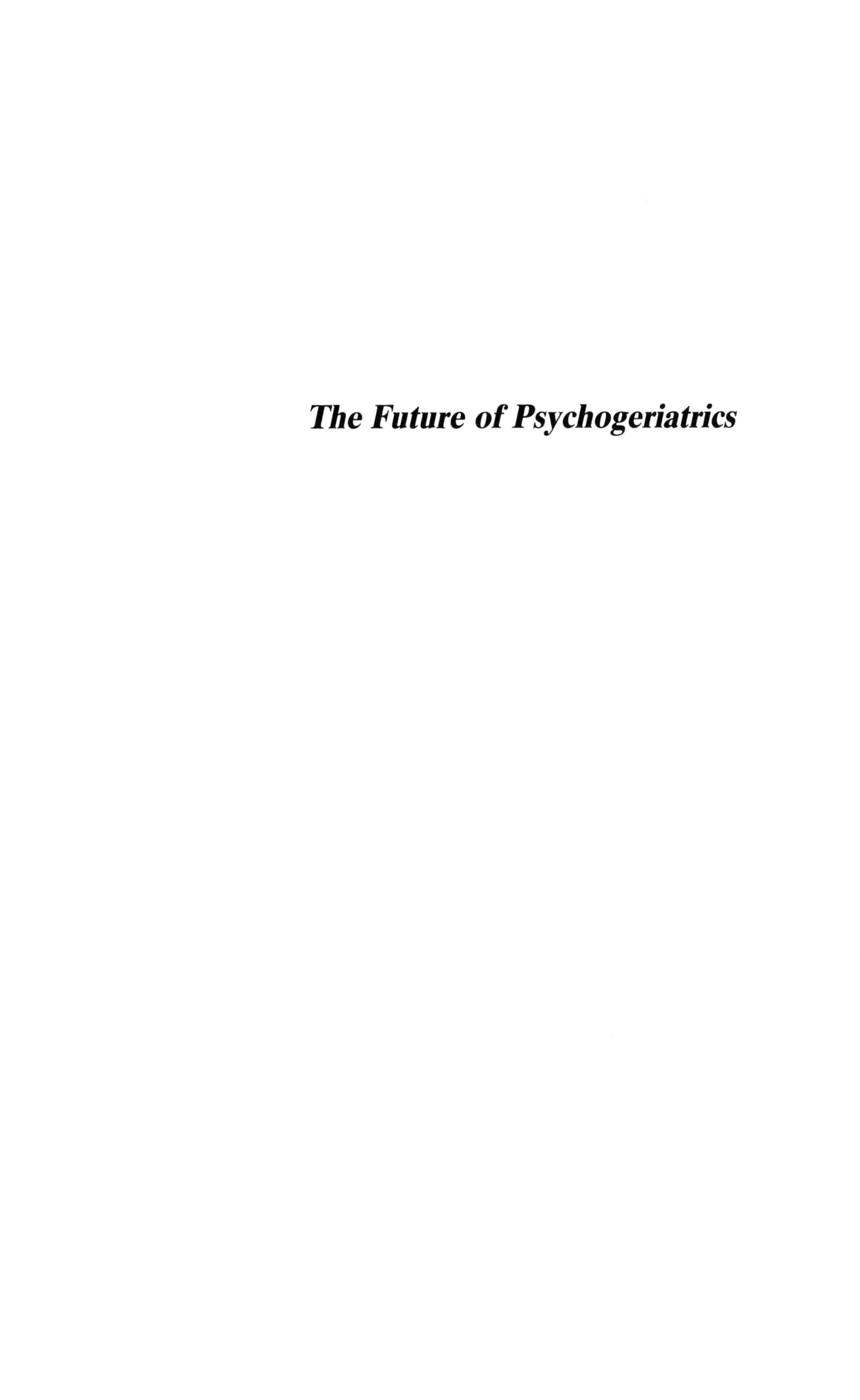

The Future of Psychogeriatrics

Future of Psychogeriatrics: A Multidisciplinary Approach with Applications for Clinical Practice

M. Bergener

Introduction

Psychogeriatrics today is to be understood as a broadly conceived psychic and pathologic science. It goes beyond the claim of being an independent, separate medical discipline and has close ties to internal medicine as well as to other medical specialties.

Distinguishing dementing processes from quantitative and qualitative cognitive changes associated with normal aging processes is one of the most important and up to now more or less unresolved problems in psychogeriatrics. Before being able to meet this requirement, we must be able to define "normal" aging processes. This is for a variety of reasons not so easy.

Empirical studies are needed that can recruit a large number of old people for their samples. But older people often suffer from somatic and/or mental impairments. If this aspect is not controlled for, it cannot be decided whether any findings of impaired performance are associated with age or with coexisting additional diseases. Furthermore, they are based mostly on data from cross-sectional studies, an approach which compares not only different age categories, but also different generations with different historical and cultural backgrounds.

Longitudinal studies have shown that intraindividual fluctuations of performance increase with age and are not infrequently more pronounced than interindividual differences. This makes it even more difficult to define standards.

Considering the characteristics of available tests and measurements for use in the elderly, it is not surprising that a patient's performance might be impaired in one study and improved on follow-up. Such difference in results can be, in the elderly more than in younger persons, much more closely related to circadian fluctuations, the weather, or other situational factors, and this can clearly reduce the reliability of a test.

For these reasons repeated assessments are needed for a differential diagnostic distinction of normal from pathological processes.

Apart from conventional test methods, we should consider especially the criterion-oriented methods which do not assess an individual's performance in comparison to his age group, but are oriented to rank order of abilities needed to cope with particular demands. Unfortunately, very few of these techniques do exist and we should welcome research in this area. A variety of psychodynamic constellations are obscured by the tangible and distinct symptoms of both functional and organic disorders.

Bergener, Reisberg (Eds.)
Diagnosis and Treatment
of Senile Dementia
© Springer-Verlag Berlin Heidelberg 1989

Interdisciplinary Foundations of Psychogeriatrics

The interdisciplinary foundations of psychogeriatrics present particular difficulties. Although in theory there is little dispute about a close relationship between psychogeriatrics, psychology and sociology, the degree of cooperation in practice between these disciplines is more or less minimal.

Interdisciplinary cooperation and multidimensional diagnostics and therapy are still in need of suitable methodologies. We observe a tendency to neglect clinical observation and decription. The extent of the consequences depends upon the structures underlying the system to be investigated. Even though fashion usually proves to be short-lived, it seems that the depreciation of descriptive clinical research has not been overcome yet. In addition, it is illusory to believe that the exclusive reliance on the forces of technology will provide substantial insight into the complex systems of concern here.

Multidimensional diagnostics as defined by E. Kretschmer (1957) should not be restricted to the itemization of each and every factor involved in the pathogenesis of an illness in like and equal manner, while at the same time doing away with overall diagnostic classification. Such an approach can present problems for a number of different reasons. For one, using the example of psychoses with mixed endogenous and organic symptoms it is evident that in multidimensional diagnoses it is easy to overestimate the relevance of cerebro-organic factors. For instance, investigators have found cerebro-organic symptoms in nearly all cases of depressive and paranoid psychoses occurring after middle age, but in hardly any psychoses of purely endogenous origin. In such cases, the diagnosis is often based on clinical findings, the pathognomonic relevance of which are ambiguous, particularly in later life, or on psychopathological characteristics and psychoexperimental investigations in which accuracy in differentiating between organic and endogenous symptoms remains a matter of dispute.

Moreover, multidimensional diagnoses can erroneously give the impression of providing insight into the structure, relationships, and relevance of pathogenetic factors. Yet such insight cannot be derived from the analysis of an individual case, but only from a comparison of large series of observations. This kind of approach rests on an unambiguous definition and description of the dependent variables, i.e., the bringing together of illnesses with similar symptoms and course into a uniform diagnostic concept.

However, these facts present us with a definite chance and challenge to adopt new methods and more suitable approaches. Immense obstacles have to be expected which can only be overcome through joint, cooperative efforts of biologists, physicians, psychologists, and sociologists. Together they could work out new approaches to current problems in research as well as in clinical practice. Expecially when dealing with depression, paranoia, psychosomatic disorders and dementia, and above all when confronted with the incurably ill and dying, the need for innovation becomes more and more obvious.

With increasing age the combination of several pathological symptoms becomes more and more likely. The resulting illness is always the result of extremely variable interferences and interactions. This is because of the complex ways in which constitutional, "endogenous", organic as well as situational, psychoreactive, and biographic factors come together to affect a particular person's psychopathological condition. The conflict situation actually experienced may, for example, in many cases not be the exclusive determining factor. More decisive in others could be the resulting responses which themselves are influenced considerably by the specific personality structure. Thus, psychological response according to personality structure, not the disease itself, is indicative.

This multifactorial etiology is a major aspect of psychic disorders in old age. Another important factor is related to the close interactions between mental and somatic diseases.

The various pathogenetic elements that are involved in the multifactorial etiology influence the individual symptoms just as they determine the course of the disease. It is frequently difficult to say which factors are important for the onset of the illness in a particular patient. In rare cases it is not even possible to make a definitive diagnosis. But in no case is one particular element alone the deciding factor.

The difficult and often decisive task in psychogeriatrics is to consider *all* the pathogenetic factors and then weigh their current relevance so that one can establish whatever therapeutic strategies are necessary. When it comes to diagnosis, importance should only be given to analyses that give *equal priority* to all findings, is still being attached to single findings. The evaluation of a single finding is just as dissatisfying for a comprehensive systematic diagnosis as is a thermometer for assessing an infectious disease.

Classification

The multiaxial classification systems, such as the *Diagnostic and Statistical Manual of Mental Disorders* (DMS-III) and the *International Classification of Diseases* (ICD 9), emphasize multifactorial etiology (Roth, 1983; Strömgren, 1983). They represent a major contribution not only in theoretical or in scientific terms, but also in clinical practice, for in addition to providing a purely descritive classification, they consider in particular physical, psychosocial, and personality factors.

Yet, however important these multiaxial systems are today, their true value will not be evident until a more systematic investigation of the relationship between the main clinical diagnostic groups and the entries on these different axes has been made in large-scale comparative studies. This is no doubt one of the most urgent tasks facing psychogeriatric research today.

The Essentials of Psychogeriatric Assessment and Diagnosis

In the following I would like to present some thoughts on functional diagnosis, or more accurately, comprehensive assessment, which in psychogeriatrics must be patient-oriented if really it should lead to adequate intervention. It is obvious that too much attention is given to the assessment of deficits. Diagnostic questions should therefore not merely be directed to discovering impairments and the extent of losses. In many cases the search would be positive, but important information would be lost with such a purely psychopathometric analysis. Instead, we should also be asking what abilities and capacities are intact and where are previously little used or unused resources to compensate for the illness-associated deficits.

This kind of extended diagnosis is an assessment which should not just include abnormal and pathological changes. The goal is to tap all available sources of information to give the most comprehensive picture of the patient's abilities as possible. No selection takes place; everything is of interest. Of course, we are interested in deficiency areas, but the search for intact functions and for potential resources and skills is just as relevant.

Psychologists have approached the problems of measuring cognitive decline in a number of ways and with varying success. One such attempt has been to devise a definitive diagnostic test which helps the clinician to differentiate between dementia and, for example, depression complicated by cognitive impairment. Miller (1977) has suggested that this search is akin to the medieval alchemist's search for the philosopher's stone and with as little likelihood for success. His prophecy has been largely fulfilled, for tests initially regarded as definitive have generally failed to cope with the surely impossible task of identifying a condition like dementia which varies in severity and affects patients of widely varying premorbid personalities (Blessed 1985).

This by no means says, however, that psychopathology has lost its importance when it comes to gathering information about psychoses in old age. Despite the fact that clinical diagnostics has increasingly shifted its emphasis to neurological and neuro-physiological techniques and objective general medical methods, a number of psychopathological studies have still been carried out in recent years, making a closer differentiation of psychoorganic syndromes possible and thus bringing to light some aspects of psychogeriatric illnesses which had previously been neglected. I should like to mention two such approaches, namely, the structural analytic and the psychometric approach. Note that the term "structural analysis" is used here not in the sense of an insight into the complex structure of pathogenetic factors, but should be seen rather as an attempt to understand the interactions between symptoms and their interconnection, to trace the countless performance deficits back to common elementary disorders and to recognize the relationships of the complex organic brain syndrome and the different environmental situations. The advantage of such a structural analysis is that it contributes to a better understanding and a clearer differentiation of psychoorganic syndromes by demonstrating the difference between epiphenomena that appear to have a similar structure, e. g., memory disturbances in senile dementia and Alzheimer's disease or the internal relationship between psychopathological symptoms that appear at first glance to be unrelated. Examples of such symptom aggregates that deserve closer study are the interactions that can exist between the amnestic psychosyndrome and organic dysfunctions (aphasias, apraxias, agnosias) and between the latter and psychomotor and motor disorders. Much has been neglected in this respect in dementia research of recent years.

Rating scales can, of course, present problems. They can lend an illusion of scientific accuracy which can be quite misleading. To be useful, they must first be valid; they must measure symptoms of real relevance for the disorder under examination. Nevertheless, rating scales have made a real contribution to the assessment of mentally ill old people. They can correct misconceptions; on the other hand, they cannot take the place of comprehensive clinical investigations. The growing number of rating scales is more a problem here than a solution. The question is how to use which scale and when.

Many of the psychometric methods available today suffer from the fact that their validity is still disputed, that they are not accurate enough when it comes to detecting milder forms of organic brain syndrome, and that they can no longer be used in advanced stages of organic psychoses in later life. Another disadvantage is that they can never portray the organic deficits to their full extent, but either measure only individual functions or represent the qualitative structure of intellectual degeneration as far as the given composition of the battery of tests allows. Yet in the long run, reliable results can only come from a multidimensional analysis of performance and behaviour, which uses psychometric methods to arrive at a uniform record of as many disturbances as possible and thus fulfills the conditions for the application of correlative statistical methods.

It is easy to see that the result cannot at the same time be the psychogeriatric diagnosis. In any case we need both, assessment and diagnosis. While a premature psychogeriatric diagnosis may hide the danger of neglecting assets of the person relevant for treatment planning, the comprehensive assessment should provide a more adequate picture of the patient's overall functioning at one or more particular times.

Preparing recommendations in this important field of clinical research and practice could be one of the most significant tasks of international and interdisciplinary cooperation in psychogeriatrics, defined, for example, as one of the goals of the International Psychogeriatric Association.

Research of Evaluation and Efficiency – More than Research Tactics

The request to offer more and better services to the elderly will be increasing in the years to come. Not only the larger number of older people, but especially the growing demands will result in problems that in all likelihood will exceed the existing dimensions by far (Arie 1983; Vladeck 1988; Williamson 1988). In the fields of gerontology and geriatrics diagnosis and therapy of old age infirmities have essentially improved. In particular strategies, overlapping of the borders of conventional disciplines has played a major role. However, we need clear, worldwide accepted concepts in order to ensure care for the increasing number of sick old people.

Although first efforts can be recognized and guidelines have been formulated, the ineffectiveness of traditional care systems has become more and more obvious. Outdated and poorly organized care structures with deficiencies in quantity and quality in the medical as well as the social fields prevent the use of efficient methods in treatment and care. Only a drastic turn in curative medicine can lead us out of the dead-end street – a change turning the present organization of public health services upside down – thereby moving the emphasis from inpatient treatment to prevention and outpatient services. Before the still prevalent and obligatory care structures in medicine have been discarded no fundamental change can be achieved, nor will it be possible to really change our attitude and views towards these issues.

In order to meet our goals, investigations in the areas of efficiency of care and evaluation will be of increasing importance (Bergener et al. 1986; Bergener and

Kranzhoff 1989). Positive results of any decisions depend upon the extent of systematic research into the further development of geriatric care systems. Again and again, we have to be aware of the danger that strategic research might turn into tactical research. Therefore we are forced to walk a tightrope. Only a high degree of objectivity will lead to success.

Bearing in mind the multimorbidity of old age, early diagnosis and treatment of diseases of old age has to be made on the basis of multidisciplinary activities. Different presentations of diseases are usually caused by the coexistence of infirmities, and each kind of disability calls for a different kind of intervention. Furthermore, the inteference of somatic and psychic elements makes the situation all the worse.

We have to make every effort to ensure that the demand for multidimensional diagnosis does not remain an empty shell. In the development of instruments for investigations, unexpected difficulties which are not merely induced by methods, or which may be deduced from the complexity of the object to be investigated, repeatedly come up. In many ways they are the consequence of the investigator's traditional self-image.

Therefore, the search for interdisciplinary cooperation still meets with considerable reservation. This is a serious obstacle and prevents the progress absolutely essential to making old age more than just a kind of appendix, but years full of life. This guideline was formulated by the American Society of Gerontology many years ago. Yet its requirements have still not been accomplished in many fields of gerontology. This is the heavy burden that everybody concerned bears, yet it represents the challenge which is the object of our discussions.

Pharmacologic and Psychopharmacologic Research

Experimental strategies in clinical-pharmacological as well as pharmacopsychological research have not yet led to success as expected. Nonhomogeneous and, in some cases, even inconsistent research, illustrate the dilemma. Where as some groups regard experimental design as indispensible, other groups view this as having sacrificed pharmacopsychology to the general principle that the efficacy of a drug can be proven when simultaneously an actual need for efficacy exists. Up to now, no studies have been undertaken to examine to what extent the measurement of drug efficacy may be biased by the measuring technique, that is, that the instrument influences the object to be measured (Gebert et al. 1983). Supposedly, the effects of experimental design change the results of testing drug efficacy. Under certain adverse conditions these results may even be terminated or simulated. Systematic investigation of these issues still has to be carried out in order to answer this questions.

Multidimensional measurements must be regarded as indispensible for future pharmacopsychiatric and pharmacopsychological research – multivariate not only in the employment of different psychological measurement techniques, above all, multidimensional through inclusion of psychic, physiological, and/or biochemical measurements. Arising discrepancies should be given special attention as they give an indication of the effects of each technique.

Another problem still remains unsolved: The multivariable techniques employed in therapy research are impracticable for clinics since they require more patients than usually are available. Bearing in mind the numerous illnesses (multimorbidity) and the variablity of symptoms (polysymptomatology) in old age, we have to confront this problem to ensure that the subgroups of patients we work with show homogeneous symptoms. It becomes even more difficult to form homogeneous subgroups when diagnostic criteria are not compatible. Today, the use of objective measuring methods – standardizing and validated investigation techniques – has not been generally acknowledged. Long-term studies employing extensive multivariate methods do require cooperation within a multicenter environment of preferably international dimensions and a considerable investment of time and money.

One of the most important aims of such joint activities is to define rational therapeutic practice, taking into account the large range of climatic and social realities. This kind of research work should not fail for financial reasons. Otherwise, I am afraid, we will not be able to gain public support for the steadily growing amount of new drugs for the aged. Even though in many places more or less expensive projects are carried out, without worldwide therapy research, issues of national concern, such as efficacy, cannot be settled.

In psychogeriatrics the problems in therapy research are particularly serious. The use of psychometric techniques is beset with difficulties arising from interaction between psychic and somatic phenomena. However, the main difficulty is caused by the special kind of psychic symptoms which evade any standardized diagnosis through testing. Although not sufficient, a fundamentally new methodology of examination and measurement is a prerequisite. In this respect clinical psychophysiology will obtain particular importance as it is defined as a multidimensional science with the objective of revealing the multivariate relationship between both physiological parameters and psychic processes – that is to say, psychopathological syndromes.

During the aging process the probability increases that pathologic symptoms acquired earlier in life will come together, thus leading to a reduction of parenchymatous activities in various organs and organ systems (Hesse and O'Malley 1987). In this way, the general ability to adapt and to compensate is increasingly reduced. Even more important is the interaction between age and disease such that it may be rather difficult, if not impossible, to distinguish the beginning of an illness from the process of normal physiological aging.

Bearing such considerations in mind, it would appear that initial steps in gerontopharmacology are recognizable. Nevertheless, a methodology for investigation is required in which biological, clinical, psychological, and psychophysiological aspects are equally taken into account. In this respect therapy research is an example of interdisciplinary strategies that have impact on basic research as well as on clinical practice.

In patients with cognitive dysfunctions the need for new and better drugs poses particular problems. Since it is often impossible to obtain informed consent, it is important to assess the risk: benefit ratio thoroughly in advance. On the other hand, only through better knowledge in psychogeriatric medicine in general will it be possible to achieve a more efficient, careful, and restricted use of drugs. This urgent research, and the training of the necessary personnel, are high-priority tasks in psychogeriatrics. In assessing the risk and the benefit of drug research one must also consider in advance the character of the study under consideration as either a therpeutic or a nontherapeutic study and also whether the subjects participating might benefit from the study or not.

With more knowledge about the use of drugs, they will probably be used more carefully and restrictedly, but probably also more efficiently (Gottfries and Hesse 1989). For the evaluation of drug therapy, therefore, more parameters broader in range have to be assessed and compared, e. g., as in the research work of the Cologne group. This prerequisite leads in a first phase to the development of a research strategy with very complex experimental studies. In a second phase, these complex settings have to be evaluated and simplified as far as possible. This is all the more necessary since the great number of parameters assessed will make it necessary to include a great number of patients in the study, and therefore, problems in data management and data interpretation can arise. It must, however, be stressed that the development of simple plans has to go through the stage of complex research concepts.

More progress brings more risks – risks that come into existence as a consequence of continuous technical involvement in medicine ("high tech" medicine), as well as a consequence of more effective drugs. To be sure, pharmacotherapy will, in the future, retain its functional importance only if it satisfies the common standards of ethics and reliability. Correct medical treatment cannot be proven by success alone. As we all know, a sick person can be cured because, or in spite of treatment, just by accident, or due to his or her belief in a recovery.

Any of these interpretations is possible. And also, the fact that recovery has been predicted does not necessarily mean that the answer to the question – either the diagnosis or the treatment – has been correct.

Research in Dementia – A Predominantly Interdisciplinary Task

The clinical term "dementia" has a long and changing pathography. The notion of dementia as a disease by itself can no longer be sustained. On the contrary, we have to deal with a pathologically defined syndrome that can be reversible as well as irreversible, independent of the respective basic disease. The specific difficulty of clinical diagnosis is that the psychopathological findings alone do not permit conclusions to be drawn about the basic disease.

In dementia research, all efforts are more or less directed toward further progress in basic research, but that is not enough. Only morphological, genetic, biochemical, *and clinical investigations together* might be able to find a new approach which will reveal the heterogeneous etiology and pathogenesis. Still, there is a lack of clarity about the pathopsychological alterations leading to dementia which is not only restricted to the subcellular and biochemical field. Now, as before, it is unclear whether only gradual degrees and different localizations of one basic disease are concerned or whether different processes are involved, leading to a continuous general cerebral disorganization (Bergener and Hesse 1987).

It should not be left unsaid that the age of the patient does not represent a dinstinction between the various forms of dementia, rather age modifies the presentation of a dementing process in different stages of life.

It is possible that the forms of dementia described by Alzheimer are based on different classifiable processes, leading via metabolic defects in protein synthesis, to vascular wall alterations with changing intensity and clear variation and with well-discernible histotopographic dispersion patterns. If these correspond to different clinical courses, the correspondence still has to be clarified and not only because of the therapeutic consequences. Undoubtedly, age influences many basic processes; this, however, does not mean that age by itself is a causal component (Bergener 1983). I hope that future research will lead to a fundamentally new classification of organic brain processes, not only in old age.

Research in dementia is another field of psychogeriatric medicine requiring world-wide interest. Great efforts have been and still are being made to illuminate the darkness. Vast numbers of single investigations have led to results which are not at all satisfactory (Meier-Ruge 1987; Gottfries 1986; Winblad et al. 1986). Now, as before, the nosologic entity of the Alzheimer syndrome and other types of dementia have not become clear yet, essential problems of case identification still remain unsolved.

All the findings described in the last 20 years agree that Alzheimer's disease cannot be seen as a single nosological unit, but that it is more likely a common final pathway of various pathological processes, the different causes of which have not yet been found. We are trying to understand what Alzheimer's disease is; a number of different branches of science provide us with bits of knowledge. But so far they resemble pieces from different puzzles. It is vital that interdisciplinary research approaches now piece the knowledge from Alzheimer research together to form an overall picture. This is the only way of finally solving the puzzle of Alzheimer's disease. What is necessary now is to find the "optic chiasm" (Helander 1983) in Alzheimer research.

In the future, clinical research will once more play an important role in attaining this goal. We must find strategies for real interdisciplinary cooperation. We must also find the necessary instruments and methods of diagnosing Alzheimer's disease in its earlier stages, at a point when treatment can at least be expected to ameliorate or even cure the symptoms. But diagnosis of the initial stages of the disease still proves to be an almost insurmountable obstacle. Promising approaches were adopted at the beginning of the 1980s (Reisberg 1985).

Yet all this is not enough as long as we do not know how Alzheimer's disease becomes manifest. Are the psychopathological signs indeed the first symptoms of the disease? Or are these to be found in another organic system outside the brain? Before these and other questions can be answered it is important to develop clinical investigative methods that will open new paths in clinical diagnostics.

At this point we can repeat the conclusions drawn by Alois Alzheimer in his original article in 1907:

Alles in allem genommen haben wir hier offenbar einen eigenartigen Krankheitsprozeß vor uns. Solche eigenartigen Krankheitsprozesse haben sich in den letzten Jahren in größerer Anzahl feststellen lassen. Diese Beobachtung wird uns nahe legen müssen, daß wir uns nicht damit zufrieden geben sollen, irgend einen klinisch unklaren Krankheitsfall in eine der uns bekannten Krankheitsgruppen unter Aufwendung von allerlei Mühe unterzubringen. Es gibt ganz zweifellos viel mehr psychische Krankheiten, als sie unsere Lehrbücher aufführen. In manchen solchen Fällen wird dann eine spätere histologische Untersuchung die Besonderheit des Falles feststellen lassen. Dann werden wir aber auch allmählich dazu kommen, von den großen Krankheitsgruppen unserer Lehrbücher einzelne Krankheiten klinisch abzuscheiden und jene selbst klinisch schärfer zu umgrenzen.*

---

* All things considered we are obviously dealing with a peculiar disease process in its own right. In recent years, many more such peculiar disease processes have been noticed. This observation should suggest to us that we should not be content to painstakingly force clinically unclear observations into one of the disease categories familiar to us. Without a doubt, there are many more psychiatric illnesses than those listed in our textbooks. In some instances the uniqueness of the case will be revealed by subsequent histological examination. Then we will gradually arrive at the stage where we will be able to separate individual diseases from larger textbook categories and provide a more precise clinical definition.
Translation: B. Vollhardt, M. D., Cologne

Conclusion

Mental breakdown in old age is characterized by clinically recognizable patterns of disorder. The major varieties were described in the beginnings of psychiatry as a science more than 50 years ago. Some of these clinical syndromes respond to treatment and it follows that accurate diagnosis is essential. When a disorder is complicated by disability, then an estimate of the severity of this disability, how it progresses over time, and responds to treatment, forms an important part of the clinical evaluation. On the other hand, psychogeriatrics has often to deal with changes that are difficult to influence or are indeed beyond repair. For those of us working in this field it is important that we offer our patients something more than just a promise of cure that we are unable to keep. Many of them have to do without something that they need to function normally. We can help to make use of other skills which were undeveloped before. A diagnostic method that looks only at deficits and has been designed from a psychopathometric point of view cannot do enough in this respect. To be sure, a turn about here will be one of the major issues for future research in psychogeriatrics. It is a big task and a great challenge and one we should accept!

Let us work to fulfill the requirements of this challenge with all our strength and abilities, with the courage to set our feet on new grounds. Let us accept criticism and opposition as well as set-backs. Let us avoid resignation when expectations and hopes are replaced by disillusion. Let us face the challenge with all our courage to take the chance.

References

Alzheimer A (1907) Über eine eigenartige Erkrankung der Hirnrinde. Allg Zschr Psychiat 64: 146–148

Arie THD (1983) Organization of services for the elderly: implications for education and patient care – experience in Nottingham. In: Bergener M (ed) Geropsychiatric dignostics and treatment. Springer Publishing, New York, pp 189–195

Bergener M (1983) Etiology, pathogenesis, and classification of senile and presenile dementias. In: Bergener M (ed) Geropsychiatric diagnostics and treatment. Springer Publishing, New York, pp 77–83

Bergener M, Kranzhoff EU, Husser J (1986) Contributions to a multi-level model of intervention in psychogeriatrics. In: Bergener M, Ermini M, Stähelin HB (eds) Academic, London, pp 263–291

Bergener M, Hesse C (1987) Research on Alzheimer's disease in German-speaking countries, Alzheimer Dis Assoc Disorders 1: 193–199

Bergener M, Kranzhoff EU (1989) Evaluating psychogeriatric treatment. Springer Publishing, New York

Blessed G (1985) Measurement in psychogeriatrics. In: Arie THD (ed) Recent advances in psychogeriatrics, vol I. Churchill Livingstone, Edinburgh, pp 141–159

Gebert A, Kohnen R, Lienert GA (1983) A methodological contribution to multivariate geronto-psychology. In: Bergener M (ed) Geropsychiatric diagnostics and treatment. Springer Publishing, New York, pp 144–152

Gottfries CG (1986) Nosological aspects of differential typology of dementia of Alzheimer type. In: Bergener M, Ermini M, Stähelin HB (eds) Dimensions in aging, Academic, London, pp 207–217

Gottfries CG, Hesse C (1989) Pharmacotherapy in psychogeriatrics – an update. In: Bergener M, Finkel SI (eds) Clinical and scientific psychogeriatrics. Springer Publishing, New York

Helander J (1983) Multidimensional aspects of aging: Psychology. In: Bergener M (ed) Geropsychiatric diagnostics and treatment. Springer Publishing, New York, pp 12–23

Hesse C, O'Malley K (1987) Drug therapy in the elderly-biochemical, pharmacological, and clinical considerations. In: Bergener M (ed) Psychogeriatrics – an international handbook. Springer Publishing, New York, pp 362–376

Kretschmer E (1957) Die mehrdimensionale Struktur der Schizophrenie mit Bezug auf ihre Psychotherapie. Z Psychother 7: 387–394

Meier-Ruge W (1985) Neurochemistry of the aging brain and senile dementia. In: Gaitz CM, Samorajski T (eds) Ageing 2000, Vol I. Springer, Berlin Heidelberg New York Tokyo, pp 101–112

Miller E (1977) Abnormal ageing: the Psychology of senile and presenile dementia. Wiley, New York

Reisberg B (1985) A guide to Alzheimer's disease (revised edn) Free Press, MacMillan, New York

Roth M (1983) Multidimensional diagnostics in gerontopsychiatry. In: Bergener M (ed) Geropsychiatric diagnostics and treatment. Springer Publishing, New York, pp 125–138

Strömgren E (1983) Methodological considerations on the design of longitudinal studies. In: Bergener M (ed) Geropsychiatric diagnostics and treatment. Springer Publishing, New York, pp 165–172

Vladeck BC (1988) Hospitals, the elderly, and comprehensive care. In: Eisdorfer C, Maddox GL (eds) The role of hospitals in geriatric care. Springer Publishing, New York, pp 35–48

Williamson J (1988) The distinctive role of the hospital in the care of the elderly in the United Kingdom. In: Eisdorfer C, Maddox GL (eds) The role of hospitals in geriatric care. Springer Publishing, New York, pp 49–81

Winblad B, Wallace W, Hardy J, Fowler C, Bucht G, Alafuzoff J, Adolfsson R (1986) Neurochemical, genetic and clinical aspects of Alzheimer's disease. In: Bergener M, Ermini M, Stähelin HB (eds) Dimensions in aging. Academic, London, pp 183–203

An Overview: Current Knowledge and Needs

What is New and what is Necessary in Dementia Research?

C. A. SHAMOIAN

Our knowledge of dementias and specifically of the dementia of the Alzheimer's type (DAT) has, since the 1950s, increased exponentially. During the past 30 years the focus of research has shifted progressively from initial studies of the incidence and prevalence of DAT, to more sophisticated diagnostic and therapeutic investigations. These have included the study of not only the neurochemical abnormalities, but also of the role of central nervous system (CNS), neurohormones, neurotransmitters, and receptors in the etiology, biology, and treatment of DAT [20]. However, the understanding of abnormal changes requires a knowledge of normal brain aging. In a recent abstract, Khachaturian [12] noted that:

> At present, the process of normal brain aging is relatively poorly understood. There exist no consistent established biological markers for what consttutes "normal" cognitive impairment and memory loss with advancing years nor are the neurophysiological or the anatomical alterations that accompany normal aging well enough understood to provide a firm base for determining "abnormal" changes.

Thus one of the major needs of this area of scientific endeavor is to clearly establish, especially at the first signs of a cognitive change, what is considered "normal" or "abnormal." Currently this can only be accomplished retrospectively or by following the course of the individual longitudinally.

The rate of advancement of knowledge in this area of study is determined in part by the development and applications of new technology. Examples of this include positron emission tomography (PET) and magnetic resonance imaging (MRI) in the study of both normal and abnormal brain structure and function [5, 11, 24]. Likewise the development and application of sophisticated immunological techniques has advanced the understanding of specific CNS receptors and the probing of genetic markers [16–18].

The use of in vitro methods utilizing extra neural tissues, including red blood cells, granulocytes, lymphocytes, platelets, and fibroblasts, has led to the interesting and provocative hypothesis that DAT is not an illness restricted to the CNS, but that "at the cellular or molecular level, this disease may be systemic" [3, 10]. The importance of this hypothesis is in the potential of studying DAT at various stages by using easily obtained peripheral tissues. A recent study by Baker et al. [1] utilizing cultured skin fibroblasts from DAT patients emphasizes this point. All DAT cells, in appropriate in vitro conditions, stained for paired helical filaments whereas none of the control cells manifested this property [1]. These findings support the hypothesis that DAT may be a systemic illness and provide the basis for a diagnostically important test [1, 3].

Bergener, Reisberg (Eds.)
Diagnosis and Treatment
of Senile Dementia
© Springer-Verlag Berlin Heidelberg 1989

Should these findings be replicated, a critical laboratory test would be available to confirm a clinical diagnosis of DAT which, even to the present day, in the early stages of the illness is difficult to make with any degree of accuracy and confidence. A critical need exists for a biological marker sufficiently sensitive and specific to DAT to assist in making or confirming the diagnosis in the early stages of the illness. Of importance is the study of Davies et al. [23], who identified in the brains of patients with Alzheimer's disease a protein (Alz 50), virtually restricted to neurons involved in the formation of plaques and neurofibrillar tangles. Alz 50 has been detected in cerebrospinal fluid of DAT patients and not normals, has been found in both familial and sporadic cases of DAT, and has been suggested as a precursor to tangle formation [7]. Although this potential biological marker and other promising candidates, such as the cultured skin fibroblast test, require additional studies, this approach to the study of DAT is indeed exciting and promising.

Many studies of the biology and therapeutics of DAT have included not only patients of differing degress of severity of illness but also familial and sporadic cases. These uncontrolled variables may account, in part, for the conflicting and equivocal data in the literature. To minimize these effects, one approach is to utilize longitudinally a validated clinical staging of DAT such as reported by Reisberg [14]. Just as important is the identification of biochemical subtypes of DAT [4, 15]. Deficiencies of neurotransmitters other than acetylcholine, have been reported and may depend upon the age of the DAT patient. Thus studies utilizing clinical staging and biochemical subtypes of DAT may lead to a less equivocal understanding of the efficacy of various therapeutic drugs. Also the need to study familial and sporadic cases separately bears on this issue. The biology, and possibly, the pharmacotherapy of the two may be quite distinct. Of great clinical importance have been the recent studies reporting the localization of a genetic defect on chromosome 21 in the familial cases of Alzheimer's disease [16]. Also the gene coding for β amyloid peptide has been localized to chromosome 21. This protein is found in different tissues of various species, suggesting that it has been conserved throughout the evolutionary process [17].

The findings of these studies raise a number of important research issues, which, to mention just a few, include: Is the gene which causes familial DAT identical to the one for the β amyloid peptide? What is the "normal" role of β amyloid peptide, and what regulatory mechanisms fail, resulting in its "abnormal" role? What is the "normal" role of the Alzheimer's gene, and what regulatory mechanisms fail, resulting in the manifestation of the disease? Now that familial and sporadic cases can be clearly differentiated, are the biology and therapeutics of the familial type different from those of the sporadic cases? These are research issues for the coming years.

The pharmacological treatment of DAT cognitive deficits have used the traditional neuronal synaptic model, with the majority of therapeutic trials focusing on the acetylcholinergic system [6]. Of the more recent promising drugs, tetrahydroamino acridine (THA), a cholinesterase inhibitor, has been the center of controversy and is currently undergoing a multicenter study [19]. The data from these trial studies are currently not available. THA is structurally similar to 4-aminopyridine which is known to enhance calcium influx. 4-Aminopyrodine has been reported as having a minimal therapeutic effect on cognitive functions of Alzheimer's patients [21]. To be emphasized is that a calcium deficiency has been reported in a number of diseases in which plaques and neurofibrillar tangles are common, including parkinsonian dementia of Guam, amyotrophic lateral sclerosis, and Down's syndrome [2, 8]. Peterson et al. [13] reported a decreased calcium uptake by cultured skin fibroblasts from patients with Alzheimer's disease. From similar studies, Gibson et al. [9] have concluded that:

> It sccms possible that there is a subgroup of demented patients who have a generalized, perhaps, genetically determined, abnormality in cellular calcium homeostasis. Although the deficit may be too subtle to be clinically significant in non-neural tissues; by the latter part of the life span, it may be capable of leading to the premature death of particular populations of neurons.

Supporting a role for calcium in Alzheimer's disease, a recent report suggested that brain calcium channels in patients with Alzheimer's disease are different from controls and hypothesized an abnormal CNS calcium metabolism in the disease [22]. Based on such studies and the accumulating data on the role of calcium and second messengers in the acquisition of memory, the study of drugs modulating calcium channel activity may be a fruitful approach to the pharmacological treatment of DAT.

References

1. Baker AC, Ko LW, Young O et al. (1988) Studies of "neuronal" and "Alzheimer" antiqens in skin cells. Alzh Dis Assoc Dis Int J 2: 178
2. Barlow PJ, Sylvester PE, Dickerson JWT (1981) Hair trace metal levels in Down syndrome patients. J Ment Defic Res 25: 161–169
3. Blass JP, Hanin I, Barclay L et al. (1985) Red blood cell abnormalities in Alzheimer disease. J Am Geriatr Soc 33: 401–405
4. Bondareff W, Mountjoy CQ, Roth M (1982) Loss of neurons of origin of the adrenergic projection to cerebral cortex (nucleus locus coeruleus) in senile dementia. Neurology 32: 164–168
5. Chase TN, Foster NL, Fedio P et al. (1984) Regional cortical dysfunction in Alzheimer's disease as determined by positron emission tomography. Ann Neurol 15 (Suppl): 5170–5174
6. Davies P (1985) Is it possible to design rational treatments for the symptoms of Alzheimer's disease? Drug Dev Res 5: 69–76
7. Finch C (1987) Biochemical markers in the diagnosis of the dementias. NIH Consensus Development Conference-differential diagnosis of dementing diseases (Program and Abstracts). pp 87–91
8. Gajdusek DC (1985) Hypothesis: interference with axonal transport of neurofilament as a common pathogenic mechanism in certain diseases of the central nervous system. N Engl J Med 312: 714–719
9. Gibson GE, Nielsen P, Sherman KA, Blass JP (1987) Diminished mitogen-induced calcium uptake by lymphocytes from Alzheimer patients. Biol Psychiatry 22: 1079–1086
10. Gibson GE, Sheu KR, Blass JP et al. (1988) Reduced activities of thiamine-dependent enzymes in the brains and peripheral tissues of patients with Alzheimer's disease. Arch Neurol 45: 836–840
11. Johnson KA, Mueller S, Walshe TM et al. (1987) Cerebral perfusion imaging in Alzheimer disease-use of single photon emission computed tomography and iofetamine hydrochloride I 123. Arch Neurol 44: 165–168
12. Khachaturian ZS (1988) The future of Alzheimer's disease research, Alzh Dis Assoc Dis Int J 2: 154
13. Peterson C, Gibson GE, Blass JP (1985) Altered calcium uptake in cultured skin fibroblasts from patients with Alzheimer's disease. N Engl J Med 312: 1063–1065

14. Reisberg B (1986) Dementia: a systematic approach to identifying reversible causes. Geriatrics 41: 30–46
15. Rossor MN, Iversen LL, Reynolds GP, Mountjoy CQ; et al. (1984) Neurochemical characteristics of early and late onset types of Alzheimer's disease. Br Med J 288: 961–964
16. St George-Hyslop PH, Tanzi RE, Polinsky RJ et al. (1987) The genetic defect causing familial Alzheimer's disease maps on chromosome 21. Science 235: 885–890
17. Selkoe DJ, Bell DS, Podlisny MB (1987) Conservation of brain amyloid proteins in aged mammals and humans with Alzheimer's disease. Science 235: 873–877
18. Sheu KF, Kim YT, Blass JP et al. (1985) An immunochemical study of the pyruvate dehydrogenase deficit in Alzheimer's disease brain. Ann Neurol 17: 444–449
19. Summers WK, Majovski LV, Marsh GM et al. (1986) Oral tetrahydroamino acridine in long term treatment of senile dementia, Alzheimer's type. Science 315: 1241–1245
20. Thienhaus OJ, Hartford JT, Skelly MF, Bosmann HB (1985) Biologic markers in Alzheimer's disease. J Am Geriatr Soc 33: 715–726
21. Wesseling H, Agoston S, Van Dam GBP et al. (1984) Effects of 4-aminopyridine in elderly patients with Alzheimer's disease. N Engl J Med 310: 988–989
22. Williams RG, Oibo JA, Ibok I et al. (1988) Brain calcium channel binding sites – Alzheimer's disease and controls. Alz Dis Assoc Dis Int J 2: 246
23. Wolozin BL, Pruchnicki A, Dickson DW, Davies P (1986) A neural antigen in the brains of Alzheimer's patients. Science 232: 648–650
24. Zoler ML (1986) Alzheimer's disease: new imaging techniques show diagnostic promise. J Geriatr 41: 91–94

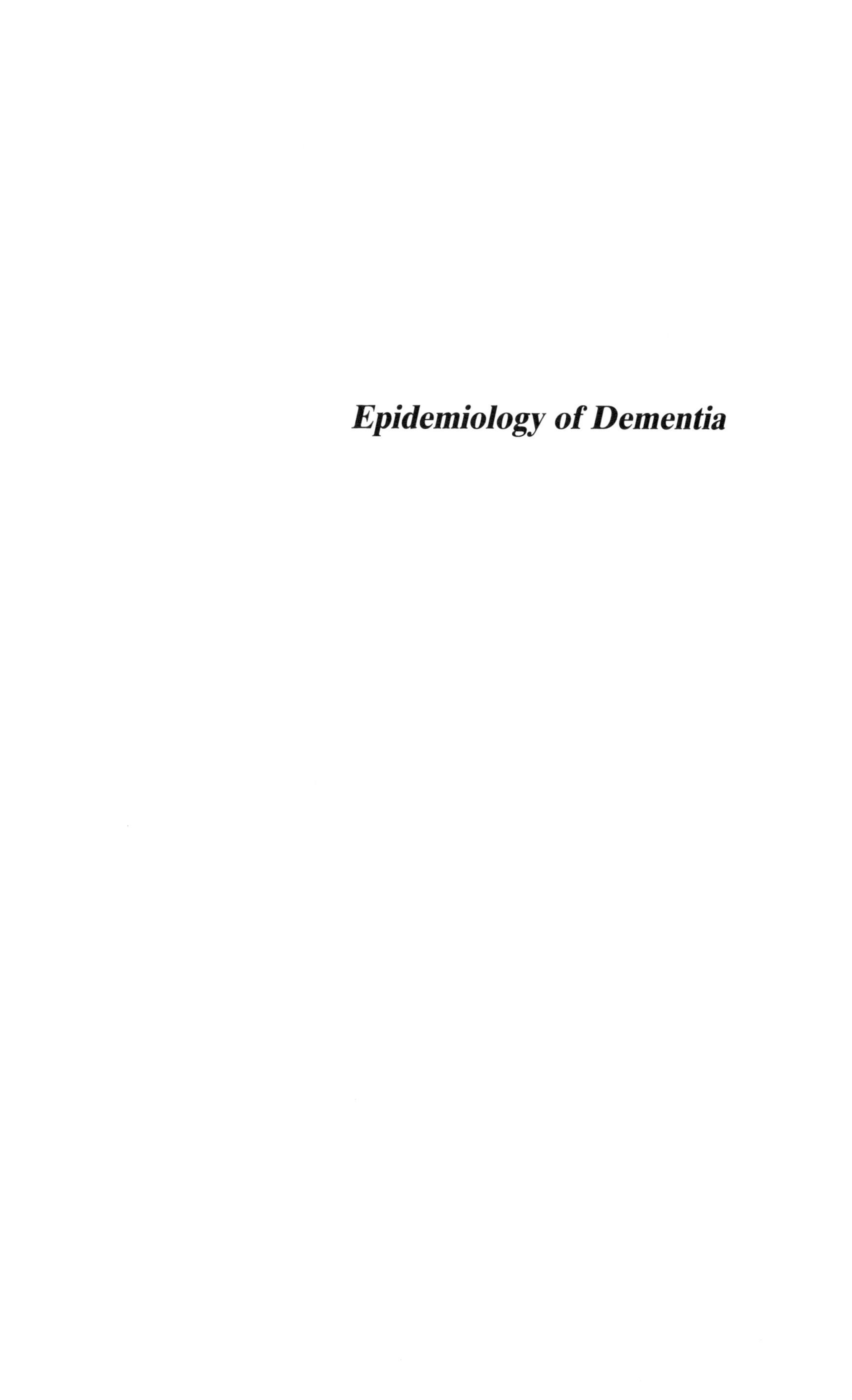

Epidemiology of Dementia

Epidemiological Study on Age-Associated Dementia in Japan

K. Hasegawa, and Y. Imai

Introduction

Recently we have seen a very substantial increase in knowledge about the epidemiology of age-associated dementia. Since the large-scale gerontopsychiatric epidemiological survey carried out in the Tokyo metropolitan area by Hasegawa et al. (1979) in 1974, there have been about 11 similar surveys on age-associated dementia supported by local governments throughout Japan.

The report of the Ministry of Health in Japan summarized the results of these studies as follows. First, the average prevalence rate in the community of dementia was 4.8%, and it appeared to increase with advancing age. Secondly, there was a substantially higher prevalence of vascular dementia than of senile dementia of the Alzheimer type (SDAT), which is the opposite to what had been found in Western studies.

The purpose of this article is to present results of a epidemiological study carried out in Kawasaki city, a suburb of Tokyo, in 1985, to confirm earlier findings regarding the prevalence of dementia in the aged in Japan and to obtain information concerning the living conditions of those in the community. The prevalence of the various etiological types of dementia in Japan was then compared with the prevalene in Western countries.

Subjects

This survey was carried out in Kawasaki city, a suburb of Tokyo. The total population in Kawasaki city was approximately 1.1 million and the population aged 65 and over was 69349 (total aged over 65, 6.5%) on 1 July 1984. The total sample comprised 1800 subjects randomly selected from 69349 elderly persons.

Procedure for Survey

The survey consisted of two parts. The primary survey was of the general health status of the sample of 1800 respondents by means of a semistructured interview conducted by lay raters. The period of the primary survey was 20 days from 28 August 1984. In

Bergener, Reisberg (Eds.)
Diagnosis and Treatment
of Senile Dementia
© Springer-Verlag Berlin Heidelberg 1989

the secondary survey, the 330 subjects who were screened out from those in the primary survey as possibly having mental illness were interviewed individually by a small team comprising a psychiatrist and a psychologist at home during 3 months from 1 November 1984, to 31 January 1985. They both undertook a psychiatric examination of each subject and evaluated the physical condition by means of a semistructured interview.

The criteria for dementia were based on DSM-III (American Psychiatric Association 1980). It is not always easy, even for experienced psychiatrists, to differentiate dementia etiologically, especially in a field survey. To lessen the risk of diagnostic misclassification, strict criteria were employed to diagnose senile dementia and vascular dementia (Table 1). Clinical staging of dementia was determined according to the criteria shown in Table 2, which were modified from those of Hughes et al. (1982).

In addition, a simple memory scale called Hasegawa's Dementia Scale (HDS) (Hasegawa 1983) was also used. The full score on the scale is 32.5. Scores of less than 20 may be indicative of mild mental deterioration, whereas scores below 10 may be regarded as indicative of severe intellectual deterioration.

Table 1. Clinical diagnostic criteria for dementia

Senile dementia

Neither history nor symptoms of suspected cerebrovascular accidents
No focal neurological symptoms or signs such as paralysis, sensory loss, or pseudobulbar palsy
Severe and/or progressive intellectual impairment with less marked physical disability

Vascular dementia

Clear onset following cerebrovascular accidents, often with focal neurological symptoms and signs
Typical clinical features of lacunar dementia

Table 2. Clinical criteria for the severity of dementia

Healthy:	No memory loss or slight occasional forgetfulness. Full orientation. Independent function at usual level of everyday life. Full capability for self care
Mental decline:	Mild consistent forgetfulness. Inability to recall relatively unimportant data and parts of an experience. Full orientation. Independent function at usual level in daily life
Mild dementia:	Occasional inability to recall recent events. Disorientation for time. Mild impairment in problem-solving. Difficulty with independent function at usual level in everyday life. Decrease in initiative. Occasional prompting for personal care
Moderate dementia:	Usual inability to recall recent events. Disorientation in time and place. Definite impairment in problem-solving. Requires assistance in dressing, hygiene, and keeping personal effects
Severe dementia:	Severe memory loss – new material rapidly lost. Orientation to person only. Severe impairment in handling problems. Inability with independent function outside home. Requirement for much help with personal care
Very severe dementia:	Severe memory loss – only fragments remain. Full disorientation. Inability to make judgements. Inability to maintain self-care without constant assistance

Results

The distributions of sex and age of the subjects in the primary survey were quite similar to those of the total population aged 65 and over in Kawasaki city. No significant differences were found. In the primary survey, results were collected for 1607 of the 1800 subjects (89.3%). Owing to death, and to inaccessibility for other reasons, only 294 subjects were actually interviewed from among the 330 subjects selected from the sample of 1607 (89.1%).

Prevalence of Dementia. Sixty-seven aged persons were suffering from dementia. The prevalence rate of dementia was 4.7% when corrected for the 36 persons dropping out at the secondary survey. Table 3 shows the prevalence rate according to sex and age. The rate was slightly higher in females than in males, and increased with advancing age. Furthermore, it was shown to increase greatly in the older age groups of 85 years and over (18.7%) (Fig. 1).

Table 3. Prevalence of dementia in the elderly in the community (%)

	Age (years)					Total
	65–69	70–74	75–79	80–84	85+	
Male	2.8	3.0	5.5	5.8	19.6	4.1
Female	–	4.4	7.0	15.9	18.2	5.2
Total	1.3	3.8	6.4	11.9	18.7	4.7

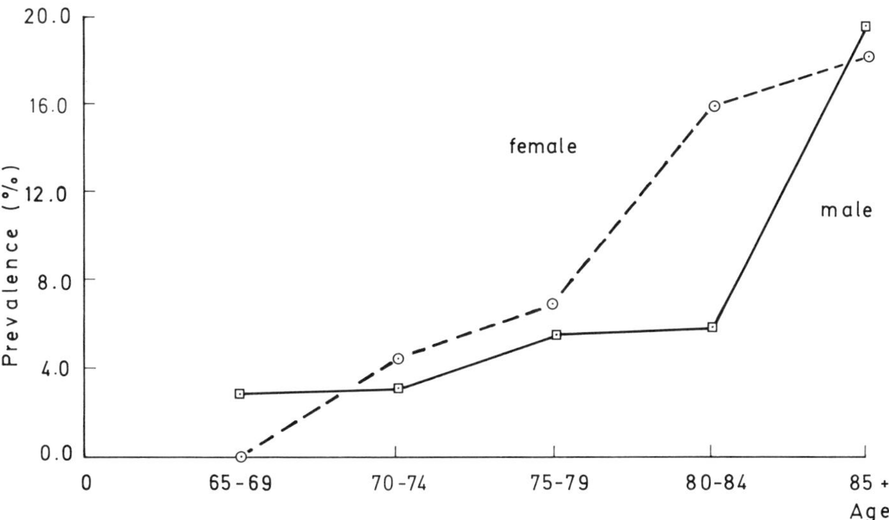

Fig. 1. Prevalence of senile and vascular dementia by age and sex

Table 4. Etiological classification of dementia by sex and age

Sex/age (years)	n	Etiological classification (%)		
		Senile dementia	Vascular dementia	Unclassified dementia
Male	26	11.5	73.1	15.4
Female	41	43.9	29.3	26.8
65–69	7	0	100.0	0
70–74	16	25.0	62.5	12.5
75–79	16	37.5	56.3	6.3
80–84	16	43.8	18.8	37.5
85+	12	33.3	16.7	50.0
Total	67	31.3	46.3	22.4

Etiological Classification of Dementia. The proportion of senile dementia was 31.3% and of vascular dementia, 46.3%; unclassified dementia accounted for 22.4%, as shown Table 4. Senile dementia was much less frequently diagnosed than vascular dementia in all age groups except those of 80 years and over. Vascular dementia was predominant in males, but senile dementia was more frequent in females. Although the diagnosis of unclassified dementia might include senile dementia or vascular dementia, it was difficult to discriminate those types of dementia in the field survey. Unclassified dementia also included dementia due to other causes.

Severity of Dementia. The results suggested that 43.3% of the aged with dementia living in the community were mildly demented, 35.8% were moderately demented, and 17.9% and 3.0% were severely and very severely demented respectively (Table 5). With respect to severity of dementia, no marked differences were found between the three types of dementia.

Activity of Daily Life. Among the aged with dementia, 42% were almost bedridden in their daily life, 33% were moderately active at home, and 25% were almost completely independently mobile. Of patients with senile dementia, 28% were almost

Table 5. Severity of dementia by sex and age

Sex/age (years)	n	Severity of dementia (%)			
		Mild	Moderate	Severe	Very severe
Male	26	61.5	19.2	19.2	0
Female	41	31.7	46.3	17.1	4.9
65–69	7	71.4	14.3	14.3	0
70–74	16	43.8	18.8	31.3	6.3
75–79	16	37.5	50.0	12.5	0
80–84	16	37.5	43.8	12.5	6.3
85+	12	41.7	41.7	16.7	0
Total	67	43.3	35.8	17.9	3.0

bedridden. On the other hand, of the elderly with vascular dementia, 64.5% were bedridden, i. e., twice as many as in the senile dementia group.

Previous and Present Physical Illness. Of the aged with dementia, 91% had previous illnesses. Cerebrovascular disorders were the most frequent previous disorders (49.2%), and the high frequency of hypertension (32.8%) was to be expected. There was a significantly higher frequency of cerebrovascular disorders in men (72.0%) than in women (33.3%).

As many as 86.6% of the aged with dementia had physical illnesses, while 52.3% of the aged without dementia had physical complications. The frequencies of hypertension and cerebrovascular disorders were notable (37.9% and 48.3%, respectively).

Psychiatric Symptoms and Behavior Disorders. The psychiatric symptoms other than memory impairment and disorientation in the demented elderly included loss of spontaneity, which was the most frequent (13.4%), and delirious states (10.4%). Sleep disorders, persecutory ideas, and hallucinations were each found in 6.0% of the demented elderly.

Of the aged with dementia, 38.8% had behavior disorders. The most frequent problem encountered was disturbed behavior during the night (14.9%). Other behavior disorders found included screaming in a loud voice, careless handling of the fire, and wandering at home; the frequency of each of these behaviors was 7.4% of the demented elderly.

Hasegawa's Dementia Scale (HDS). According to clinical criteria for the severity of dementia, mean scores on the HDS in mild, moderate, severe, and very severe dementias were 20.3, 10.9, 3.6, and 1.0 respectively. The mean score for those with senile dementia was lower than that for those with vascular dementia (11.7 vs. 16.8).

Discussion

Prevalence of Dementia in the Aged

There have been many surveys of the prevalence of dementia in the aged and the great majority have been reported from Scandinavia, northern Europe, North America, and Japan.

This gerontopsychiatric epidemiological study was carried out in Kawasaki city in 1984. The prevalence of dementia in the aged, i. e., those over the age of 65 years was 4.7%. This result coincides quite well with the prevalence rates reported from two other surveys in Tokyo, which noted prevalence rates of 4.5% and 4.6% respectively (Hasegawa et al. 1979; Karasawa et al. 1982). Table 6 shows results from 11 recent large scale epidemiological studies in Japan. The prevalence of dementia in the aged in the community in Japan obtained from all the investigations, if the highest and lowest are excluded, is approximately 4%–5%. The studies used methodologies similar to that of the Kawasaki study. As mentioned previously, the report of the Ministry of Health declared that the prevalence of dementia in the aged in Japan was

4.8%. Therefore, in 1985 there were about 600000 people aged 65 years or over with dementia in Japan, although the population aged 65 years and over in Japan was about 12 million.

It is difficult to compare the prevalence rates of dementia in the elderly found in Japan with those found in Western countries, because studies have used different methods and diagnostic criteria for dementia and the characteristics of sample populations have been different. Therefore, overall prevalence rates have a very wide range of values – from 0.5% (Lin 1953) to 14.0% (Parsons 1965). With regard to the age

Table 6. Comparison between Japanese and Western epidemiological studies of the aged with dementia

Area Investigated (source)		Year	No. of subjects	Prevalence %	Etiological classification			Ratio VD/SD[a]
					Senile demen-tia	Vascular demen-tia	Unclassi-fied demen-tia	
Tokyo metropolis	(1)	1974	4716	4.5	25.8	59.9	14.3	2.3
Sashiki village (Okinawa pref.)	(2)	1975	708	3.8	27.6	65.5	6.9	2.4
Tokyo metropolis	(3)	1980	4502	4.6	12.6	36.4	51.0	2.9
Yokohama city	(4)	1982	2287	4.8	21.8	34.7	43.5	1.6
Ohyama machi[b] (Tottori pref.)	(5)	1982	1236	4.4	40.7	49.2	10.1	1.2
Osaka pref.	(6)	1983	1844	4.3	36.4	50.3	13.3	1.4
Aichi pref.	(7)	1983	3106	5.8	42.0	48.1	9.9	1.1
Hosini village[c] (Fukuoka pref.)	(8)	1983	782	3.5	28.6	48.2	23.2	1.7
Kanagawa pref.	(9)	1983	1507	4.8	24.3	41.4	34.3	1.7
Toyama pref.	(10)	1985	1327	3.0	56.7	36.7	6.6	0.6
Kawasaki city (present study)		1985	1607	4.7	31.3	46.9	22.4	1.5
Newcastle, UK	(11)	1964	297	6.4	42.0	39.0	19.0	0.9
Sweden	(12)	1964	2979	1.3	60.3	39.7	–	0.7
Kilsyth, UK	(13)	1970	808	8.3	71.2	22.7	6.1	0.3
Finland	(14)	1980	8000	6.7	54.4	40.0	6.0	0.7
Baltimore, USA	(15)	1985	590	6.1	32.8	45.9	21.3	1.4

[a] VD/SD: The ratio of senile dementia to vascular dementia
[b] Aged 60 years and over
[c] Includes institutionalization

Sources: (1) Hasegawa et al. (1979). (2) Makiya (1978). (3) Karasawa et al. (1982). (4) Department of Public Welfare: Report on the sociomedical condition of the aged with dementia in the community (in Japanese), Yokohama City Office, Yokohama, 1982. (5) Takahashi and Fukuda (1984). (6) Department of Public Welfare, Osaka Prefecture Office: Report on the health condition of the aged in the community. Osaka Prefecture Office, Osaka, 1984. (7) Department of Public Welfare, Aichi Prefecture Office: Report on the health condition of the aged. Aichi Prefecture Office, Aichi 1984. (8) Mental Health Center, Fukuoka Prefecture: Report on the health condition of the aged living in the agricultural area (in Japanese). Fukuoka Mental Health Center, Fukuoka, 1983. (9) Hasegawa et al. (1986). (10) Department of Public Welfare, Toyama Prefecture Office: Report on the health condition of the aged in the community. Toyama Prefecture Office, Osaka, 1985. (11) Kay et al. (1964). (12) Aksson et al. (1969). (13) Broe et al. (1976). (14) Sulkava et al. (1985). (15) Folstein et al. (1985).

distribution of dementia, Broe and associates (1976) demonstrated a sharp increase in prevalence with age. Overall in Japanese studies the prevalence appeared to increase with advancing age (65–69, 1.2%; 70–74, 2.7%; 75–79, 4.9%; and 85 or over, 19.9%) and it was shown that the prevalence of senile dementia increased more sharply with age than did that of vascular dementia. Two British surveys (Kay et al. 1964; Broe et al. 1976) yielded results showing a higher prevalence of Alzheimer's disease in women. Also, studies in Finland (Molsa et al. 1982; Sulkava et al. 1985) and in Sweden (Akesson 1969) have produced similar results. As stated previously, in the Kawasaki study, senile dementia was more frequent in women, while vascular dementia was more frequent in men. In recent Japanese surveys, the sex-specific prevalence of senile dementia was similar to that of European studies.

Etiological Classification of Dementia

There is a marked difference between the prevalence of senile dementia and vascular dementia in northern Europe and that in Japan (Table 6). The characteristic finding of Japanese studies was that the prevalence of vascular dementia exceeded that of the senile dementia. This was also found in the Kawasaki study. As is well known from previous work by Kay et al. (1964), Akesson (1964), Broe et al. (1976), and Sulkava et al. (1986), the prevalence SDAT appeared to be higher than that of vascular dementia. Recently, Folstein and associates (1985) reported some of the results of the NIMH Epidemiologic Catchment Area Program and revealed that the prevalence rates of senile, vascular, and unspecified dementias were 2.0%, 2.8%, and 1.3% respectively. Although the total prevalence rate of dementia seems slightly higher than that in Japan, the rates of senile and vascular dementia are quite similar to those reported in Japan. However, this was rather exceptional. Generally, the ratio of the prevalence of SDAT to that of vascular dementia has been above 1.0 in Japanese studies, which is in contrast to Western studies which, apart from the Baltimore study, give ratios below 1.0 (Table 6).

There are several possible explanations for this finding. First, there are no internationally accepted diagnostic criteria for the two major types of dementia that can be used for research purposes. Also, the clinical distinction between SDAT and vascular dementia has not been demonstrated to be accurate, nor have clinical criteria been shown to correlate well with post-mortem neuropathology (Liston and La Rue 1983). A second explanation is that cerebrovascular disorders, which occur at a high rate in the Japanese population, affect the older age group before they have a chance to develop senile dementia and this leads to an increased prevalence of apparent vascular dementia but an artificially lowered rate of senile dementia. Thirdly, the present result might suggest that aged Japanese people are less susceptible to or have less constitutional or environmental factors disposing towards SDAT.

At present there is no evidence to support either the second or the third hypothesis. Further extensive longitudinal studies using cross-comparative methodology in community settings or precise case control studies are required to clarify the difference in the prevalence of dementia. It must also be emphasized that internationally standardized diagnostic assessments for senile dementia should be developed that are suitable for use in field studies.

Actual Condition of the Aged with Dementia in the Community

Most studies have reported a category of mild dementia which affected from 2.6% (Kay et al. 1970) to 21.9% (Parsons 1965) of all persons with dementia, a wide range. Although there is no code for mild dementia in DSM-III, it is quite important for early diagnosis of senile dementia to evaluate mildly demented states. The definitions of mild dementia by Nielsen (1962) and Kay et al. (1964) appear to correspond more closely to benign senescent forgetfulness in Kral's (1962) taxonomy of dementia. In the Kawasaki study, the clinical criteria for the severity of dementia used were modified from those of Hughes et al. (1982). These criteria were also used in the Kanagawa study by Hasegawa et al. (1986) in 1983. In the Kawasaki study (1984) the prevalence of mild dementia was 1.8%, similar to the 1.9% found in the Kanagawa study. Therefore, the prevalence of mild dementia in the population aged 65 years and over in Japan might be almost 2.0%. On the other hand, the prevalence of severe and very severe dementia was almost half that of mild dementia. Sulkava et al. (1985) reported the prevalence of all types of severe dementia as 1.8% in a Finish study population aged 30 years and over. It is difficult to compare the Kawasaki study with the Finish study, because the latter included the elderly in institutions and the subjects were younger than those in the Kawasaki study.

A general deterioration of physical functions was observed among many of the demented aged with the advancement of dementia. In the Kawasaki study, 42% were almost bedridden, whereas only 7.0% of the nondemented aged were confined to bed. About 50% of the aged with dementia suffered from various degrees of incontinence, as compared with 0.9% of the nondemented elderly. In the Kawasaki study, almost all the aged with dementia had physical illnesses, hypertension and cerebrovascular disorder being the most frequent. Although some investigators (Schoenberg et al. 1985; Sulkava et al. 1983; Peck et al. 1973) found that most deaths in people with dementia were due to respiratory or cardiovascular disease, in the aged with dementia there is an interaction with other conditions predisposing to early death such as bedridden incontinence and physical illness.

The behavioral disturbance in the demented elderly including institutionalization, responsible for a significant amount of family stress and burden. In the Kawasaki study, 38.8% of the elderly with dementia had behavior problems. Families caring for demented elderly people wished to have them admitted to an institution or hospital if they manifested marked behavioral problems such as nocturnal confusion or constant aggressiveness. However, they did not wish to have the aged person admitted if the main symptoms of were merely those of simple dementia without behavioral problems. Thus, the control or the treatment of behavioral problems is very important if the demented aged are to remain at home.

The proportion of the demented elderly needing constant care increased with the progression of dementia. Heavy physical, psychological, and economic burdens are imposed on the families, who often admitted that there were problems within the families: these included the difficulty in house keeping, physical and mental exhaustion, the economic burden, and intrafamilial discord.

Overall, the findings suggest that both physical and psychological care are required for the aged with dementia. Furthermore, in order to provide better nursing care, individual needs must be met adequately, not only through public health policy but also through the resources of the private sector such as self-help groups in the community. We need urgently an integrated network of social and medical services for the community.

Conclusion

This epidemiological study of age-related dementia in a population selected randomly from the population at risk aged 65 years and over was carried out in Kawasaki city in 1984. The study disclosed that the prevalence of dementia in the aged was 4.7%. The prevalence of vascular dementia appeared higher than that of senile dementia. This finding is in agreement with other recent epidemiological studies in Japan, and may be characteristic of the prevalence of aged-related dementia in Japan. In the future, it might be interesting to confirm the finding using internationally accepted criteria for the diagnosis of senile dementia and to compare the results of studies in Western nations with those in Japan. The families taking care of the aged with dementia suffered a heavy burden. The authors wish to emphasize the urgent need for an integrated social and medical care system in the community and the need to take care of the family caregivers in the community.

References

Aksson HO (1969) A population study of senile and arteriosclerotic psychoses. Hum Hered 19: 546–566

American Psychiatric Association (1980) Diagnostic an statistical manual of mental disorder, 3rd ed. APA, Washington DC

Broe GA, Akhtar AJ, Andrews GR, Caird FI, Gilmore AJJ, McLennan WJ (1976) Neurological disorders in the elderly at home. J Neurol Neurosurg Psychiatry 39: 362–366

Folstein M, Anthony JC, Parhad I, Duffy B, Gruenberg EM (1985) The meaning of cognitive impairment in the elderly. J Am Geriatr Soc 33: 228–235

Hasegawa K (1983) The clinical assessment of dementia in the aged: a dementia screening scale for psychogeriatric patients. In: Bergener M (ed) Aging in the eighties and beyond. Springer Publishing, New York, p 207–218

Hasegawa K, Iwai S, Amamoto H, Satou H, Shukutani K, Homma A, Yung M, Karasawa A, Kawashima K, Yamada O (1979) An epidemiological study on psychiatric disorders in the elderly (in Japanese). In: The commemorative publication for Professor Shinfuku. Tokyo Jikei University School of Medicine, Department of Psychiatry, pp 342–354

Hasegawa K, Homma A, Imai Y (1986) An epidemiological study of age-related dementia in the community. Int J Geriatr Psychiatry 1: 45–55

Hughes CP, Berg L, Danziger WL, Coben LA, Martin RL (1982) A new clinical scale for the staging of dementia. Br J Psychiatry 140: 566–572

Karasawa K, Kawashima K, Kawahara H (1982) Epidemiological study of the senile in Tokyo metropolitan area. Proceedings of World Psychiatric Association regional symposium. Japanese Society for Psychiatry and neurology, Tokyo, pp 285–289

Kay DWK, Beamish P, Roth M (1964) Old age mental disorders in Newcastle upon Tyne. Part I: a study of prevalence. Br J Psychiatry 110: 146–158

Kay DWK, Bergmann K, Foster EM, McKechnie AH, Roth M (1970) Mental illness and hospital usage in the elderly: a random sample followed-up. Comp Psychiatry 11: 26–35

Kral VA (1962) Senescent forgetfulness: benign and malignat. Can Med Ass J 86: 257–260

Lin T (1953) A study of the incidence of mental disorder in Chinese and other cultures. Psychiatry 16: 313–336

Liston EL, La Rue A (1983) Clinical differentiation of primary degenerative and multi-infarct dementia: a critical review of the evidence. Biol Psychiatry 18: 1467–1484

Makiya H (1978) An epidemiological investigation on the psychiatric disorders of the old age in Sashiki-village in Okinawa prefecture (in Japanese). Keio J Med 55: 503–512

Molsa PK, Marttila RJ, Rinne UK (1982) Epidemiology of dementia in a Finnish population. Acta Neurol Scand 65: 641–652

Nielsen J (1962) Geronto-psychiatric period prevalence investigation in a geographically delimited population. Acta Psychiatr Scand 38: 307–330

Parsons PL (1965) Mental health of Swansea's old folk. Br J Prevent Soc Med 19: 43–47

Peck A, Wollock L, Rodstein M (1973) Mortality of the aged with chronic brain syndrome. J Am Geriatr Soc 21: 264–270

Schoenberg BS, Anderson DW, Haerer AF (1985) Severe dementia: prevalence and clinical features in a biracial US population. Arch Neurol 42: 740–743

Sulkava R, Haltia M, Paetau A, Wikstrom J, Polo J (1983) Accuracy of clinical diagnosis in primary degenerative dementia: correlation with neuropathological finding. J Neurol Neurosurg Psychiatry 46: 9–13

Sulkava R, Wikstrom J, Aromaa A, Raitasalo R, Lehtinen V, Lahtela K, Palo J (1985) Prevalence of severe dementia in Finland. Neurology 35: 1025–1029

Takahashi K, Fukuda M (1984) Epidemiology of dementia in the agricultural area (in Japanese). Geriatr Med 22: 1119–1122

Risk Factors for Dementia: A Review of Hypotheses and Current Epidemiological Evidence

M. R. Eastwood, and S. L. Rifat

Introduction

"Cogito, ergo sum," Decartes' famous dictum, underlines the particular horror of a dementing illness. A state of mindlessness, when it represents an irreversible deterioration from previously competent, adult mental function, must constitute one of the most tragic of human conditions.

The brain is a uniquely complex structure, weighing around 1500 g in the prime of life. Normally 40% of this mass is lost by the ninth decade, mainly from the frontal and temporal lobes. The brain receives 40% of the body's blood supply and is relatively immune to oxygen starvation. However, it is subject to deterioration either gradually, through primary parenchymal disease, or abruptly, through cessation of blood supply. In either event, such critical faculties as intelligence, memory and judgement become impaired and thinking muted.

The clinical and pathological features of dementia and the complexities of differential diagnosis are addressed in depth by others at this workshop. The specific focus of this paper is a review of the epidemiological evidence pertaining to risk factors for dementia syndromes. However, it must be appreciated that this evidence is partial and limited by the diagnostic and prognostic difficulties already alluded to.

Types of Dementia

Dementia of Alzheimer's type (DAT) and multi-infarct dementia (MID), as characterized by clinical and neuropathological changes, are the common forms of dementia. However, the distribution of dementias by type remains uncertain and likely varies between populations and over time. Since DAT is idiopathic and MID is known to be due to vascular disease, the differentiation is critical. The stroke rate has fallen in this century, especially with the introduction of hypotensive agents in the past 20 years, and the prospect is for a further reduction in MID rates. In contrast, the prospects for DAT, if projections are realized, are dismal.

Bergener, Reisberg (Eds.)
Diagnosis and Treatment
of Senile Dementia
© Springer-Verlag Berlin Heidelberg 1989

Projected Prevalence

Ineichen (1987), in a review of 20 studies, reported a range of prevalence figures for dementia from 2.5% to 24.6%. He made the conservative estimate that DAT afflicts 1% of the population 65–74 years of age and 10% of those over 75. Using point prevalence ratios provided by Broe et al. (1976), 2.4% for ages 65–74, 10.9% for ages over 75, and United Nations demographic estimates, Rocca et al. (1986) estimated for the years 1980 and 2000 the prevalence of Alzheimer's disease for several developed countries. Percentage increase in expected prevalence over this 20-year period ranged from lows of 9% for France and 11.8% for Great Britain (where only small increases in the proportions of population over 65 are anticipated) to increases of 40% in Italy and the United States and over 75% in Japan (where anticipated increases in population age are greater).

Methods of Analysis

In addition to providing descriptive data such as prevalence and incidence rates, there are classical analytical epidemiology methods for evaluating the significance and strength of association between illness and exposure or other precursor factors. The principal research designs of analytic epidemiology are the retrospective, or case-control method, and the prospective, or cohort, method. Each has its strengths and weaknesses. The case-control design, which compares individuals with known outcome on history of exposure, is suitable for studying uncommon diseases and a large number of potential risk factors. However, this method requires careful definition of cases and suitable controls and is dependent upon available information. Validity and reliability of exposure data are often questionable, and the order of events is an issue (i. e. was the exposure a cause or an effect of the disorder?). The cohort method, which follows individuals known to be well at the time of exposure, more closely mimics the experimental approach, but this requires knowledge of critical exposures and may need a long follow-up of many individuals. As a cohort study is generally more exacting and expensive, it is usually reserved for a second stage of research, while the case-control study is often used for hypothesis formulation or a "fishing expedition". It should be noted that all of the current epidemiologic evidence pertaining to risk factors for DAT is derived from either descriptive population survey research or studies using a case-control design.

Risk Factors for Dementia

Risk factors for MID, Korsakoff's and other specific dementias are relatively well defined. In contrast, risk factors for DAT remain speculative and largely hypothetical. Regardless of their putative nature, there are several risk factors for which some evidence is available. These can be considered under the headings: demograpic factors; genetic factors; virology and immunology; toxicology; and non-specific factors which have been investigated.

Demographic Factors

Age, gender and social status are variables which have been examined principally by contrasting descriptive data of populations on whom prevalence or incidence data have been collected.

Age is the variable most consistently related to the dementias. Jorm et al. (1987) in his meta-analysis of 22 different studies showed that prevalence and age were consistently related, with estimated prevalence doubling every 5.1 years up to age 95. This was despite study differences in methodology and with no ready explanation. Further, the limited data on age-specific incidence support the contention that the increase is age related (Henderson 1986; Schoenberg 1986).

Dementia is not consistently related to gender. Jorm et al. (1987) found that the rate of DAT was higher in women, but that that of MID was equal in the sexes, albeit with little age- and sex-specific information for MID. Schoenberg (1986) argued that both prevalence and incidence rates for both dementia (i. e. all types) and clinically diagnosed Alzheimer's disease are greater for women than for men, even after adjusting for the greater longevity of women (Ineichen 1987).

There is some evidence for racial differences, on which Professor Hasegawa may elaborate in his presentation here. Jorm et al. (1987) suggests that MID is more common than DAT in Japan and the Soviet Union while DAT with onset in the senium is considered the commonest type of dementia in Western studies. The source of these differences, if real, is likely the greater risk for MID in populations with higher rates of hypertension and completed cerebrovascular accident rather than differential risk for DAT. Higher age-specific incidence rates for clinically diagnosed DAT with early onset (i. e. ages 40–60) among Israelis of European and American than of Afro-Asian birth, however, requires another explanation (Rocca et al. 1986; Schoenberg 1986).

Socio-economic status (SES) has been little studied, apart from the Epidemiological Catchment Area studies in the United States (Weissman et al. 1986) and a West German investigation by Cooper (1984). In the United States, where skin colour and SES remain confounded at the population level, there appeared to be greater prevalence of cognitive impairment among non-Whites (e. g. Blacks, Hispanics). Cooper also reported higher rates of cognitive impairment within the West German lower classes. Interpretation of SES effects is problematic, as the associations between illness and opportunity may be a complex web of causation from cradle to grave. Moreover, as standardized methods of screening for dementia at the population level are subject to cultural, educational and language biases, contrasts between different classes may be entirely unfair.

Genetic Factors

Since the seminal work of Sjörgren et al. (1952) and Larsson et al. (1963) there has been considerable research on the genetics of dementia. As Kay noted in 1986, however, the existing evidence is incomplete and often conflicting. Heritability of DAT has been studied by examining for clustering of disease in families, including the special case of twin studies, and by investigation for evidence of chromosomal abnormalities (e. g. association with Down's syndrome, maternal age effects, fecundity of DAT cases and controls).

Clusters of dementia within some families have been well documented. However, there are two apparently opposing interpretations. Heston and co-workers (1981) found familial risk to vary with age of onset and severity of illness in the proband, with risk for families of DAT cases with onset after 70 no greater than in families with no dementing illness. This pattern seems to imply polygenic inheritance. Conversely, familial cases also have been used as evidence for an autosomal dominant condition, with age-dependent penetrance (Mohs et al. 1985; Breitner et al. 1986a, b). By their method, the calculated risk for first-degree relatives of DAT cases approximates 50% by age 90, with achieved risk determined by longevity. Given current life expectancy, only about 30% of "at risk" relatives would develop a dementing disorder, i. e. 15% of the first-degree relatives of a case. This figure of 10%–15% is typically the observed rate of dementia among relatives of DAT probands.

Comparison of concordance in monozygotic and dizygotic twin studies is a classic method of examining for genetic contribution; however, in DAT research we have conflicting reports. Kallmann (1953), examining a total of 58 twin pairs, described over 40% concordance for dementia among monozygotic twins and 8% concordance in dizygotic twins. A more recent study by Nee et al. (1987), with 22 twin pairs, found approximately 40% concordance for both monozygotic and dizygotic twins. Clearly the definitive twin study remains to be done.

As those with Down's syndrome surviving to middle age typically develop clinical and pathological signs of DAT, a link with chomosomal abnormalities has been considered in DAT. This has been investigated by examining for an excess of Down's syndrome in families of DAT probands, with variable results. It appears that where the series is large, there is a statistically significant excess (Heston et al. 1981); however, the frequency of Down's syndrome is sufficiently low that case-control studies have not had adequate statistical power to detect a moderate odds ratio. Only one study of the converse, examining for an excess of DAT in families of Down's syndrome probands, has been located in the literature (Yatham et al. 1988). The authors of this study acknowledged methodological problems (e. g. confirmation of Alzheimer's disease diagnosis, small number of probands, compounded by 52% response rate); however, they interpreted their findings as further support for the association between Down's snydrome and Alzheimer's disease with onset before age 65.

As maternal age has been associated with trisomy-21 and other chromosomal abnormalities, it has also been examined in DAT case-control studies. Cohen et al. (1982) originally reported a significant maternal-age effect, with mean age of mother at birth of DAT cases higher than in population controls. Subsequently, other investigations (e. g. Corkin et al. 1983; English and Cohen 1985) failed to find such effect, or found only a greater proportion of cases born to mothers aged over 40 (Amaducci et al. 1986).

Possible effects of chomosomal abnormalities also have been examined in terms of foetal wastage and fecundity. DAT cases appear not to differ from controls in size of birth family nor in own reproductive history and to have been slightly more fertile than their normal siblings (Amaducci et al. 1986; Ridley et al. 1986; White et al. 1987).

Virology and Immunology

Changes in immune function with normal ageing have been well documented. These changes include both a decline in cellular and humoral immune response to foreign antigens and an increase in autoantibodies to many tissues, including brain tissue. These are well reviewed by Meredith and Walford (1979), Hausman and Weksler (1985), and Hulette and Walford (1987). Evidence of exaggerated immune function changes in patients with DAT has been more equivocal (Hulette and Walford 1987). While some investigators have reported significant differences between individuals with DAT and age-matched controls in immunoglobulin levels, these have been in the direction both of elevated and of depressed levels. Cellular immune function appears intact in DAT cases relative to age-matched controls. Autoantibodies to CNS appear to increase normally with ageing, and whether these are at greater titre or show more affinity for brain tissue in DAT has not been established.

Infectious agents (e. g. herpesvirus, cytomegalovirus and the scrapie agent) have been examined by antigen and antibody titres, genomic sequencing and comparisons of ultrastructural changes. Attempts have also been made to transmit infection through direct injection of DAT tissues into experimental animals. The first reports of a successful transmission experiment could not be replicated, even using materials from the same subjects. However, a report appeared in summer 1988 of the induction of spongy encephalopathy (Creutzfeldt-Jacob disease changes) following injection of tissues from asymptomatic relatives of DAT patients into hamsters (Manuelidis et al. 1988). Although any evidence of transmission is tantalizing at this stage, the exact meaning of this result is unclear and requires further investigation and replication.

Epidemiological research has not provided evidence of an infectious agent. While DAT does cluster in some families, there does not appear to be an increased risk for spouses, nor is there other evidence of the space or time clustering associated with infectious disease. Case-control studies which have included questions regarding medical history have not found evidence of increased frequency of report of viral diseases (e. g. herpes, meningitis, poliomyelitis) nor more common immune disorders (e. g. allergies, arthritis) among cases than controls.

Toxicology

Aluminium is the suspected agent in dialysis dementia, a condition affecting certain patients on renal dialysis in regions where alum is in high concentrations in the water supply (Davies 1986). Extreme concentrations of aluminium have been found in the brain tissue of patients dying with dialysis dementia, and the clinical progression, although more rapid, is similar to that in DAT. Additionally, animal models of chronic aluminium encephalopathy have been demonstrated. A third line of evidence is the finding of focal elevated concentrations of aluminium in the brains of autopsied DAT patients, relative to age-matched controls. Aluminium in the brains of DAT patients and normal controls appears confined to the nuclei of neurons undergoing degenerative change rather than widespread throughout the cytoplasm, as is found in dialysis dementia (Crapper McLachlan 1986).

Criticisms of the aluminium hypothesis have focused on the dissimilarities between induced aluminium encephalopathy and DAT (Wisniewski et al. 1986; Foncin 1987). Differences have been noted in the ultrastructure of damaged neurons, and questions raised regarding the modes of aluminium entry into brain tissue, given the lack of elevated Al^+ in CSF, serum and hair of DAT patients (Shore and Wyatt 1983). In vitro and experimental animal evidence, however, has indicated that aluminium metabolism and manifestation of aluminium encephalopathy are affected by a variety of factors (e. g. route and rate of delivery, species and dose of aluminium compound, concentrations of zinc, calcium and magnesium, age and species of animal). Whether or not aluminium is a causal factor in DAT, the evidence from experimental aluminium encephalopathy has further demonstrated the complex variability of metal metabolism.

There is some epidemiological evidence regarding the aluminium hypothesis. First, the distribution of aluminium (the third most common element and the most common metal on earth) would fit with the apparent lack of geographical clustering of DAT. Second, results of recent Norwegian ecological studies (Flaten 1986; Vogt 1986) have been interpreted as evidence that acidification of drinking water and resultant increased bioavailability of aluminium are associated with higher rates of DAT. Third, antiperspirants, antacids and some analgesics (e. g. buffered aspirin) contain aluminium chloride and aluminium hydroxides. While case-control studies which have examined for differences in use of these products resulted in non-significant odds ratios, there are major difficulties in obtaining a reliable surrogate report for history of use of common agents. Work in progress in Seattle (A. Graves, personal communication, 1988) may provide refinements of this methodology.

The retrospective cohort method of study may be useful here, as groups which differ in history of documented exposure may be contrasted on current and future outcome measures. An example of this is a study that we are now conducting in northern Ontario on men aged 60–70 who have been occupationally exposed to aluminium over a 35-year period. Such exceptional exposures may provide a better means of testing the aluminium hypothesis than is provided by a case-control study. Other examples of good cohorts for study may be series of patients with gastritis or arthritis on chronic antacid or analgesic therapy.

Traditionally, Korsakoff's dementia is associated with alcohol excess. Additionally, liver disease may contribute to dementia, and alcohol-induced cerebrovascular disease may lead to multi-infarct dementia. It has been found in Toronto by Carlen and Wilkinson (1981) that heavy drinkers have more cerebral atrophy than controls. King (1986) discovered that 21% of patients with Alzheimer's disease at a special clinic at Johns Hopkins University had been heavy drinkers. The figure was 40% in those over 80, with the sexes affected equally. Despite the known association between alcohol consumption and dementia, alcohol use has been little studied in connection with DAT. This is due to the necessity of excluding other potentially "sufficient" causes of dementia from series of cases in case-control studies. One exception is the study that we currently have underway in northern Ontario, in which the case definition is one of alcoholism. A striking problem of such research is acquiring reliable consensual information from relatives.

As pointed out in a recent review (Clarkson 1987) the nervous system is the principal target for many toxins, including the metals manganese, lead, mercury and tin. Metals were among the earliest recognized neurotoxins; however, the exact mechanisms of even lead and methylmercury toxicity are not well defined. Although it is known that lead inhibits haem synthesis, compromising metabolic processes in the brain, it is now suspected that lead also interferes with membrane transport and binding of calcium ions. Likewise, methylmercury is known to cause focal damage in the adult brain and more severe and wide-spread damage in early developmental stages. Recent evidence indicates that microtubules are destroyed by methylmercury. Solvents (e. g. paint thinners, dry-cleaning fluids, fuels and antifreeze) are also known neurotoxins. One question about known neurotoxins is whether they may act as precursors by damaging the blood brain barrier or as vehicles for other agents.

A point to be made regarding all known or suspected neurotoxic agents is that to date there has been no reported evidence of clustering of DAT cases within an occupational group, nor evidence from case-control studies that known exposures to suspect agents are more frequent among cases.

History of prior head injury has been one of the few risk factors to appear significant with any consistency across case-control studies. Of six studies which examined for this factor between 1984 and 1987, the frequency of reported prior head injury (resulting in a loss of consciousness but with apparent full recovery of function) ranged from 5% to 26% in cases. Odds ratios ranged from 2.0 to 11.5, and although statistically significant in only three of the six studies, they reflected greater frequency of prior head injury among cases than controls in all six.

Non-specific Factors

Despite the frequent perception of family members that bereavement of other loss may have precipitated the dementing illness, such life events have rarely been systematically examined. Amaducci and co-workers in Italy included a range of life events in their case-control study of DAT (e. g. unplanned pregnancies, death of an intimate, loss of valuable objects, legal difficulties) but found no consistently significant effects.

As with life events, premorbid personality has been subject to little study. Again, Amaducci et al. (1985) included items describing types A and B personality and found no differences between cases and controls in the descriptions provided by relatives. There is, however, some evidence that individuals with DAT have a more frequent and more recent history of depressive symptoms, including treated depression, than control subjects. This has been interpreted as evidence that depressive symptoms may be among the earliest signs of a dementing illness.

Case-control studies examining for increased risk associated with previous medical conditions have provided conflicting evidence. Heston et al. (1981) reported significantly more frequent leukaemia, as well as Down's syndrome, in families of DAT patients than expected from population data. Researchers conducting case-control studies, however, have not replicated these results. Thyroid disease was reported as a risk factor among women in one case-control study (Heyman et al. 1984), but was not a significant factor in later studies (Small et al. 1985; Shalat et al. 1987; Amaducci et al. 1986).

Conclusions

In summary, there are few risk factors for DAT which have been supported by epidemiological evidence. It is clear that the differentiation of dementias by type, particularly the distinction between DAT and MID, is critical, There may be reason to distinguish further between DAT with early and with late onset. As Henderson (1986) noted, most of the epidemiological evidence from case-control studies has applied to early-onset disease. From prevalence and incidence data, however, we can see that advancing age is the strongest risk factor for dementia.

Other risk factors for which there is supporting evidence include familial cases, female gender, possibly altered aluminium metabolism and history of prior head injury. Evidence on these and other risk fractors which have been considered is less than clear, partly due to difficulties with methodology. Descriptive studies cannot address causality, and case-control studies are particulary sensitive to selection and recall biases. Also, given the small numbers in most of the reported case-control studies of DAT, there has been insufficient statistical power to detect moderate risks associated with events of low frequency.

Epidemiology may yet play a key role in identifying the causes of dementia of Alzheimer's type, and the work continues.

References

Alfrey AC, Legendre GR, Kaehny WD (1976) The dialysis encephalopathy syndrome possible aluminium intoxication. N Engl J Med 294: 184–188

Amaducci LA, Fratiglioni L, Rocca WA, Fieschi C et al. (1986) Risk factors for clinically diagnosed Alzheimer's disease: a case-control study of an Italian population. Neurology 36: 922–931

Breitner JCS, Folstein MF, Murphy EA (1986) Familial aggregation in Alzheimer dementia. I. A model for the age-dependent expression of an autosomal dominant gene. J Psychiatr Res 20 (1): 31–43

Breitner JCS, Folstein MF, Murphy EA (1986) Familial aggregation in Alzheimer dementia. II. Clinical genetic implications of age-dependent onset. J Psychiatr Res 20 (1): 45–55

Breitner JCS, Silverman JM, Mohs RC, Davis KL (1988) Familial aggregation in Alzheimer's disease: comparisons of risk among relatives of early- and late-onset cases, and among male and female relatives in successive generations. Neurology 38: 207–212

Carlen PL, Wilkinson DA, Holgate RC, Wortzman G (1979) Computed otmography scans of alcoholics; cerebral atrophy, science 204: 1238

Chandra V, Philipose V, Bell PA, Lazaroff A, Schoenberg BS (1987) Case-control study of late onset "probable Alzheimer's disease", Neurology 37: 1295–1300

Clarkson TW (1987) Metal toxicity in the central nervous system. Environ Health Perspect 75: 59–64

Cohen D, Eisdorfer C, Leverenz J (1982) Alzheimer's disease and maternal age. J Am Geriatric Soc 30: 656–658

Cooper B (1984) Home and away: the disposition of mentally ill old people in an urban population. Soc Psychiatry 19: 187–196

Corkin S, Growdon JH, Rasmussen SL (1983) Parental age as a risk factor in Alzheimer's disease. Ann Neurol 13: 674–675

Corsellis AN (1986) The transmissibility of dementia. Br Med Bull 42: 111–114

Crapper McLachlan DR (1986) Review: aluminium and Alzheimer's disease. Neurobiol Aging 7: 525–532

Davis I (1986) Aluminium, neurotoxicology and dementia. Rev Environ Health 6 (1–4): 251–296

English D, Cohen D (1985) A case-control study of maternal age in Alzheimer's disease. J Am Geriatric Soc 33: 167–169

Fitch N, Becker R, Heller A (1988) The inheritance of Alzheimer's disease: a new interpretation. Ann Neurology 23: 14–19

Flaten TP (1986) An investigation of the chemical composition of Norwegian drinking water and its possible relationships with the epidemiology of some diseases. Thesis Institutt for Uorganisk Kjemi, Norges Tekniske Hogskole, Universitetet I, Trondheim

Foncin JF (1987) Alzheimer's disease and aluminium. Nature 326: 846

French LR, Schumann LM, Mortimer JA, Hutton JT, Boatman RA, Christians B (1985) A case-control study of dementia of the Alzheimer type. Am J Epidemiol 121 (3): 414–421

Hausman PB, Weksler ME (1985) Changes in the immune response with age. In Finch CD, Schneider EL (eds) Handbook of the biology of aging, 2nd edn. Van Nostrand Reinhold, New York, pp 414–432

Henderson AS (1986) The epidemiology of Alzheimer's disease. Br Med Bull 42: 3–10

Heston LL, Mastri AR, Anderson E and White J (1981) Dementia of the Alzheimer type: clinical genetics, natural history and associated conditions. Arch Gen Psychiatry 38: 1085–1090

Heyman A, Wilkinson WE, Stafford JA, Helms MJ, Sigmon AH, Weinberg T (1984) Alzheimer's disease: a study of epidemiological aspects. Ann Neurol 15: 335–341

Hulette CM, Walford RL (1987) Immunological aspects of Alzheimer disease: a review. Alzheimer Dis Assoc Disorders 1 (2): 72–82

Ineichen B (1987) Measuring the rising tide: how many dementia cases will there be by 2001? Br J Psychiatry 150: 193–200

Jorm AF, Korten AE, Henderson AS (1987) The prevalence of dementia: a quantitative integration of the literature. Acta Psychiatrica Scand 76: 465–479

Kallmann FJ (1953) Heredity in health and mental disorder. Norton, New York

Kay DWK (1986) The genetics of Alzheimer's disease. Br Med Bull 42: 19–23

King MB (1986) Alcohol abuse and dementia. International Journal of Geriatric Psychiatry, 1 (1): 31–36

Larsson T, Sjögren T, Jacobson G (1963) Senile dementia: a clinical sociological and genetic study. Acta Psychiatrica Scand 39 (Suppl 167): 1–259

Manuelidis EE, De Figueiredo JM, Kim JH, Fritch WW, Manuelidis L (1988) Transmission studies from blood of Alzheimer disease patients and healthy relatives. Proc Nat Acad Sci USA 85: 4898–4901

Meredith PJ, Walford RL (1979) Autoimmunity, histocompatibility and aging. Mech Ageing Dev 9: 61–77

Mohs RC, Breitner JCS, Silverman JM, Davis KL (1987) Alzheimer's disease: morbid risk among first degree relatives approximates 50% by 90 years of age. Arch Gen Psychiatry 44: 405–408

Mortimer JA, French LR, Hutton JT, Schuman LM (1985) Head injury as a risk factor for Alzheimer's disease. Neurology 35: 264–267

Nee LE, Eldridge R, Thomas CB, Katz D, Thompson KE, Weingartner H, Weiss H, Julian C, Cohen R (1987) Dementia of the Alzheimer type: clinical and family study of 22 twin pairs. Neurology 37: 359–363

Perl DP (1985) Relationship of aluminium to Alzheimer's disease. Environ Health Perspect 63: 149–153

Ridley RM, Baker HF, Crow TJ (1986) Transmissible and non-transmissible neurodegenerative disease: similarities in age of onset and genetics in relation to aetiology. Psychol Med 16: 199–207

Rocca WA, Amaducci LA, Schoenberg BS (1986) Epidemiology of clinically diagnosed Alzheimer's disease. Ann Neurol 19: 415–424

Schoenberg BS (1986) Epidemiology of Alzheimer's disease and other dementing illnesses. J Chron Dis 39 (12): 1095–1104

Shalat SL. Seltzer B, Pidcock C, Baker EL (1987) Risk factors for Alzheimer's disease: a case-control study. Neurology 37: 1630–1633

Shore D, Wyatt RJ (1983) Aluminium and Alzheimer's disease. The J Nerv Ment Dis 171 (9): 553–558

Sjögren T, Sjögren H, Lindgren AGH (1952) Morbus Alzheimer and Morbus Pick. Acta Psychiatr Neurol Scand (Suppl 82): 1–152

Small GW, Matsuyama SS, Komanduri R, Kumar V, Jarvik LF (1985) Thyroid disease in patients with dementia of the Alzheimer type. J Am Geriatric Soc 33: 538–539

Vogt T (1986) A study of the relationship between aluminium in drinking water and Alzheimer's disease in southern Norway. Paper presented at the second conference of the Society for Human Ecology, Bar Harbor, Maine, October 1986

Weissman M, Myers JK, Ross CE (eds) (1986) Community surveys of psychiatric disorders. Rutgers University Press, New Brunswick

Wisniewski HM, Moretz RC, Igbal K (1986) No evidence for aluminium in etiology and pathogenesis of Alzheimer's disease. Neurobiol Aging 7: 532–535

Whalley LJ, Carothers AD, Collyer S, De Mey R, Frackiewicz A (1982) A study of familial factors in Alzheimer's disease. Br J Psychiatry 140: 249–256

White JA. McGue M and Heston LL (1986) Fertility and parental age in Alzheimer disease. J Gerontology 41 (1): 40–43

Yatham LN, McHale PA, Kinsella A (1988) Down's syndrome and its association with Alzheimer's disease. Acta Psychiatr Scand 77: 38–41

Neuropathologic and Neurochemical Aspects of Dementia

Alzheimer's Disease – Histopathological, Neurochemical and Molecular Biological Aspects*

A. NORDBERG, A. ADEM, R. ADOLFSSON, I. ALAFUZOFF, N. LÅNGSTRÖM, L. NILSSON-HÅKANSSON, B. WALLACE, and B. WINBLAD

Introduction

The most common type of primary dementia is commonly referred to as Alzheimer's disease, senile dementia of Alzheimer type (AD/SDAT), where AD refers to the early onset form (before age 65) and SDAT to the late onset form (after age 65). AD/SDAT which is the most prevalent disease causing progressive dementia in old age constitutes about 50%–70% of the dementias seen at autopsy (Tomlinson 1980). The prevalence is considered to be less than 5% for definite cases of dementia in people 65 years and older, but rises dramatically with increasing age and is about 35% at 90 years. The essential features of AD/SDAT are an insidious onset with gradual progression, involving loss of intellectual abilities such as memory, abstract thinking, judgement, and other cortical functions, as well as changes in personality and behavior (Roth 1955, 1985; Slater and Roth 1970). Vascular, multi-infarct dementia (MID) which is considered to account for at least 15% of the total number of dementia cases seen at autopsy (Tomlison 1980; Adolfsson and Forsgren 1984) is characterized by an abrupt onset, a stepwise and fluctuating progression with rapid changes that early in the course of the disease leave some of the intellectual function relatively intact (Hachinski et al. 1974, 1975). The MID patients often have variable cerebrovascular risk factors. Similar to AD/SDAT, disturbances in memory, abstract thinking, judgement, impulse control, and personality are common. In addition, focal neurological signs and symptoms are present.

Histopathological Aspects of AD/SDAT

The histopathological diagnostic hallmarks of AD/SDAT are the presence of neurofibrillary tangles (Tomlinson 1980; Terry and Davies 1980) and senile/neuritic plaques (Tomlinson 1980; Gibson 1983). Plaques and tangles are also found in normally aged brain, but to a far less degree. In the brains of patients suffering from AD/SDAT an accentuation of tangles and plaques is observed in the temporoparietal lobe and the posterior cingulate gyrus and hippocampus (Brun and Englund 1981).

---

* This work was supported by the Swedish Medical Research Council, Swedish Tobacco Company, Stiftelsen för Gamla Tjänarinnor, Osterman's fund, and Stohne's fund.

Bergener, Reisberg (Eds.)
Diagnosis and Treatment
of Senile Dementia
© Springer-Verlag Berlin Heidelberg 1989

The diagnostic hallmark for MID is the presence of macro- and microscopic infarcts in cortical and subcortical areas (Tomlinson et al. 1968, 1970) and perivascular serum protein deposits (Alafuzoff et al. 1985). In certain cases of dementia a separate histopathological group AD/MID with a coexistence of degenerative (plaques, tangles) and vascular changes has been characterized (Alafuzoff et al. 1987). Since the pathology in the AD/MID is not merely a linear combination of the pathology found in AD/SDAT and MID, it probably represents a separate dementia type (Alafuzoff et al. 1987).

For the definitive diagnosis of AD/SDAT both a clinical and a histopathological diagnosis is required. In a recent study (Adolfsson et al. 1988) the clinical diagnoses of a nonselected series of patients using the Diagnostic and Statistical Manual of Mental Disorders' (DSM-111) criteria were compared with the histopathological diagnoses found later at autopsy. The patients were assigned to one of five groups according to clinical diagnosis of AD/SDAT, probable AD/SDAT, MID, probable MID, or possible MID (Adolfsson et al. 1988). A comparison of the clinical and histopathological diagnoses revealed a rather poor correlation. Thus, the clinical diagnosis of 12 out of 21 AD/SDAT patients was histopathologicaly verified and likewise, 5 out of 7 MID patients. This is in agreement with the observations made by Todorov et al. (1975). The findings point to the need for comprehensivee longitudinal studes to ascertain the different subgroups.

Neurochemical Aspects of AD/SDAT

Neurochemical studies on AD/SDAT have mostly been performed in human brain tissue obtained at autopsy. The studies indicate deficiencies in several transmitter systems such as acetylcholine (ACh), noradrenaline (NA), dopamine (DA), serotonin (5-HT), and some peptides (for review see Hardy et al. 1985; Gottfries 1985). Because neurosurgery is seldom carried out in patients with dementia, the amount of tissue obtained from biopsies is probably very small and the use of autopsy tissue will continue. Recently, in vitro functional neurotransmitter methods using human postmortal brain tissue have been developed (for review see Dodd et al. 1988) which give valuable information. Neurotransmitter levels, neurotransmitter-related enzyme activities, and radioligand-binding densities were until recently the only measurements available in autopsy tissue. Now new techniques will make it possible to measure presynaptic transmitter uptake, release, and postsynaptic responses to receptor stimulation. There is growing evidence that AD/SDAT might be a more general disease confined not only to the brain. Interest has therefore recently focused on peripheral tissue elements such as blood cells (Adem et al. 1986a, b; Gibson et al. 1987; Zubenko et al. 1987) and skin cells (fibroblasts; Peterson et al. 1986, 1988). Hopefully, easily obtained human peripheral tissue can be used as a model system for studying CNS transmitter processes. In the future in vivo brain imaging techniques such as positron emission tomography (PET) will probably be important reseach tools. Figure 1 illustrates different tissues and techniques which can be used for neurotransmitter studies in AD/SDAT.

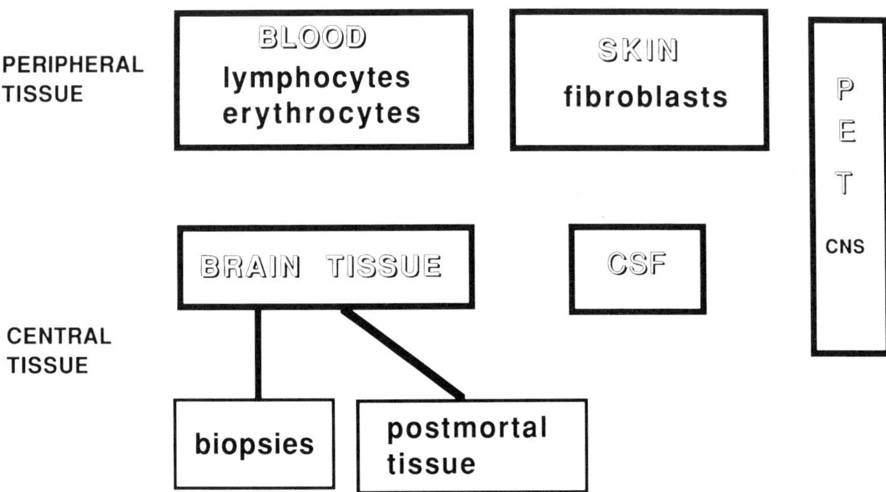

Fig. 1. Different tissues and techniques which can be used for neurotransmitter studies in AD/SDAT

Cholinergic Receptors on Peripheral Lymphocytes

The presence of muscarinic and nicotinic cholinergic receptors have been identified on human lymphocytes (Adem et al. 1986a, b). When cholinergic receptor sites on lymphocytes were measured in a group of AD/SDAT patients and a group of MID patients, a significant decrease in the number of nicotinic receptors was found in the AD/SDAT group (Fig. 2), while there was no change in the MID group compared with controls. A similar decrease in muscarinic receptors was also found in the AD/SDAT group (Adem et al. 1986b). When institutionalized AD/SDAT patients were compared with noninstitutionalized AD/SDAT patients (presumably with less severe forms of the disease) the decrease in number of nicotinic receptors on lymphocytes was only observed in the institutionalized group (Nordberg et al. 1987). Longitudinal studies are now in progress to further investigate receptor changes in a larger group of patients with an emphasis on genetic predisposition of the disease as well.

Positron Emission Tomography Studies in AD/SDAT

Positron emission tomography (PET) studies in AD/SDAT patients have mostly been performed using labeled deoxyglucose. Glucose abnormalities have been reported to occur early and most severely in the temporal and parietal cortex (Friedland et al. 1985; Duara et al. 1986; Jagust et al. 1988). There have been very few attempts to study neurotransmitter receptors in vivo in the bain of AD/SDAT patients (for review see Meyer et al., this volume). A technique to study by PET the uptake of 11C-nicotine and thereby the nicotinic receptors in human brain has recently been developed (Nybäck et al. 1988). Since the number of high affinity nicotinic receptors

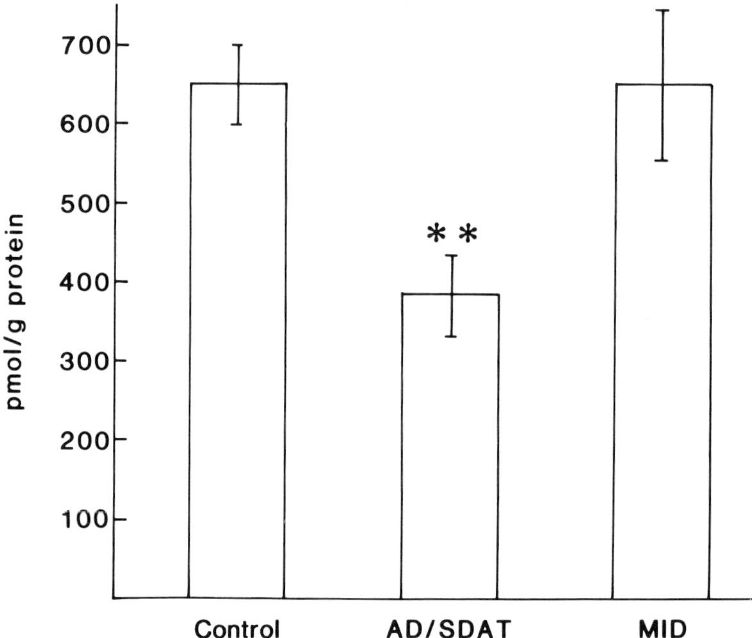

Fig. 2. [^{3}H]-nicotine binding in human lymphocytes from AD/SDAT, MID, and control patients. Mean ± SE; ** $P < 0.01$

are decreased in cortical postmortem brain tissue from AD/SDAT patients (Whitehouse et al. 1986; Nordberg and Winblad 1986), the use of PET to study brain nicotinic receptors in AD/SDAT patients and age-matched controls might be a promising new technique.

Dynamic Transmitter Action in the Brains of AD/SDAT Patients

Until recently, neurochemical studies on AD/SDAT were restricted to the measurement of enzymes, neurotransmitters, and receptor binding sites. There is now a growing body of evidence showing that metabolically and functionally active preparations can be obtained from human brain after considerable postmortem delay. By freezing the tissue slowly in an isosmotic solution, storing it at $-70°C$, and thawing it rapidly on the day of experiment, metabolic and functionally active synaptosomal preparations can be obtained (Hardy et al. 1983). Using this technique uptake and release of several transmitters have been investigated in the brains of control and AD/ SDAT patients (for review see Dodd et al. 1988). The agonal state of the tissue is significant. Normally viable preparation from control human brain can be obtained up to 24 h postmortem if the subject has died suddenly. In AD/SDAT where death is often slow the tissue is less viabile, which means that cell respiration declines faster in AD/SDAT tissue compared with control tissue (Wester et al. 1985). Functional studies on human postmortem brain tissue will provide valuable information on the properties of neurotransmitter uptake, release, and metabolism.

We have developed an in vitro model which allows measurement of synthesis and release of ACh from human brain slices (Nilsson et al. 1986). When human brain tissue with short postmortem delay is incubated with labeled choline, the calcium-dependent potassium-evoked release of labeled ACh can be investigated. As shown in Fig. 3 the release of ACh is markedly enhanced when the potassium concentration is increased from 5 to 35 mM and lowered in the absence of calcium (calcium-dependent release process) in cortical slices from both control and AD/SDAT patients. The potassium-evoked release of ACh is markedly diminished in AD/SDAT cortical tissue when compared with control tissue (Nilsson et al. 1986). This in vitro release model has been used to investigate the underlying neurochemical mechanisms of the acetylcholinesterase (AChE) inhibitors physostigmine and tetrahydroamino-acridine (THA) in brain tissue from AD/SDAT patients. In cortical tissue from controls both AChE inhibitors decrease the release of ACh, while in AD/SDAT tissue they restore the release to the control level (Nilsson et al. 1987). The decreased release of ACh in control tissue can be explained by a negative feedback mechanism mediated via presynaptic muscarinic autoreceptors. To further evaluate the mechanism by which the AChE inhibitors facilitate the release of ACh in AD/SDAT patient cortical tissue, different nicotinic and muscarinic receptor antagonists, have been added to the test system. Figure 4 illustrates the effects of the antagonists in tissue from AD/SDAT patients. The nicotinic antagonist mecamylamine counteracts the effect of THA on ACh release, while it has no effect in control tissue. The muscarinic

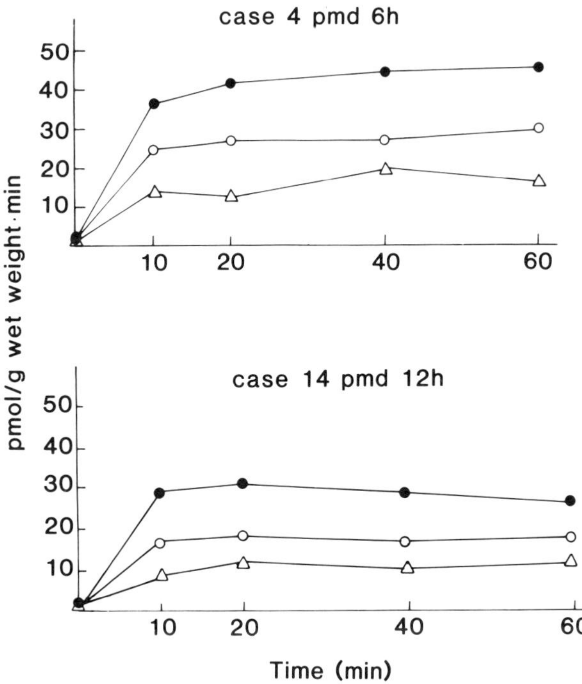

Fig. 3. In vitro release of [^{3}H]-ACh in control *(top)* and AD/SDAT *(bottom)* frontal cortex in the presence of 5 mM K$^+$ *(open circles)*, 35 mM K$^+$ *(solid circles)*, and 35 mM K$^+$ without Ca^{2+} *(triangles)*. pmd, postmortem delay

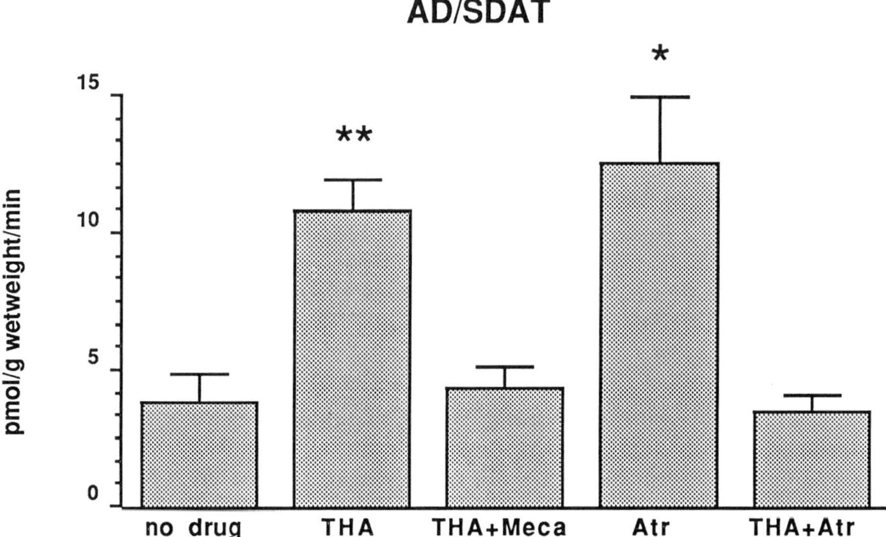

Fig. 4. Effect of THA 10^{-4} M *(THA)*, THA 10^{-4} M plus mecamylamine 10^{-5} M *(THA + Meca)*, atropine 10^{-6} M *(Atr)*, and THA 10^{-4} M plus atropine 10^{-6} M *(THA + Atr)* on in vitro release of [^{3}H]-ACh in AD/SDAT frontal cortex. Mean $\pm$ SE, ** $P < 0.01$; * $P < 0.05$

antagonist atropine increases the release of ACh in brain tissue from both control and AD/SDAT patients. This effect is due to a blockade of presynaptic muscarinic autoreceptors which seem to be present also in AD/SDAT tissue (Fig. 4). When atropine and THA is added together in our release system the effect on ACh release is abolished (Fig. 4). These findings indicate that both muscarinic and nicotinic receptors must be directly/indirectly involved in the mechanism of the AChE inhibitors in AD/SDAT brain; this is also supported by ligand-binding studies (Nordberg et al. 1988). These investigations illustrate the importance of using AD/SDAT brain tissue instead of rat brain or human control brain tissue for studying the effect certain drugs may have in AD/SDAT.

Molecular Biological Aspects of AD/SDAT

Certain families in which AD/SDAT is prevalent exhibit an autosomal dominant mode of disease transmission (Larsson et al. 1963, Heston et al. 1981, Nee et al. 1983). In order to determine the genetic component of AD/SDAT great attempts have been made to identify the abnormal gene(s) responsible for the disease. The gene coding for the amyloid protein has been shown to be encoded by a gene on chromosome 21 (Kang et al. 1987; St. George-Hyslop et al. 1987). However, the mutation found in the amyloid protein gene is probably not the primary defect causing familial AD (Breckenhoven et al. 1987; Tanzi et al. 1987). A reduced amount of total RNA and/or total mRNA has been found in AD/SDAT brains (Mann 1984; Sajdel-Sulkowska and Marotta 1984; Taylor et al. 1986). In order to further investigate the mechanisms responsible for changes in gene expression in AD/SDAT brain, polysomes were isolated. A reduced amount of cytosolic polysomes were isolated from frontal cortices of the brains of AD/SDAT patients compared with age-matched controls (Winblad et al. 1986; Långström et al. 1988, unpublished). The relative rates of mRNA translation by the AD/SDAT brain polysomes compared to control polysomes indicated a reduced protein synthesis in the AD/SDAT frontal cortex (Långström et al. 1988, unpublished). This might be a mechanism by which gene expression is impaired in AD/SDAT.

Conclusions

The lack of agreement between clinical diagnosis and histopathological examination highlights the need for improved diagnostic resolution. The uncertainty as to whether AD and SDAT represent a continuum or heterogenous disorders needs further investigation. Examination of patients from a longitudinal point of view must be stressed. We also must look for and try to find diagnostic markers. Peripheral blood elements and skin cells (fibroblasts) might be valuable tissues in neurochemical and molecular biological studies as well as using the PET technique for examination of the brain. New neurochemical techniques are developing which enable us to measure not only transmitter content, enzyme activity, and receptor number in postmortem brain tissue, but also will allow us to focus on functional, physiological mechanisms in diseased brain tissue. These techniques will hopefully also enable us to study the effect certain drugs may have in AD/SDAT tissue.

References

Adem A, Nordberg A, Slanina P (1986a) A muscarinic receptor type in human lymphocytes: a comparison of ^{3}H-QNB binding to intact lymphocytes and lysed lymphocyte membranes. Life Sci 38: 1359–1368

Adem A, Nordberg A, Bucht G, Winblad B (1986b) Extraneural cholinergic markers in Alzheimer's and Parkinson's disease. Prog Neuropsychopharmacol Biol Psychiatry 10: 247–257

Adolfsson R, Forsgren L (1984) Clinical views on the diagnoses Alzheimer's disease and multiinfarct dementia (in Swedish) Lakartidningen 81: 3919–3924

Adolfsson R, Alafuzoff I, Winblad B (1988) Histopathological validation of the DSM-III criteria in Alzheimer type dementia and multi-infarct dementia. Acta Neurol Scand (in press)

Alafuzoff I, Adolfsson R, Grundke-Iqbal I, Winblad B (1985) Perivascular deposits of serum proteins in cerebral cortex in vascular dementia. Acta Neuropathol (Berl) 66: 292–298

Alafuzoff I, Iqbal K, Friden H, Adolfsson R, Winblad B (1987) Histopathologic criteria for progressive dementia disorders; clinical – pathological correlation and classification by multi-variate data analysis. Acta Neuropathol (Berl) 74: 209–225

Van Broeckhoven C, Genthe AM, Vandenberghe A, Horsthemke B, Backhoven H, Raeymaekers P, van Hul W, Wehnert A et al. (1987) Failure of familial Alzheimer's disease to segregate with the Ah-amyloid gene in several European families. Nature 329: 153–155

Brun A, Englund E (1981) Regional pattern of degeneration in Alzheimer's diesease: neuronal loss and histopathological grading. Histopathology 5: 549–564

Dodd PR, Hambley JW, Cowburn RF, Hardy JA (1988) A comparison of methodologies for the study of functional transmitter neurochemistry in human brain. J Neurochem 50: 1333–1345

Duara R, Grady C, Haxby J, Sundaram M, Cutter NR, Heston L, Moore MSW, Schlageter N, Larsson S, Rapoport SI (1986) Positron emission tomography in Alzheimer's disease. Neurology 36: 879–887

Friedland RP, Budinger TF, Koss E, Ober BA (1985) Alzheimer's disease: anterior – posterior and lateral hemispheric alterations in cortical glucose utilization. Neurosci Lett 53: 235–240

Gibson GE, Nielsen P, Sherman K, Blass JP (1987) Diminished mitogen-induced calcium uptake by lymphocytes from Alzheimer patients. Biol Psychiatry 22: 1079–1086

Gibson PH (1983) Form and distribution of senile plaques seen in silver impregnated sections in the brain of intellectually normally elderly people and people with Alzheimer type dementia. Neuropathol Appl Neurobiol 9: 379–389

Gottfries CG (1985) Alzheimer's disease and senile dementia: biochemical characteristics and aspects of treatment. Psychopharmacology 86: 245–252

Hachinski VC (1979) Relevance of cerebrovascular changes to mental function. Mech Ageing Dev 9: 173–183

Hachinski VC, Lassen NA, Marshall J (1974) Multi-infarct dementia, a cause of mental deterioration in the elderly. Lancet II: 207–210

Hachinski VC, Ihift LD, Zilhka E, Du Boulay GH, Mc Allister VL, Marshall J, Russel RW, Symou L (1975) Cerebral blood flow in dementia. Arch Neurol 32: 632–637

Hardy JA, Dodd PR (1983) Metabolic and functional studies on post-mortem human brain. Neurochem Int 5: 253–266

Hardy JA, Adolfsson R, Alafuzoff I, Bucht G, Marcusson J, Nyberg P, Perdahl E, Wester P, Winblad B (1985) Transmitter deficits in Alzheimer's disease. Neurochem Int 7: 545–563

Heston LL, Mastri AR, Anderson VE, White J (1981) Dementia of the Alzheimer type: Genetics, natural history and associated conditions. Arch Gen Psychiatry 38: 1085–1090

Jaqust WJ, Friedland RP, Budinger TF, Koss E, Ober B (1988) Longitudinal studies of regional cerebral metabolism in Alzheimer's disease. Neurology 38: 909–912

Kang J, Lemaire H-G, Unterbeck A, Salbaum JM, Masters CL, Grzeschik K-H, Multhaup G, Beyreuther K, Muller-Hill B (1987) The precursor of Alzheimer's disease amyloid A4 protein resembles a cell-surface receptor. Nature 325: 733–736

Larsson T, Sjögren T, Jacobson G (1963) Senile dementia. Acta Psychiatr Scand 39 [Suppl 167]: 1–259

Mann DMA (1984) Alzheimer's disease as a disorder of nerve cell protein synthesis. Brain Pathology 1: 269–287

Nee LE, Polinsky RJ, Eldridge R, Weingartner H, Smallberg S, Eberg M (1983) A family with histologically confirmed Alzheimer's disease. Arch Neurol 40: 203–208

Nilsson L, Nordberg A, Hardy J, Wester P, Winblad B (1986) Physostigmine restores ^{3}H-acetylcholine efflux from Alzheimer brain slices to normal level. J Neural Transm 67: 275–285

Nilsson L, Adem A, Hardy J, Winblad B, Nordberg A (1987) Do tetrahydroaminoacridine (THA) and physostigmine restore acetylcholine in AD/SDAT brains via nicotinic receptors? J Neural Transm 70: 357–368

Nordberg A, Winblad B (1986) Reduced number of ^{3}H-nicotine and ^{3}H-acetylcholine binding sites in the frontal cortex of Alzheimer brains. Neurosci Letters 72: 115–119

Nordberg A, Adem A, Nilsson L, Winblad B (1987) Cholinergic deficits in CNS and peripheral non-neuronal tissue in Alzheimer dementia. In: Dowdall M, Hawthorne J (eds) Cellular and molecular basis of cholinergic function. Ellis-Howard, Chichester, p 858–868

Nordberg A, Nilsson L, Adem A, Hardy J, Winblad B (1988) Effects of THA on acetylcholine release and cholinergic receptors in Alzheimer brains. In: Giacobini E, Becker R (eds) Current research in Alzheimer therapy. Taylor and Francis, New York, p 247–257

Nybäck H, Nordberg A, Långström B, Halldin C, Hartvig P, Åhlin A, Schwan C.G., Sedvall G (1988) Attempts to visualize nicotinic receptors in the brain of monkey and man by positron emission tomography. In: Nordberg A, Fuxe K, Holmstedt B, Sundwall A (eds) Nicotinic receptors in the CNS – their role in synaptic transmission. Prog Brain Research Elsevier (in press)

Peterson C, Ratan CR, Shelanski ML, Goldman JE (1986) Cytosolic free calcium and cell spreading decrease in fibroblasts from aged and Alzheimer donors. Proc Natl Acad Sci USA 83: 7999–8001

Peterson C, Ratan RR, Shelanski ML, Goldman JE (1988) Altered response of fibroblasts from aged and Alzheimer donors to drug that elevate cytosolic free calcium. Neurobiol Aging 9: 261–266

Roth M (1955) The natural history of mental disorder in old age. J Ment Sci 101: 281–301

Roth M (1985) Some strategies for tacking the problems of senile dementia and related disorders within the next decade. Danish Med Bull 32 (Suppl I): 92–111

Sajdel-Sulkowska EM, Marotta CA (1984) Alzheimer's disease brain: alterations in RNA levels and in a ribonuclease-inhibitor complex. Science 225: 947–949

Slater E, Roth M (1970) Aging and the mental disease of aged. In: Mayer-Gross W, Slater E, Roth M (eds) Clinical psychiatry, vol. 3, ch 8. Bailliere, Tindall and Cassell, London p 533–560

St George-Hyslop PH, Tanzi RE, Polinsky RJ, Haines JL, Nee L, Watkins PC, Myers RH, Feldman RG, Pollen D, Drachman D, Growdon J, Bruni A, Foncin J-F, Salmon D, Frommelt P, Amaducci L, Sorbi S, Piacentini S, Stewart GD, Hobbs WJ, Conneally PM, Gusella JF (1987) The genetic defect causing familial Alzheimer's disease maps on chromosome 21. Science 235: 885–890

Tanzi RE, St George-Hyslop PH, Haines JL, Polinsky RJ, Nee L, Foncin J-F, Neve RL, McClatchey AI, Conneally PM, Gusella JF (1987) The genetic defect in familial Alzheimer's disease is not tightly linked to the amyloid protein gene. Nature 329: 156–157

Taylor GR, Carter GI, Crow TJ, Johnson JA, Fairbrain AF, Perry EK, Perry RH (1986) Recovery and measurement of specific RNA species from post-mortem brain tissue: a general reduction in Alzheimer's disease detected by molecular hybridization. Exp Mol Pathol 44: 111–116

Terry RD, Davies P (1980) Dementia of the Alzheimer type. Ann Rev Neurosci 3: 77–95

Todorov AB, Go RCP, Constantinidis J, Elston RC (1975) Specificity of the clinical diagnosis of dementia. J Neurol Sci 26: 81–98

Tomlinson BE (1980) The structural and quantitative aspects of the dementia. In: Roberts PJ (ed) Biochemistry of dementia. J Wiley, Chichester, p 15–51

Tomlinson BE, Blessed G, Roth M (1968) Observations on the brain on non-demented old people. J Neurol Sci 7: 331–356

Tomlinson BE, Blessed G, Roth M (1970) Observations of the brain of demented old people. J Neurol Sci 11: 205–242

Van Broeckhoven C, Genthe AM, Vandenberghe A, Horsthemke B, Backhovens H, Raeymackers P, Van Hul W, Wehnert A, Gheuens J, Cras P, Bruyland M, Martin JJ, Salbaum M, Multhaup G, Masters CL, Beyreuther K, Gurling HMD, Mullan MJ, Holland A, Barton A, Irving N, Williamson R, Richards SJ, Hardy JA (1987) Failure of familial Alzheimer's disease to segregate with the A4-amyloid gene in several European families. Nature 329: 153–155

Wester P, Bateman DE, Dodd PR, Edwardson JA, Hardy JA, Kidd AM, Perry RH, Singh GB (1985) Agonal status effects the metabolic activity of nerve endings isolated from postmortem human brain. Neurochem Pathol 3: 169–180

Whitehouse P, Martino AM, Antuono PG, Lowenstein PR, Coyle J, Price DL, Kellar KJ (1986) Nicotinic acetylcholine binding sites in Alzheimer's disease. Brain Res 371: 146–151

Winblad B, Wallace W, Hardy J, Fowler C, Bucht G, Alafuzoff I, Adolfsson R (1986) Neurochemical, genetic and clinical aspects of Alzheimer's disease. In: Bergener M (ed) Dimensions of aging. Academic, London, p 183–203

Zubenko GS, Cohen BM, Boller F, Malinakova I, Keefe N, Chojnacki B (1987) Platelet membrane abnormality in Alzheimer's diesease. Ann Neurol 22: 237–244

Neurochemistry of Dementia: Clinical Pathological Relationships

P. J. Whitehouse, J. R. Unnerstall, M. Tabaton, and D. J. Lanska

Introduction

The inventory of neurotransmitter systems in different dementias is expanding rapidly. Most attention has been focused on the degenerative dementias, particularly Alzheimer's disease (AD) and related disorders such as Parkinson's disease (PD) (Whitehouse et al. 1985; Price et al. 1986). In this paper, we will review some of the neurochemical changes that have been reported in AD, focusing particularly on alterations in the cholinergic and bioaminergic systems. We will then discuss several approaches that are likely to improve our understanding of the neurochemical basis of dementia and behavioral symptoms and outline some strategies to better relate neurochemical studies to molecular biology and clinical investigations.

Review of Neurochemical Changes

Most neurochemical studies in AD have focused on a limited number of brain areas, particularly the neocortex and hippocampus. The subcortical structures most investigated have been the cholinergic basal forebrain, the noradrenergic locus coeruleus and raphe nucleus, and the dopaminergic substantia nigra and ventral tegmental area (Whitehouse et al. 1985; Price et al. 1986). Table 1 summarizes the reported neurochemical abnormalities in AD in some of these brain regions. Consistent loss of somatostatin, corticotropin releasing factor (CRF), excitatory amino acid, and γ-aminobutyric acid (GABA) markers are reported in cortex. A large number of cortical systems are found to be variably affected, such as substance P and neuropeptide Y. Loss of telencephalic cholinergic markers due to degeneration of cells in the basal forebrain also occurs consistently, whereas variable changes have been reported in serotonin and norepinephrine markers. It is not known whether the inconsistency in reported neurochemical changes represents different methods and techniques used in different laboratories, or intrinsic biological variability in the disease such that some patients show changes in certain systems whereas others do not.

Recently, areas of the brain not previously systematically studied in AD have been described as showing pathology, including retina, striatum, thalamus, hypothalamus, and even white matter (Saper, in press). Neurotransmitter system abnormalities associated with cellular pathology in these areas are less well understood. Thus, the

Bergener, Reisberg (Eds.)
Diagnosis and Treatment
of Senile Dementia
© Springer-Verlag Berlin Heidelberg 1989

Table 1. Neurochemical abnormalities reported in AD

Anatomical area	Neurotransmitter
Cortex and hippocampus	Somatostatin CRF Excitatory amino acids (e. g., glutamate) GABA ? Neuropeptide Y ? Substance P
Basal forebrain	acetylcholine
Locus coeruleus	Norepinephrine ? Neuropeptide Y
Raphe nucleus	Serotonin
Substantia nigra	Dopamine

study of AD is leading to a more complicated picture of neural dysfunction than previously thought.

The neurochemistry of the degenerative disorders is also becoming more complex as more overlapping features are described among different disorders. For example, it is now clear that certain patients with PD become demented (Mayeux et al. 1981) and some, but not all, of those patients show neurofibrillay tangles and senile plaques characteristic of AD (Boller et al. 1980). Abnormalities in most of the neurochemical systems affected in AD have also been reported to occur in PD, including cortical levels of somatostatin, CRF, acetylcholine, norepinephrine, and serotonin (Whitehouse et al. 1985; Price et al. 1986). Some of these overlapping neurochemical features occur whether or not the dementia is associated with plaques or tangles. On the other hand, in other disorders such as Huntington's disease (HD) the cognitive abnormalities seem to have a different biological basis; in HD most attention has been focused on the caudate nucleus and its role in cognition and motor performance.

Clinical Pathological Correlation

In PD, understanding the relationship between brain structures and motor symptoms led to the development of effective therapies. Since this initial success, investigators have tried to associate neurochemical systems with cognitive impairment in PD and other degenerative disorders. Claims have been made that dysfunction in several neurotransmitter systems forms the primary basis of the cognitive symptoms in AD. It seems obvious that pathology in a number of different brain regions contributes to the cognitive impairment. The task for the future is not to identify single systems that can explain all the symptoms, but rather to understand the interactions between neuronal loss in different systems and the complex patterns of dysfunction in intellectual abilities.

Despite the fact that appropriate criticism has been voiced concerning too exclusive a focus on cholinergic mechanisms, it is still the case that abnormalities in cholinergic systems are most closely related to the cognitive impairment. Pathology in non-cholinergic systems in the hippocampus and cortex is undoubtedly equally or more important in producing the cognitive symptoms, but the neurotransmitter circuitry of these regions is exceedingly complex. The evidence for the important role of acetyl-choline comes from both animal and human studies (Price et al. 1986; Whitehouse et al. 1985). In animal studies, either stimulation or experimental lesions of basal forebrain neurons and the administration of drugs that either block or enhance the activity of the system have profound effects on cognitive abilities, particularly learn-ing and memory. Moreover, in human subjects, drugs with anticholinergic properties are particularly prone to causing confusion, particularly in elderly patients with or without dementia. Moreover, although the effects are modest and inconsistent, cholinomimetic drugs such as anticholinesterases can improve cognition in AD in some circumstances. In most clinical pathological studies, the strongest correlations found between biological measures and behavior are between cholinergic markers in brain and severity of dementia shortly before death.

Renewed attention is being paid to other aspects of the clinical symptomatology in AD; notably, the psychiatric symptoms. For years, psychiatrists have proposed that abnormalities in bioaminergic systems (norepinephrine and serotonin) relate to psychiatric syndromes in intellectually intact patients such as depression and schizo-phrenia. In our studies, hallucinations and affective symptoms are common in AD (GSA abstract), and it is well known that the raphe and serotonergic systems are consistently but variably affected in the disorder (D'Amato et al. 1987; Zweig et al. 1988). We have found very preliminary evidence that patients with more affective symptoms may have more severe alterations in bioaminergic markers (Zweig et al. 1988). The major support for the bioaminergic theory of psychiatric illnesses in the absence of dementia lies in the effects of drugs in both producing and eliminating psychiatric symptoms. Drugs that deplete bioamines may cause depression, and drugs that block the reuptake and, therefore, enhance the action of serotonin and norepinephrine are used in treating depression. Norepinephrine can produce a clini-cal syndrome which resembles paranoid schizophrenia and lysergic acid diethylamide (LSD), which acts on serotonergic systems, can produce hallucinations.

Although work on developing drugs that improve the cognitive symptoms in AD is slow, rapid advances are being made in developing compounds which may be useful to treat the psychiatric symptoms in AD. Novel tranquilizers (anxiolytics) such as Busperone may be useful if they cause minimal sedation and tolerance does not develop to the extent that it does with benzodiazepines. New major tranquilizers such as Clozapine may be useful in the elderly if they produce fewer extrapyramidal side effects than currently available compounds. Antidepressants which are more selective in their action on neurotransmitter systems such as fluoxetine have fewer anti-cholinergic properties and may be less likely to cause confusion in elderly subjects. An understanding of the biological basis of psychiatric symptoms in these illnesses may lead us to develop more effective therapies for the behavioral symptoms. These behavioral symptoms are probably more major contributors to stress on our health care system than the cognitive symptoms. Both family caregivers and caregivers in institutional settings report that wandering, agitation, depression, and psychotic features lead to greater difficulties in management than do the purely cognitive symptoms.

Problems in Approaches to Clinical – Pathological Correlation

Our understanding of the biological basis of dementia is rudimentary. In order to improve our understanding of these brain-behavior relationships, we need to consider some of the problems with clinical assessment, postmortem biological measures, and attempts to relate the clinical and pathological data.

Clinical Assessment. Most attempts to correlate severity of dementia with pathological data have used brief mental status instruments. For the most part, these instruments do not allow quantitative separation of the different aspects of cognition, and are insensitive to the early changes in cognitive function. Moreover, these tests may not be true interval scales, making parametric statistical tests difficult. More recent efforts have avoided the use of simplistic rating scales and have attempted to relate specific behavioral functions to pathological measurements in particular brain regions.

Pathological Analysis. The assessment of biological changes in the brains of patients with dementia is fraught with difficulty. A number of variables need to be taken into account including the cause of death, the patient's drug history, post-mortem delay in refrigerating and freezing tissue, and length of time the tissue is stored. Currently, pathological assessment is often only semiquantitative. A variety of new techniques (immunocytochemistry, receptor autoradiography, in situ hybridization) allow creating images in auotpsy tissue of the distribution of biological markers, including neurotransmitters and their receptors, other proteins, and nucleic acids (RNA and DNA). New computer systems should permit quantifying these images in ways not previously possible by manual methods (Whitehouse et al. 1985).

Relating Clinical and Pathological Data. The major problem in understanding brain-behavior relationships lies in correlating the clinical and pathological data which are often obtained by different groups of researchers at widely different points in time. Most biological studies are based on a single set of measurements made at autopsy late in the disease process. Relating measurements to behavioral variables which have been assessed serially through the course of the illness is difficult. Clinical-pathological correlation is furhter limited by inadequacies of our models of normal cognition.

Statistical Problems. Even when relationships are established between behavioral and biological data, it is important to consider the possibility of artifactual associations. Appropriate statistical tests need to be used to determine that the likelihood that the association occurred by chance is small. Many studies involve few subjects and both clinical and biological measures may have considerable variability, which makes it difficult to detect variance which links the two levels of description. Several confounding factors can affect the apparent clinical-pathological correlation. Particularly notable is the effect of age, since many of the same neurochemical systems are affected in normal aging in the absence of intellectual impairment. Systematic biases in assessing the demented and control groups need to be watched for carefully, particularly in aspects of history taking and recording of observations and staging.

A statistically significant correlation does not establish a causal association. Several criteria can be helpful in distinguishing causal and indirect associations, including strength of the association, coherence with existing knowledge, temporality of the anatomical and behavioral observations, rating of effect (i. e., dose-response relationship), modification of the effect by some agent such as a drugs, and experimental reproduction of the disease.

Look to the Future

The establishment of clinical-pathological correlations in dementia can be enhanced by improving both the biological and behavioral measures. Attempts are being mounted in different parts of the world to follow longitudinally groups of clinically assessed patients whose brains are examined in a standardized way at death. The National Institute of Aging's Alzheimer's Disease Research Centers (NIA ADRCs) represent such a coordinated effort in the United States. Neurochemical studies of dementia will also be more valuable if links are made to our growing understanding of the pathophysiology of the disease and molecular mechanisms of cell death. If the genetic abnormality in HD on chromosome 4 can be linked to abnormalities in excitatory neurotransmitters and potential toxins, we can begin to explain the selective vulnerability of neural systems in the striatum. In AD, our understanding of the molecular biology of neurofibrillary tangles and amyloid in senile plaques is increasing dramatically. Perhaps the amyloid precursor protein is related to a growth factor that selectively affects the functioning of specific populations of cells and their characteristic neurotransmitter. In PD, much excitement has been created by the development of the MPTP model. In this model, both animal subjects and human drug abusers have developed PD through exposure to a drug that appears to selectively impair dopaminergic systems.

Thus, the way to improve our understanding of the clinical pathological correlates in dementia is threefold: First, we must improve our modeling and assessment of normal human cognitive abilities and our descriptions of how cognition is affected in dementia. Second, we must develop better quantitative methods for assessing critical aspects of brain function at both the molecular and systems neuroscience level. Third, we must develop large data bases and more sophisticated statistical models to relate the biological and behavioral measures. These studies should not only help us understand how the brain disease causes clinical symptoms but also lead to the development of more effective therapies.

Acknowledgements. The authors thank Pierluigi Gambetti, M.D., Steve Younkin, M.D., Ph.D., George Perry, Ph.D., Mark Palmert, Ph.D., and Todd Golde, Ph.D., for their contributions to this work. Research was supported in part by Alzheimer Disease Research Center grants (NIMH #MH-43-444-01 and Ohio Department of Aging #ADR-2)

References

Boller F, Mizutani T, Roessmann U, Gambetti P (1980) Parkinson disease, dementia, and Alzheimer disease: Clinicopathological correlations. Ann Neurol 7: 329–335

D'Amato RJ, Zweig RM, Whitehouse PJ, et al (1987) Aminergic systems in Alzheimer's and Parkinson's disease. Ann Neurol 22: 229–236

Kalaria JN, Mitchell MJ, Harik SI (1987) Correlation of 1-methyl-4-phenyl-1, 2, 3, 6-tetrahydropyridine neurotoxicity with blood-brain barrier monoamine oxidase activity. Proc Natl Acad Sci USA 84: 3521–3525

Martin JB, Gusella JF (1986) Huntington's Disease pathogenesis and management. Seminars in Medicine of the Beth Israel Hospital, Boston 315: 1257–1276

Mayeux R, Stern Y, Rosen J, Leventhal J (1981) Depression, intellectual impairment, and Parkinson disease. Neurology 31: 645–650

Palmert MR, Golde TE, Cohen ML, Kovacs DM, Tanzi RE, Gusella JF, Usiak MF, Younkin LH, Younkin SG (1988) Amyloid protein precursor messenger RNAs: differential expression in Alzheimer's disease. Science 241: 1080–1084

Perry G, Friedman R, Shaw G, Chau V (1987) Ubiquitin is detected in neurofibrillary tangles and senile plaque neurites of Alzheimer disease brains. Proc Natl Acad Sci USA 84: 3033–3036

Tabaton M, Whitehouse PJ, Perry G, Davies P, Autilio-Gambetti L, Gambetti P (1988) Alz 50 recognizes abnormal filaments in Alzheimer disease and progressive supranuclear palsy. Ann Neurol 24: 407–413

Price DL, Whitehouse PJ, Struble RG (1986) Cellular pathology in Alzheimer's and Parkinson's diseases. TINS 9: 29–33

Saper CB (1988) Chemical neuroanatomy of Alzheimer's Disease. In: Iversen SD, Iversen LL, and Sanyo SH (eds). Biology of Alzheimer's Disease, Vol 20. Plenum Press, New York

Whitehouse PJ, Loats HL, Price DL (1985a) New approaches in quantitative neuropathology. In: Shagass C, et al. (eds) Biological psychiatry, pp 1385–1387

Whitehouse PJ, Struble RG, Hedreen JC, et al. (1985b) Alzheimer's disease and related dementias: Selective involvement of specific neuronal systems. Crit Rev Clin Neurobiol 1: 319–339

Whitehouse PJ and Unnerstall JR (1988) Neurochemistry of dementia (abstract). Alzheimer Disease and Associated Disorders: An International Journal. 2: 159

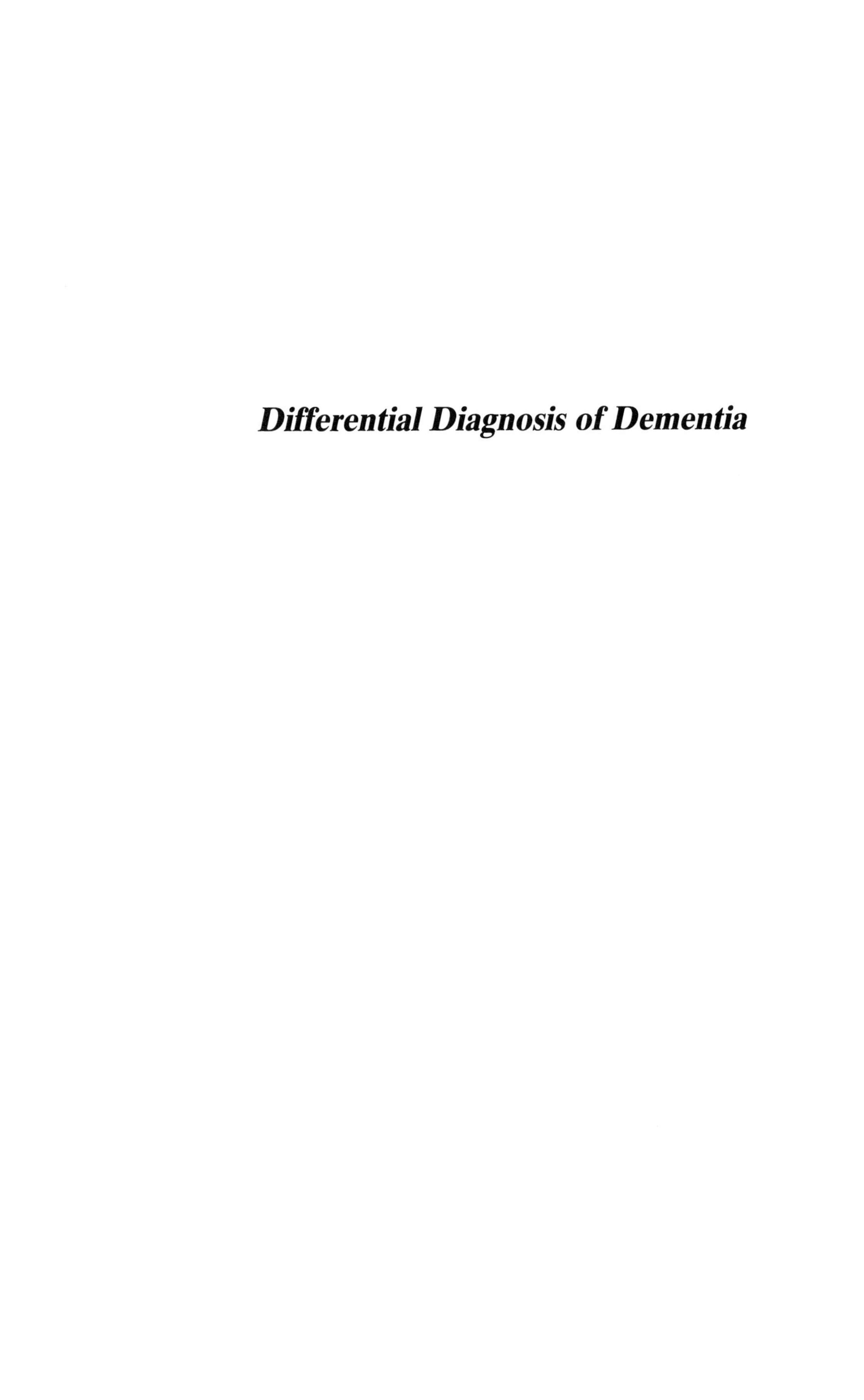

Differential Diagnosis of Dementia

Depression Versus Dementia:
Further Evidence from the Liverpool Outcome Studies*

J. R. M. Copeland, I. A. Davidson, C. D. Neal, M. E. Dewey,
and C. McWilliam

Introduction

The US/UK Diagnostic Project (Copeland et al. 1975) showed that the high preponderance of dementia over depression recorded among United States compared to United Kingdom hospital admissions disappeared when standardised methods of interview and diagnosis were used. Gurland et al. (1976) showed that patients with depression who had paranoid symptoms were those most likely to be mis-diagnosed as having dementia. But some mis-diagnosis due to a proportion of depressions being associated with organic features continues to present clinical problems in spite of improved diagnostic techniques. Follow-up studies of clinically diagnosed dementia have recorded cases of good recovery where the diagnosis of dementia had been given to cases suffering from depression (Nott and Fleminger 1975; Ron et al. 1979). Cohen et al. (1982) attributed the cognitive impairment in depression mainly to lack of motivation and attention, and McAllister (1981) could not demonstrate that it had any special pattern, or that it differed from that found in dementia.

The relationship of dementia to depression remains obscure. Post (1962) found no evidence that depression was a prodromal symptom of dementia, although the latter could on occasion provoke the former. The term "pseudo-dementia" is now used where a functional mental illness tends to simulate dementia of organic cause. But organic pathology could underline some depressions. In a series of studies using computed tomography Jacoby and colleagues demonstrated that some depressions of old age were associated with enlargement of the brain ventricles and increased risk of dying (Jacoby and Levy 1980; Jacoby et al. 1981). A number of physiological methods have been tried for distinguishing between the two conditions, including the dexamethasone suppression test, average evoked responses and the event-related potential component P 300, with only moderate degrees of success.

Standardised interviews and diagnoses using computer methods examined against outcome now allow for a more accurate investigation of the prevalence of these disorders and for some refinement in clinical differentiation.

* This research was supported by grants from the Wellcome Trust and the Mersey Regional Health
Authority Research Committee, United Kingdom.

Bergener, Reisberg (Eds.)
Diagnosis and Treatment
of Senile Dementia
© Springer-Verlag Berlin Heidelberg 1989

Method

In this paper we examine the clinical relationship of depression to dementia and its prevalence using data derived from the application of the Geriatric Mental State – AGECAT (GMS-AGECAT) Package to community- and hospital-based samples of elderly persons. The GMS-AGECAT Package consists of
a) the GMS itself (Copeland et al. 1976; Gurland et al. 1976), a semi-structured standardised interview for those aged 65 and over, derived in part from the Present State Examination (Wing et al. 1974),
b) the History and Aetiology Schedule for an informant, and
c) the AGECAT computerised diagnosis.

The edition of the GMS used in the study was GMSA, the community version, derived from the main schedule by a series of discriminant function analyses between diagnostic groups, cases and non-cases, covering the onset of the illness, family history, the subject's own past history of mental and physical illness, some putative risk factors for dementia, a more extensive investigation of organic type behaviour, alcohol abuse and head injury. The data are computer-processed to produce the AGECAT diagnostic system (Copeland et al. 1986; Dewey and Copeland 1986).

This system condenses 157 symptom components into 38 symptom subclusters which in turn are assembled under eight diagnostic clusters according to their importance for determining the certainty of diagnosis for that cluster. Each subject is assigned to a level of confidence of diagnosis from 0 to 6 on each diagnostic cluster. Clusters are then compared, level for level, according to a hierarchy starting with organic disorders, including depression and ending with anxiety. Each subject emerges with a main diagnosis, an alternative if appropriate, the levels of confidence on all eight clusters, levels on 19 symptom profiles of illness as well as scores for quick case identification. The levels of diagnostic confidence for dementia and depression have been shown to equate well with levels of severity of illness. Of the levels 0–5, level 3, 4 and 5 are identified by psychiatric raters as the case levels (we term these "syndrome cases"), and 1 and 2 as subcase levels ("syndrome subcases"). Where a "syndrome case" or "subcase" is also the primary diagnosis, it is termed a diagnostic (syndrome) case or subcase. Thus a subject may be a diagnostic case of depression with (syndrome) case or subcase organic disorder or vice versa. To simplify the nomenclature we tend to refer to syndrome cases and subcases simply as cases and subcases. The depression cluster is divided into depressive psychosis (equivalent to endogenous depression) and depressive neurosis (equivalent to reactive depression). The system thus allows not only for a primary differential diagnosis but also identifies levels of co-morbid states, making it suitable to examine dementia with co-morbid depressive levels and depression with co-morbid organic levels.

The validity of the AGECAT diagnosis has been tested against psychiatrists' diagnosis on over 1000 hospital and community cases. Kappa values of agreement between psychiatrists' diagnoses using DSM-III criteria are in excess of 0.80 for organic disorders and 0.76 for depression (Copeland et al. 1986, 1988).

Data from two studies are reported. The first, a random community sample of 1070 persons aged 65 and over living in Liverpool, in their own or residential homes but not in hospital, derived from general practitioners' lists. All subjects were interviewed by para-medical staff specially trained in the GMS-AGECAT Package (Copeland et al. 1987). The second study was a consecutive series of 101 admissions aged 65 and over to the psychogeriatric wards of a district general hospital serving a catchment area population. They were from an area adjacent to Liverpool.

Results

Prevalence of Dementia with Depression

Table 1 shows the AGECAT primary diagnosis of dementia (diagnostic cases) associated with co-morbid depression (syndrome case and subcase levels). Approximately one-quarter of the diagnostic cases of dementia in the community are associated with subcase and a further 20% with case levels of depression of one type or another. However, just over half the community diagnostic cases of dementia have no associated depressive levels. In terms of the full sample of 1070 subjects, only 1.1% of the elderly population are diagnostic cases of dementia associated with case levels of depression.

In the hospital series almost two-thirds of the diagnostic dementias have associated levels of subcase depression, while similar proportions to the community sample are associated with case levels of depression. Of all the hospital admissions 9% are diagnostic cases of dementia associated with case levels of depression.

Table 1. Prevalence of AGECAT primary dementia (case level) with depression (subcase and case levels)

AGECAT depression levels	Community[a]			Hospital[b]		
	n	De-mentia %	Full sample %	n	De-mentia %	Full sample %
Subcase	14	25.5	1.3	30	61.2	29.8
Case						
Depressive neurosis	9	16.3	0.9	7	14.4	7.0
Depressive psychosis	2	3.6	0.2	2	4.0	2.0
No case level	30	54.6	2.8	10	20.4	9.9
Total	55	100.0	5.2	49	100.0	48.7

[a] Liverpool Longitudinal Community Study ($n = 1070$)
[b] Nantwich Hospital Study ($n = 101$)

Prevalence of Depression with Organic Levels

Table 2 shows the AGECAT diagnostic depression cases associated with organic subcase and case levels, so called pseudo-dementias.

Almost 15% of depressive neurotic diagnostic cases in the community are associated with subcase organic levels, while for depressive psychosis the figure is 32.2%.

Table 2. Prevalence of AGECAT primary depressions (case level) with organic symptoms (subcase and case levels)

AGECAT organic levels	Community[a]				DN + DP	Hospital[b]				DN + DP
	Depressive Neurosis (DN)		Depressive Psychosis (DP)		Full sample	Depressive Neurosis (DN)		Depressive Psychosis (DP)		Full sample
	n	%	n	%	%	n	%	n	%	%
Subcase										
O 1	7	7.9	5	16.1	1.1	0	0.0	1	5.8	1.0
O 2	6	6.7	5	16.1	1.0	1	8.3	4	23.5	5.0
Case										
O 3	0	0.0	4	12.9	0.4	0	0.0	0	0.0	0.0
No case	76	85.4	17	54.9	8.7	11	91.7	12	70.7	22.7
Total	89	100.0	31	100.0	11.2	12	100.0	17	100.0	28.7

[a] Liverpool Longitudinal Community Study ($n = 1070$)
[b] Nantwich Hospital Study ($n = 101$)

There are no diagnostic cases of depressive neurosis associated with syndrome case levels of organic disorder because, at this level, organic disorder would automatically override depressive neurosis to become a diagnostic case. However, nearly 13% of the diagnostic cases of depressive psychoses have associated organic case levels. These true pseudo-dementias amount to no more than 0.4% of the full sample. The community prevalence is therefore very small. Even if all the depressive diagnostic cases associated with *any* organic level are added together, they amount to no more than 2.5% of the full community random samples. Of the remaining depression diagnostic cases in the community, 8.7% have no organic case levels.

In the hospital admission series, only 8.3% of depressive neurosis diagnostic cases entering the hospital are associated with subcases of organic disorder, compared to nearly 30% of depressive psychosis cases. Surprisingly, there were no subjects in the hospital series in whom diagnostic case level depression was associated with case level organic disorder. Diagnostic cases of depression as a whole accounted for 28.7% of the consecutive admissions, but only 17 of these were of depressive psychosis. However, with community prevalence of only 4 pseudo-dementia cases out of 31 depressions, it is, after all, less surprising that in the hospital there are none out of 17 cases.

Association Between Dementia and Depression with Increasing Levels of Illness-Severity

Contrary to expectation, as the level of dementia rises from diagnostic case level 3 to 4 (roughly from serious memory problems with some disorientation in time to more serious disorientation in place and person), it is found that 12 out of 20 cases are associated with depressive levels of some kind at level 3, but 27 out of 29 such cases at level 4. Thus organic diagnostic levels appear, in the hospital series, to be associated with more, rather than less, expression of depression symptoms as the dementia progresses (p < 0.02). This cannot be explained as a tendency to affirm all functional symptoms indiscriminately, because the prevalence of neurotic levels appears to diminish.

As the levels of diagnostic depression increase, they, in turn, tend to be associated with more organic levels. At depression level 3 only one of the nine hospital admissions with depression was associated with an organic level. At level 4, seven such cases were associated with organic levels out of 20, but this does not reach statistical significance.

Do the Clinical Pictures of Dementia with Depressive Symptoms and Depression with Organic Symptoms Differ?

Here we use the symptom profiles derived from the GMS by a factor-analytical study (Gurland et al. 1976). Figure 1a shows the symptom profile for diagnostic cases of dementia with case level depression, and Fig. 1b for diagnostic cases of depression with case and subcase organic levels. The overall profiles emphasize the similarity of the clinical pictures. Only two scores are significantly different, that for somatic dysfunction (complaints of appetite and weight loss, and sleep disturbance; $p < .01$ and that for disorientation (in time, place or person; $p < .02$).

Outcome of Co-morbid Dementia and Depression

Table 3 shows the outcome of mixed organic and depression levels as assessed by psychiatrists at a follow-up study between 1 and 3 years after initial interview. Because of the small number of cases the community and hospital samples have been combined.

Of the 19 cases with AGECAT diagnostic dementia and case level depression the outcome was unknown in five, due to refused interview or death, with inadequate documentation. Twelve were known either to have died of dementia or to be still demented at follow-up, only one had become a case of depression, and one had become "well".

Of the 32 cases of AGECAT diagnostic depression with organic levels – the pseudo-dementias – eight had unknown outcomes; one had had stereotaxic surgery for

Table 3. Outcome of mixed organic and depression levels: AGECAT diagnosis confirmed by psychiatrists at 1–3 year follow-up (community and hospital samples mixed)

Year 0: AGECAT diagnosis	1–3 Year outcome – psychiatrists' diagnosis			
	Unknown due to refusals or death	Dementia	Depression	Other, well
Primary dementia with case level depression ($n = 19$)	5	12	1	1
Primary depression with organic levels subcase and case – "Pseudo-dementias" ($n = 31$)	8	4	5	14

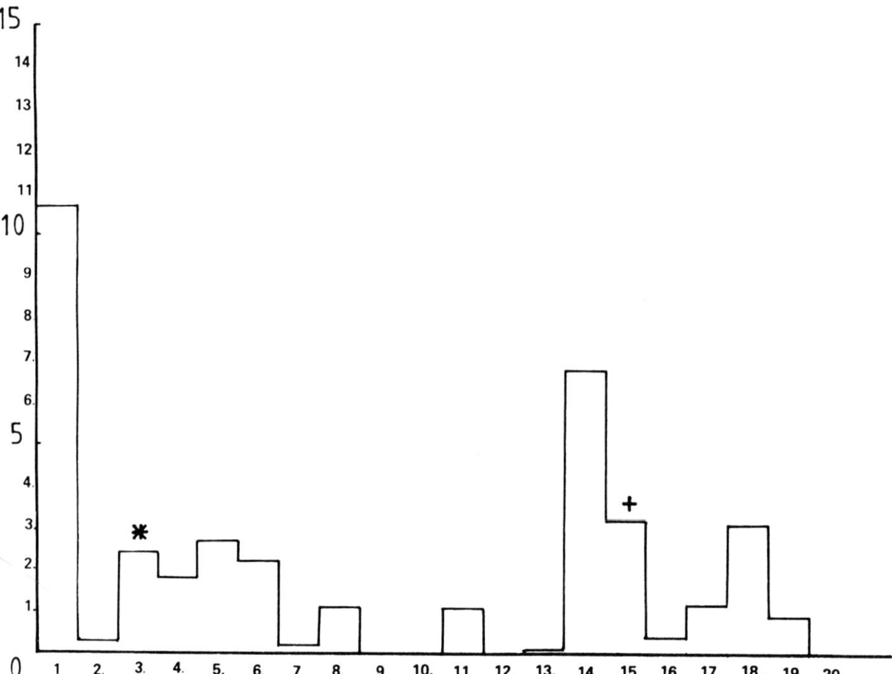

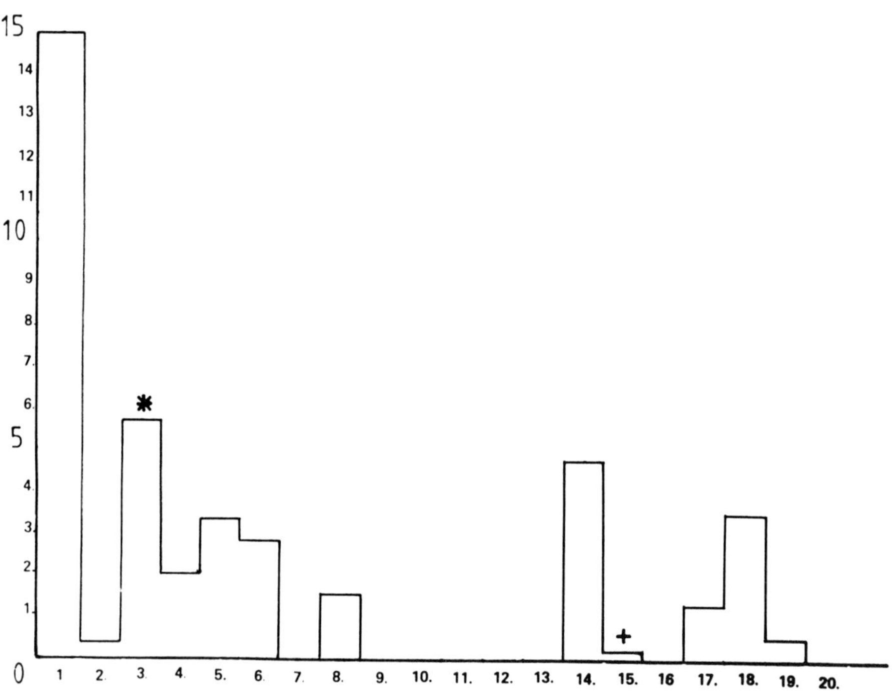

Fig. 1

Parkinson's disease and has been excluded. Five further cases were known to be depressed at follow-up, but only one of these was still associated with organic levels; fourteen had developed unrelated conditions or were entirely well, and four had become demented. Of those who developed dementia, one was said to have become an early case, one was an alcoholic dementia who had continued to drink heavily after the initial interview, and the remaining two were probably mis-diagnoses at initial interview. Thus the AGECAT diagnosis at initial interview would seem to have differentiated successfully between dementia and depression using mental state items alone.

Discussion

The overall prevalence for diagnostic cases of dementia in the Liverpool community was assessed at 5.2%, approximately half of whom were associated with subcase or case levels of depression. In the hospital series of those who were more severely ill (higher proportion at level 4), more than two-thirds of the dementia diagnostic cases had some depressive levels. There is a significant tendency for the increasing levels of severity of dementia to be associated with depressive levels. This was against expectation. It was assumed that as dementia progresses depression would become less evident, perhaps related to loss of insight. This may happen only at the most severe level of dementia, level 5 on the AGECAT system, of which there were no examples in this study.

Pseudo-dementia, defined most stringently as diagnostic case level depression with case level organic disorder is not a common condition, at 0.4% in the general population and not represented in the small hospital series. However, it is clear from both studies that some diagnostic depressions may be associated with other organic levels, and that there is a non-significant trend for such proportions to increase with the severity of the depression. This relationship by no means holds for all depressions; over 70% of depressive psychoses have no such organic levels, and even at severity level 4 as many as 13 out of 20 (65%) have no organic levels. There may be fundamental differences between depressions in those who develop co-morbid organic levels and in those who do not, such as underlying organic disease in a brain which only becomes decompensated when suffering a depressive illness. Do such cases represent early dementia, with organic disorder affecting that part of the brain responsible for a major depressive disorder, or two relatively common conditions co-existing? Is early dementia a psychological precipitant for depression? The effects of lost motivation and concentration, severe in most dementias and some depressions, may contribute to a common clinical picture. Certainly workers have found it difficult to distinguish between the cognitive changes of dementia and those of depression.

Fig. 1a, b. Profile symptom scores. *a* Cases of primary dementia (case level) with depression (case levels). *b* Cases of primary depression (case level) with organic symptoms (subcase and case levels). *1,* Depression; *2,* suicidal thoughts; *3,* somatic dysfunction; *4,* slowing; *5,* worries and tension; *6,* anxiety; *7,* obsessional; *8,* somatic concerns; *9,* hypomania; *10,* hallucinations; *11,* other perceptual distortions; *12,* disordered throught and control; *13,* paranoid ideas (delusions); *14,* impaired memory; *15,* disorientation; *16,* drug and alcohol abuse; *17,* lack of insight; *18,* poor life satisfaction; *19,* communication difficulties. *, p < 0.01; +, p < 0.02

Retarded types of depression might be expected to produce more cognitive-type symptoms. Two symptoms emerge as diagnostically helpful. "Disorientation" is rarely present in depression, even in retarded depression. "Somatic dysfunction", often associated with depression, is often absent in the early stages of dementia.

The similarity in symptom profiles explains to some extent the difficulty in distinguishing between these two conditions using symptom scales. A method using scores appears at present to be less useful than a method which uses a traditional clinical differential diagnostic approach, such as the AGECAT computer system. Here AGECAT asks questions similar to those posed by the examining psychiatrist. Are the symptoms of depression sufficient to explain the organic features, or are the organic features out of proportion to the other depressive symptoms? AGECAT answers this question by comparing the levels of dementia with the levels of depression, level for level, using one or two symptom components such as the presence of "retardation" to aid the distinction. This method appears to work reasonably well when validated against psychiatrists' diagnoses at follow-up. Outcome is shown, on the whole, to have followed the course consistent with the original AGECAT diagnosis.

The subjects with AGECAT diagnostic depressions who later became demented are interesting for further study. The case of alcoholic dementia presented in the initial interview primarily as depressed but presumably deteriorated through further drinking. One of the others had pronounced paranoid symptoms and hypochondriasis at case level. Three years later another case was still described only as early dementia. The remaining subject had progressed from level 3 to level 4 at follow-up 3 years later when the depression levels had entirely resolved.

Conclusions

We conclude that pseudo-dementias are comparatively rare in the community and even in hospital practice, and that at present a clinically based method is still the best method for differential diagnosis, but this can be more accurately undertaken by a computer. It is possible that the clinical pictures of pseudo-dementia and dementia with depressive levels resemble one another because lack of motivation and interest and failure of concentration are common to both conditions. However, more than half of the depressive cases do not develop organic symptoms even at high levels of severity of illness. This difference may be related to different clinical types of depression or to underlying occult brain disease. Further outcome studies with new imaging techniques should help to resolve the problem.

Acknowledgements. The authors would like to acknowledge the contributions of Drs. V. K. Sharma, P. Saunders, C. Sullivan, L. M. Voruganti and S. V. Manohar, who undertook much of the interviewing in the community study, and of Dr. N. Wood, Miss M. Heary, Mrs. J. Silcock, Miss C. Hensy, Mrs. J. Wood and Mrs. R. Searle, who undertook much of the initial interviewing. Our thanks are also due to Mrs. B. Ackerley for her skill in organising the interviewing, to the general practitioners in Liverpool for access to their register and to the staff of Leighton Hospital, Crewe, for their cooperation.

References

Cohen RM, Weingartner H, Smallberg SA, Pickar D, Murphy DL (1982) Effort and cognition in depression. Arch Gen Psychiatry 39: 593–597

Copeland JRM, Kelleher MJ, Kellett JM, Gourlay AJ, Barron G, Cowan DW, De Gruchy J, Gurland BJ, Sharpe L, Simon R, Kuriansky J, Stiller P (1975) Cross-national study of comparison of the diagnosis of elderly psychiatric patients admitted to mental hospitals serving Queens County in New York and the old Borough of Camberwell, London. Br J Psychiatry 126: 11–20

Copeland JRM, Kelleher MJ, Kellett JM, Gourlay AJ, Gurland BJ, Fleiss JL, Sharpe L (1976) A semi-structured clinical interview for the assessment of diagnosis and mental state in the elderly. The Geriatric Mental State Schedule. 1. Development and reliability. Psychol Med 6: 439–449

Copeland JRM, Dewey ME, Griffith-Jones HM (1986) Computerised psychiatric diagnostic system and case nomenclature for elderly subjects: GMS and AGECAT. Psychol. Med. 16: 89–99

Copeland JRM, Dewey ME, Wood N, Searle R, Davidson IA, McWilliam C (1987) Range of mental illness among the elderly in the community: prevalence in Liverpool using the GMS-AGECAT Package. Br J Psychiatry 150: 815–823

Copeland JRM, Dewey ME, Henderson AS, Kay DWK, Neal CD, Harrison MAM, McWilliam C, Forshaw D, Shiwach R (1988) The Geriatric Mental State (GMS) used in the community: replication studies of the computerised diagnosis AGECAT Psychol. Med 18: 219–223

Dewey ME, Copeland JRM (1986) Computerised psychiatric diagnosis in the elderly: AGECAT, J Microcomput Appl 9: 135–140

Gurland BJ, Fleiss JL, Goldberg K, Sharpe L, Copeland JRM, Kelleher MJ, Kellett JM (1976) A semi-structured clinical interview for the assessment of diagnosis and mental state in the elderly. The Geriatric Mental State Schedule 2. A factor analysis. Psychol Med 6: 451–459

Jacoby RJ, Levy R (1980) Computed tomography in the elderly. 3. Affective disorder. Br J Psychiatry 136: 270–275

Jacoby RJ, Levy R, Bird JM (1981) Computed tomography and the outcome of affective disorders; a follow-up study of elderly patients. Br J Psychiat 139: 288–292

McAllister TW (1981) Cognitive functioning in the affective disorders. Compr Psychiatry 22: 572–586

Nott PN, Fleminger JJ (1975) Pre-senile dementia: the difficulties of early diagnosis. Acta Psychiatr Scand 51: 210–217

Post F (1962) Significance of affective symptoms old age. Oxford University Press, London

Ron MA, Toone BK, Garralda ME, Lishman WA (1979) Diagnostic accuracy in pre-senile dementia. Br J Psychiatry 134: 161–168

Wing JK, Cooper JE, Sartorius N (1974) The description and classification of psychiatric symptoms: an instruction manual for PSE and Catego system. Cambridge University Press, London

Age-Associated Memory Impairment, Benign Forgetfulness and Dementia*

S. H. Ferris, C. Flicker, B. Reisberg, and T. Crook

This chapter has several interrelated goals. First, it will provide an overview of the changes in various aspects of memory and other cognitive functions that occur more or less on a continuum as a function of human aging and as the slowly progressing age-related changes accelerate to produce dementing disorders such as Alzheimer's disease (AD). In so doing, we will present the construct of age-associated memory impairment (AAMI) and discuss the rationale, operational criteria and scientific utility of this new term for the well-established decline in memory performance which accompanies "normal" aging. The chapter will then review some principles, concepts and criteria for developing appropriate test measures for evaluating memory and cognition in aging, AAMI and AD. Finally, some examples of new cognitive tests that are compatible with these criteria will be presented, and results from these tests will be used to illustrate the pattern of cognitive changes that occur in aging and dementia.

Overview of Cognitive Decline in Aging and Dementia

What we observe clinically in AD and, to a much lesser extent in the normal elderly, is a global cognitive impairment. One of the tasks in aging research is to determine and examine the more specific cognitive changes that are contributing to this global result. In studying aging and dementia, the primary interests in such an evaluation are memory function and other aspects of complex cognitive processing which are to some extent dependent on memory processes. However, we always must consider, take into account, or control for, the fact that a variety of other factors contribute to the global result. These include attentional processes and neural processing speed, as well as more indirect factors such as mood and motivation. Thus, a number of mutually interacting systems and processes all influence and contribute to the global outcome (Ferris et al. 1986). One of the difficulties in both research and individual assessment is to isolate a particular process for study. The relatively broad aspects of cognition influencing global outcome can be further subdivided into a whole series of subcomponents. An arbitrary list of these components is presented in Table 1. In principle we ought to be able to devise experimental tasks or clinical test measures that allow us to assess, relatively independently, each of these subprocesses.

---

* This work was supported in part by grants MH4010, AG03051, and MH29590

Bergener, Reisberg (Eds.)
Diagnosis and Treatment
of Senile Dementia
© Springer-Verlag Berlin Heidelberg 1989

Table 1. Cognitive processes and their subcomponents

Cognitive process	Subcomponents
Memory	
Primary memory (short-term; immediate)	
Secondary memory (long-term; recent)	Verbal and nonverbal/spatial memory
	Storage and retrieval
	Associative memory
	Depth of processing
	Effortful and automatic memory
	Declarative and procedural memory
Tertiary memory (remote)	Episodic and semantic memory
Language	Fluency
	Naming
Attention	General arousal
	Selective attention
	Vigilance
	Perseveration
Speed of function	Motor speed
	Perceptual speed
	Sensorimotor speed
	Central processing speed
Higher order cognition	Spatial orientation
	Constructional abilities
	Concept learning
	Problem solving
	Decision making

What aspects of cognition actually change in human aging, and what further changes occur in early dementia? In regard to dementia, the discussion will be restricted to patients with relatively early to moderate dementia because in the later stages of AD just about every aspect of mental function shows marked decline. The general results gleaned from an extensive research literature (Fozard 1985; Poon 1985) and from our own research (Flicker et al. 1986b) are summarized in Table 2. A key conclusion in summarizing what happens when we compare the effects of the aging process (young versus old subjects) and the effects of AD (elderly normals versus early dementia) is that, with only a few exceptions, the differences between aging and dementia are quantitative rather than qualitative. Thus, for sensory motor processing, attention, recent memory, and higher-level functions like concept learning and praxis, a survey of the literature indicates that there is a measurable decline when comparing young and elderly groups cross-sectionally. Of course, there is considerable variability within the elderly and the young normal groups and the group distributions overlap. Thus, while there certainly are some elderly individuals who perform better than some young subjects, overall the group means differ consistently.

Table 2. Cognitive decline in normal aging and early dementia[a]

Cognitive function	Relative performance	
	Elderly normal versus young normal	Early dementia versus elderly normal
Sensorimotor processing	Impaired	Impaired
Attention	Impaired	Impaired
Recent memory	Impaired	Impaired
Concept formation	Impaired	Impaired
Visuospatial praxis	Impaired	Impaired
Immediate memory	Unimpaired	Unimpaired
Language (syntax and phonology)	Unimpaired	Unimpaired
Language (naming)	Unimpaired	Impaired
Remote memory	Unimpaired	Impaired
Visuoperceptual abilities	Impaired	Unimpaired

[a] Adapted from Flicker et al. 1986b

But for most cognitive processes a much more dramatic decline is observed when comparing early dementia patients with elderly normals. It should be noted, however, that certain functions such as immediate memory are unimpaired in both groups. On the other hand, changes in language function may differentiate early AD from normal aging since impairments in remote memory and language do not occur in aging, but clearly occur in AD. In general, however, the basic conclusion to be drawn is that many aspects of cognition decline on a continuum between young, elderly and early AD groups. Further discussion about the extreme cognitive deficits in severe AD is beyond the scope of this chapter and is provided elsewhere in this book. However, since many normal elderly individuals show a significant decline in memory, the nature of age-associated memory impairment will be described in greater detail.

Age-Associated Memory Impairment

As indicated above, many elderly individuals suffer a decline in memory function relative to their performance as young adults. For the purpose of stimulating further research and to provide a basis for selecting subjects and evaluating potential treatment strategies, a series of conferences sponsored by the National Institute of Mental Health culminated in establishing an operational definition for the syndrome of AAMI (Crook, et al. 1986). Conceptually, the nature of AAMI is illustrated in Fig. 1. As previously mentioned, there is certainly an overlap in memory performance between the young population and the elderly population, but the elderly distribution as a whole clearly shifts toward poorer performance. Excluded from AAMI are the extreme cases where there is a malignant, progressive dementing process such as AD (approximately 5% prevalence). Such extreme cases of dementia are generally easy to distinguish from AAMI, except in borderline cases. Those individuals who perform at one SD below the average for the young population and who complain that their memory has declined are defined as meeting criteria for AAMI. Thus, individuals with AAMI are those normal elderly who have shown a meaningful degree of decline in meory (i. e. 1 SD) relative to their earlier level of function. Ideally, the proper way to identify such individuals would be to obtain at least two longitudinal assessments, one during their twenties and one in old age. In practice, however, we can obtain only the second assessment and rely on normative data for young individuals to estimate degree of change. It is assumed that the validity of this imperfect approach can be improved by also requiring significant subjective complaints that memory function has declined.

Based on initial experience in applying these criteria for subject selection, it turns out that about half of the normal elderly population fit the current definition of AAMI. Thus, as shown in Fig. 1, the memory performance of those with AAMI is below average for the elderly population as a whole. Of course, more definitive epidemiologic data on the prevalence of AAMI are needed. But the important thing to emphasize is that the concept of AAMI does not define a new entity or disease. The construct merely characterizes operationally as a syndrome the well-known fact that, as a part of normal aging, the brain and virtually all the other organs of the body show age-related changes. Furthermore, to varying degrees there are clinical and behavioral consequences of these age-related organ and brain changes. One of the behavioral consequences of the brain changes, which might or might not have an impact on one's daily life, is a decline in memory function. Examples of analogous age-related syndromes affecting other organ systems include hypertension and

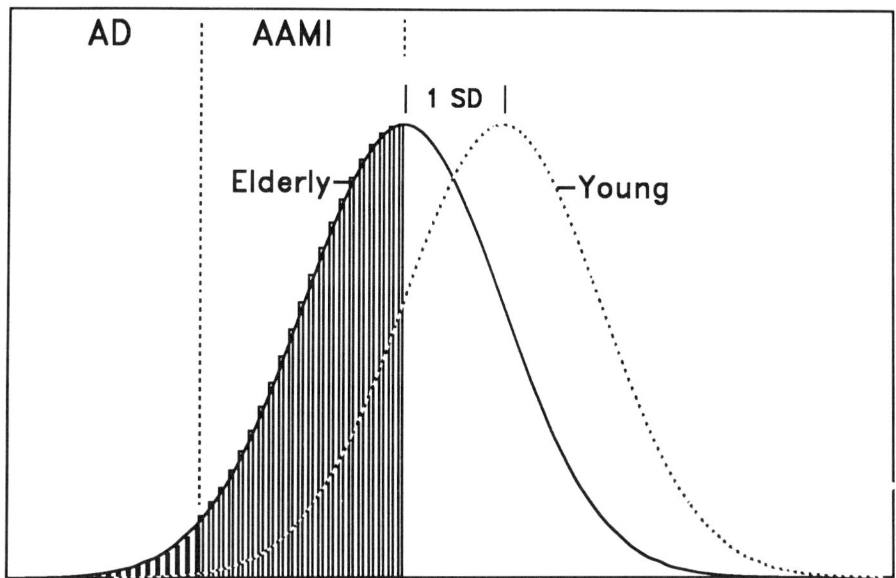

Fig. 1. Relationship of age-associated memory impairment (AAMI) to normal aging and Alzheimer's disease (AD). Standard unit normal distributions for the young and elderly populations overlap, with the elderly distribution shifted toward poorer memory performance. Normal elderly subjects with memory performance 1 SD below the mean for the young population and who do not meet criteria for AD or other dementias (about 5%) are classified as AAMI

presbyopia. In both cases the syndromes are generally due to age related biological changes, they can have significant clinical consequences, and some form of treatment is commonly recommended.

For the human brain, a variety of age-associated changes occur in structure, neurochemistry and cellular physiology (Crook et al. 1986). Some of the gross structural changes are evident *in vivo,* through neuroradiological imaging techniques (de Leon et al. 1984). AAMI is a direct and clinically relevant consequence of these brain changes. Furthermore, studies of various other vertebrate species (particularly rodents and nonhuman primates) demonstrate similar age-related biological and cognitive changes. For memory performance in particular, analogous memory tasks elicit quite similar patterns of decline in aged rats, monkeys and humans (Flicker et al. 1985). Thus AAMI is not unique to man. The goal in establishing the construct of AAMI is to define this syndrome of normal aging operationally, so that we have an objective basis for selecting research subjects for studying its epidemiology, course and clinical significance, and for attempting to do something about it through pharmacologic or other forms of intervention.

The current inclusion criteria for selecting research subjects with AAMI are summarized in Table 3 (adapted from Crook et al. 1986). It is important to emphasize that these are provisional operational criteria which have evolved through the series of consensus conferences sponsored by the National Institute of Mental Health. Thus as additional research information becomes available, a further evolution of these criteria is possible. Basically, since AAMI is an aging phenomenon, the inclusion criteria require people who are over 50 years of age, who have specific complaints of memory loss in everyday life and who show objective evidence of decline in memory performance. For both extent of memory complaint and degree of objective memory decline, the scores of normal young people provide the normative reference. There also has to be an indication that earlier in life the general level of intellectual function was quite normal, and that currently the degree of cognitive decline is not sufficient to meet criteria for dementia. Also provided in Table 3 are the specific exclusion criteria

Table 3. Age-associated memory impairment (AAMI): criteria for subject selection[a]

Inclusion criteria:
1. At least 50 years of age
2. Complaints of memory loss in everyday life
3. Scores on standardized memory tests at least one standard deviation below the mean for young adults
4. Evidence of adequate intellectual function
5. Absence of dementia; score of 24 or higher on the Mini-Mental State Examination

Exclusion criteria:
1. Disturbance of consciousness
2. Neurologic disorders associated with cognitive impairment
3. History of infective or inflammatory brain disease
4. Evidence of cerebrovascular pathology; modified Hachinski score of 4 or more
5. History of head injury
6. Depression or other major psychiatric disorder; Hamilton score of 13 or more
7. History of alcoholism or drug dependence
8. Medical disorders associated with cognitive impairment
9. Use of drugs that may affect cognitive functioning

[a] Adapted from Crook et al. 1986

for AAMI. These exclusions are the same as those typically applied in the differential diagnosis of AD. Such exclusions are needed to rule out any of the many possible reasons for the memory impairment other than normal aging. Thus we conservatively exclude subjects with specific medical and related conditions which might cause the mild memory impairment.

Distinction between AAMI, Benign Senescent Forgetfulness and AD

The term "benign senescent forgetfulness" (BSF) was proposed by Kral more than 25 years ago to describe elderly individuals with mild, but clinically significant memory impairment (Kral 1962, 1966; Kral and Muller 1966). BSF is apparently a more restricted construct which applies to a smaller subset of the elderly population who are at the more severely impaired end of the larger AAMI distribution. Thus BSF, which was never adequately described or defined operationally, may be subsumed under the broader AAMI construct. BSF appears to apply to those AAMI subjects whose degree of memory impairment approaches borderline dementia and who probably are at great risk for progressing to AD.

Although cross-sectional cognitive and neuropathological data suggest a continuum between aging, AAMI and AD, AD is clearly discontinuous with aging when longitudinal course and outcome are considered. Thus, while many of the behavioral and neurobiological hallmarks of AD also occur in aging, AD progresses fairly rapidly and the quantitative differences between AD and aging often become enormous. *In vivo* brain imaging data also indicate differences between AD and aging. For example, quantitative studies of CT scans have shown consistent structural changes (e. g., enlargement of ventricular volume) in aging and further changes (even greater ventricular volume) in AD (George et al. 1983). However, a measure of brain function – rate of glucose utilization (determined by positron emission tomography, PET) – shows a discontinuity between aging and AD. Thus no consistent changes in brain metabolism determined by PET have been found in normal aging (de Leon et al. 1987), but marked reductions occur in AD (de Leon et al. 1983). These results illustrate the fact that despite the numerous changes that occur in the aging brain, in many instances the brain has sufficient reserves so that reasonable global function and behavioral performance can be maintained. What probably distinguishes AD from aging is that in AD the brain changes progress rapidly and produce more devastating effects on brain function. There is probably a threshold phenomenon such that with varying degrees of slowly increasing brain change, overall brain function can remain fairly intact. But beyond a certain point, when the process becomes malignant and progresses rapidly as in AD, broader brain systems fail, global brain metabolism is diminished and the severe symptoms of AD become apparent.

Cognitive Assessment in Studies of AAMI and AD

In studying subjects with AAMI or AD, appropriate cognitive test measures are needed to determine patterns of cognitive decline, changes over time and effects of treatment. The guidelines outlined in Table 4 encompass the criteria we have applied

Table 4. Requirements for cognitive assessment batteries[a]

1. Sample a variety of cognitive functions
2. Sensitivity to deficits of aging or dementia
3. Difficulty range appropriate to severity of subject sample
4. Equivalent forms for repeated administration
5. Reasonable duration
6. Sensitivity to treatment effects
7. Reliability
8. Validity: construct, ecologic, neuropathologic
9. Other desirable features:
   a) Face validity
   b) Computerization
   c) Analogous to animal test models

[a] Adapted from Ferris et al. 1986

during the past 10 years in developing optimal test measures (Ferris and Crook 1983; Ferris et al. 1986, 1988).

Briefly, the battery should assess change over time or due to treatment in a wide variety of fairly specific and relevant cognitive processes which decline with age or show deficits in early dementia (e. g., see Tables 1 and 2). The tests developed must be sensitive to these cognitive changes and also must have a difficulty range which is appropriate for the elderly and for early AD patients so as to avoid floor and ceiling effects. In addition, multiple equivalent forms for repetitive testing are generally essential; the battery as a whole should not be overly long in order to avoid subject fatigue; and when used in clinical trials, the measures should be sensitive to the effects of drugs.

The traditional psychometric requirements of high reliability and validity are also paramount criteria. Reliability is opitmized through test computerization, which standardizes test administration, provides precise temporal control and latency recording and automates scoring and storage of results. Computers also facilitate meeting another desirable test criterion: improved face validity. Through the use of realistic color graphics displays and touch screen response and feedback, situations which are meaningful to the subject and simulate real-life cognitive behavior can be incorporated into tasks which assess various relevant cognitive processes. Face-valid tasks improve subject cooperation and lead to less test anxiety and greater reliability. With their increased ecological validity, improvement on such tasks in drug trials has greater clinical relevance than improvement on more abstract cognitive measures.

A final test-development criterion which we have applied to certain tasks (Flicker et al. 1984, 1987a) concerns the clinical adaptation of animal models used in preclinical studies of putative cognitive enhancing compounds. Elderly and demented humans and aged or lesioned animals show quite similar impairments when tested on their respective, but analogous memory tasks (Flicker et al. 1985). Thus the use of face-valid, computerized tasks which also are clinical analogues of preclinical memory models can greatly facilitate the transition from preclinical to clinical drug development. Two such measures are described below.

The face-valid, computerized tasks described below all meet the various criteria summarized above (Flicker et al. 1988a, 1988b; Ferris et al. 1988). The differential performance of young, elderly, and early AD patients on these measures illustrates the patterns of cognitive decline previously summarized in Table 2.

Immediate Memory

Telephone Number Recall (Crook et al. 1980). In this test the subject is presented with a three-digit area code, or a seven- or ten-digit telephone number for 5 s and is then instructed to dial the number on a dial phone. This task measures immediate memory under conditions of interference from the motor dialing response. Recall of the ten-digit number is significanlty different in young normal, elderly normal and elderly demented subjects.

Recent Memory

Verbal: *Shopping List Task* (McCarthy et al. 1981) On this task the subject is presented with a list of ten grocery items to recall. Five trials are administered, after each of which the subject is selectively reminded (Buschke and Fuld 1974) of the items not recalled. Delayed recall after 30 min is also assessed. In comparison to young normal subjects, this task elicits progressively more severe performance decrements from elderly normals and elderly demented subjects. The frequency of intrusion errors on this verbal recall task is used as a measure of perseverative tendency. Intrusion errors in patients with AD have been linked to cholinergic dysfunction (Fuld et al. 1982).

Verbal associative memory: *First-Last Name Task* (Ferris et al. 1986). This task evaluates associative memory for verbal – verbal information (first and last names). The test assesses both accuracy of recall after a single presentation of one, three, five or seven name pairs (associative span) and paired associate learning of four pairs (three presentation – recall trials and delayed recall). Both measures show progressive deficits in aging and early dementia.

Visuospatial: *Delayed Spatial Memory Task* (Flicker et al. 1984). On this task the subject is presented with a representation of a 25-room house that has common household objects in one or more rooms. After a delay interval of 0,15 or 30 s, the subject is instructed to point out (touch on the screen) the room, or rooms, that the objects were in. The subject performs the *Driving Test* described below as a distractor task during the 15- and 30-s delay intervals. The slope of the forgetting curve is progressively steeper in young normals, elderly normals, early dementia patients and advanced dementia patients. The test is conceptually and operationally similar to a delayed response task that is sensitive to scopolamine administration (Bartus and Johnson 1976) and aging (Bartus et al. 1978) in nonhuman primates.

Visual Recognition: *Visual Recognition Span* (Flicker et al. 1987a). On this task the subject is presented with a group of household objects within a 5 × 5 matrix (rooms of a house). The number of objects is progressively incremented from 1 to 25. On each trial, the subject is instructed to point out (touch) the *new* object. This test has been shown to be highly sensitive to aging and dementia. The task is also operationally analogous to the delayed non-matching to sample procedure used with nonhuman primates (Mishkin and Delacour 1975).

Facial Recognition: *Facial Recognition Task* (Ferris et al. 1980). In this test the subject is presented with a series of faces and must identify which faces are being presented for the first time and which faces are repeat presentations. The subject responds by touching a "yes" or "no" box on the screen. Repeat presentations occur at delay intervals of 0, 5, 15, 30, 120 and 300 s. The current computerized version of this task shows changes due to both age and AD (Flicker et al. 1988b).

Language

Object Naming (Flicker et al. 1987b). This test uses images of objects derived from the Boston Naming Test (Kaplan et al. 1983). One by one 20 pictures are presented on the video monitor screen and subjects are instructed to name each object. This test elicits a marked deficit from AD patients, whereas the performance of nondemented young and old subjects is not significantly different.

Object Function Recall (Flicker et al. 1987b). The subject is asked what the objects presented in the above task are used for. Any accurate contextual information is scored as correct.

Object Name Recognition (Flicker et al. 1987b). The subject is instructed to select the name of the object from a list of four words presented under the representation of the object on the video monitor.

Object Function Recognition (Flicker et al. 1987b). The subject is presented with a representation of a 25-room house. Each of the rooms in the 5×5 matrix is filled with the image of an object derived from a standardized set of pictures (Snodgrass and Vanderwart 1980). Subjects are instructed to point out (touch on the screen) the eight items that would be most useful for a particular chore (e. g., dressing). Responses are automatically recorded via the touchscreen. As with the other language tasks above, early dementia patients are impaired on this task whereas the nondemented elderly exhibit no deficit (Flicker et al. 1987b).

Concept Formation

Object Sorting (Flicker et al. 1986a). The subject is presented with the 25-room house, full of household items, and is instructed to pick out (touch on the screen) the eight items that are most alike. Alzheimer's patients are severely impaired on this task, and elderly normals perform significantly worse than young normals.

Psychomotor Speed and Attention

Driving Test (Flicker et al. 1988a). On this task a traffic stoplight, a "brake" box, and an "accelerator" box are presented on the video monitor touchscreen and the subject is instructed to press the brake box when the stoplight is red and the accelerator box when the stoplight is green. The overall time taken to shift from brake to accelerator or accelerator to brake can be divided into its release (reaction time) and travel time components. This task thus provides separate measures of sensorimotor speed (including cognitive processing speed) and pure motor speed. As in previous research (Ferris et al. 1976) results from this task indicate that psychomotor slowing occurs in aging and is more pronounced even in the earliest stages of AD.

In the context of age-related psychomotor impairment, it is relevant to mention the role of white matter lesions (WML) in the brain. These lesions, which appear as patchy, periventricular lucencies on CT scans (George et al. 1986), and their pathology are described elsewhere in this book (see Gottfries, this volume). Kluger et al. (1988), recently demonstrated that this microvessel pathology, which occurs in about 20% of the normal elderly, has clinical consequences. Specifically, two groups of normal elderly, one with and one without WML, were found to be equivalent in performance on memory and other nonmotor cognitive tests. However, on tests of psychomotor function (e. g., digit symbol, reaction time, and a computerized motor tracking task) there were marked impairments in the WML group relative to the non-WML group. These results lead to the intriguing possibility that drugs having positive effects on microvessel function (e. g., nimodipine) might reduce or prevent these age-related motor function impairments.

References

Bartus RT, Johnson HR (1976) Short term memory in the rhesus monkey: disruption from the anticholinergic scopolamine. Pharmacol Biochem Behav 5: 39–40

Bartus RT, Fleming D, Johnson HR (1978) Aging in the rhesus monkey: debilitating effects on short-term memory. J Gerontol 33: 858–871

Buschke H, Fuld PA (1974) Evaluating storage, retention and retrieval in disordered memory and learning. Neurology 11: 1019–1025

Crook T, Ferris SH, McCarthy M, Rae D (1980) The utility of digit recall tasks for assessing memory in the aged. J Consult Clin Psychol 48: 228–233

Crook T, Bartus RT, Ferris SH, Whitehouse P, Cohen GD, Gershon, S (1986) Age-associated memory impairment: proposed diagnostic criteria and measures of clinical change – report of a NIMH work group. Dev Neuropsychol 2: 261–276

de Leon MJ, Ferris SH, George AE, Christman DR, Fowler JS, Gentes C, Reisberg B, Gee B, Emmerich M, Yonekura Y, Brodie J, Kricheff II, Wolf AP (1983). Positron emission tomography studies of aging and Alzheimer's disease. Am J Neuroradiol 4: 568–571

de Leon MJ, George AE, Ferris SH, Christman DR, Fowler JS, Gentes C, Brodie J, Reisberg B, Wolf AP (1984). Positron emission tomography and computed tomography assessments of the aging human brain. J Comput Assist Tomogr 8: 88–94

de Leon MJ, George AE, Tomanelli J, Christman D, Kluger A, Miller J, Ferris SH, Fowler J, Brodie J, Klinger A, Wolf AP (1987) Positron emission tomography studies of normal aging: a replication of PET III and 18-FDG using PET VI and 11-C-2DG. Neurobiol Aging 8: 319–323

Ferris SH, Crook T (1983) Cognitive assessment in mild to moderately severe dementia. In Crook T, Ferris S, Bartus R (eds) Assessment in geriatric psychopharmacology. Powley, New Canaan, pp 177–186

Ferris SH, Crook T, Sathananthan G, Gershon S (1976) Reaction time as a diagnostic measure of cognitive impairment in senility. J Am Geriatr Soc 24: 529–533

Ferris SH, Crook T, Clark E, McCarthy M, Rae D (1980) Facial recognition memory deficits in normal aging and senile dementia. J Gerontol 35: 707–714

Ferris SH, Crook T, Flicker C, Reisberg B, Bartus RT (1986) Psychometric assessment of treatment effects. In Poon LW (ed) The handbook for clinical memory assessment of older adults. American Psychological Association, Washington

Ferris SH, Flicker C, Reisberg B (1988) NYU computerized test battery for assessing cognition in aging and dementia. Psychopharmacol Bull 24: 699–702

Flicker C, Bartus RT, Crook T, Ferris SH (1984) Effects of aging and dementia upon recent visuospatial memory. Neurobiol Aging 5: 275–283

Flicker C, Dean RL, Bartus RT, Ferris SH, Crook T (1985) Animal and human memory dysfunctions associated with aging, cholinergic lesions, and senile dementia. Ann NY Acad Sci 444: 515–517

Flicker C, Ferris SH, Crook T, Bartus RT (1986a) The effects of aging and dementia on concept formation as measured on an object-sorting task. Dev Neuropsychol 2: 65–72

Flicker C, Ferris SH, Crook T, Bartus RT, Reisberg B (1986b) Cognitive decline in advanced age: future directions for psychometric differentiation of normal and pathological age changes in cognitive function. Dev Neuropsychol 2: 309–322

Flicker C, Ferris SH, Crook T, Bartus RT (1987a) A visual recognition memory test for the assessment of cognitive function in aging and dementia. Exp Aging Res 13: 127–132

Flicker C, Ferris SH, Crook T, Bartus RT (1987b) Implications of memory and language dysfunction in the naming deficit of senile dementia. Brain Lang 31: 187–200

Flicker C, Serby M, Ferris SH (1988a) Scopolamine effects on memory, language, visuospatial praxis, and psychomotor speed in comparison with aging and dementia. (Submitted)

Flicker C, Ferris SH, Crook T, Bartus RT (1988b). Impaired facial recognition memory in aging and dementia. (Submitted)

Flicker C, Ferris SH, Reisberg B (1989). A two-year longitudinal follow-up study of cognitive function in normal aging and dementia. (Submitted)

Fozard JL (1985) Psychology of aging – normal and pathological age differences in memory. In Brocklehurst JC (ed) Textbook of geriatric medicine and gerontology. Chruchill Livingstone, Edinburgh

Fuld PA, Katzman R, Davies P, Terry RD (1982) Intrusions as a sign of Alzheimer dementia: chemical and pathological verification. Ann Neurol 11: 155–159

George AE, de Leon MJ, Rosenbloom S, Ferris SH, Gentes C, Emmerich M, Kricheff II (1983) Ventricular volume and cognitive deficit: a computed tomographic study. Radiology 149: 493–498

George AE, de Leon MJ, Gentes CI, Miller J, London E, Budzilovich GN, Ferris SH, Chase N (1986) Leukoencephalopathy in normal and pathologic aging: 1. CT of brain lucencies. Am J Neuroradiol 7: 561–566

Kaplan E, Goodglass H, Weintraub S (1983) Boston naming test. Lea and Febiger, Philadelphia

Kluger A, Gianutsos J, de Leon MJ George AE (1988) The significance of age-related white matter lesions. Stroke 19: 1054–1055

Kral VA (1962) Senescent forgetfulness: Benign and malignant. *J canad Med Assoc* 86: 257–260

Kral VA (1966) Memory loss in the aged. Diseases of the Nervous System, 27 (Suppl. I), 51–54

Kral VA, Muller H (1966) Memory dysfunction, a prognostic indicator in geriatric patients. Can Psychiatr Assoc J 11: 343–349

McCarthy M, Ferris SH, Clark E, Crook T (1981). Acquisition and retention of categorized material in normal aging and senile dementia. Exp Aging Res 7: 127–135

Mishkin M, Delacour J (1975) An analysis of short-term visual memory in the monkey. J Exp Psychol [Anim Behav] 1: 326–334

Poon LW (1985) Differences in human memory with aging: nature, causes, and clinical implications. In: Birren JE, Schaie KW (eds) Handbook of the psychology of aging, 2nd edn. Van Nostrand Reinhold, New York, pp 427–462

Snodgrass JG, Vanderwart M (1980) A standardized set of 260 pictures: norms for name agreement, image agreement, familiarity, and visual complexity. J Exp Psychol [Hum Learn] 6: 174–215

Current Problems in the Clinical Diagnosis of Vascular Dementia

G. Bono, A. Martelli, P. Merlo, M. Mauri, E. Sinforiani, and G. Nappi

Introduction

So-called chronic cerebrovascular disorders (CCVD) represent an ill-defined nosological entity which includes polymorphous clinical pictures with different pathogenesis, type and degree of morphological or functional damage, evolution and prognosis [7]. Attempts to give a better definition of this group of disorders, however, have been made during recent years for methodological reasons, particularly in the need to establish standardized admission criteria for drug trials. According to the definition commonly in use [18], patients are considered as having CCVD when meeting the following requirements:
a) history of one or more cerebrovascular episodes, including transient ischaemic attacks;
b) presence of vascular risk factors (mainly hypertension);
c) presence of focal or diffuse neurological and/or psychiatric signs;
d) positivity of instrumental examinations, such as computed tomography (CT) scan, positron emission scan or magnetic resonance imaging (MRI)
e) mild derangement of higher cerebral functions.

However, using these conditions as inclusion criteria for admitting patients in therapeutic studies results in extremely heterogeneous populations, in which different degrees of cognitive and behavioural dysfunctions (presumably) occur in association with signs and symptoms of ischaemic vascular disease [9]. Some of these patients therefore eventually present with superimposed Alzheimer's disease (AD) and cerebrovascular signs/symptoms, while some others actually fit the criteria for multi-infarct dementia (MID).

Even in its semantic aspects, the term CCVD is equivocal. The term "chronic", in fact, should indicate that the primary pathological process (i.e. cerebral ischaemia) is taking place almost continuously with progression over time, but this probably holds true only for a minority of cases [6]. Moreover, recent investigation demonstrates that cerebral blood flow rates in demented vascular patients are significantly higher than in AD subjects, even if in the latter the vascular changes are considered a secondary phenomenon to neural loss and impaired metabolic activity [22].

Another problem, as mentioned above, concerns the extreme variety of the clinical picture in different series; besides sensorimotor deficits, CCVD patients are characterized by a wide spectrum of neuropsychiatric and neuropsychological abnormalities

Bergener, Reisberg (Eds.)
Diagnosis and Treatment
of Senile Dementia
© Springer-Verlag Berlin Heidelberg 1989

ranging from minor changes in mood/personality (possibly associated with impairment of memory, verbal and visuo-spatial abilities), to overt dementia. Clear-cut correlations between these alterations and the site or the extent of vascular damage, however, seem to exist only for the so-called (subacute) post-stroke mood disorders [6]; in addition, the existence of distinct cognitive/behavioural profiles for vascular and non-vascular dementias is also still debated [4, 6].

The general term MID therefore seems preferable to that of CCVD for the definition of a large majority of the above patients.

The current diagnostic criteria for MID [1, 15] stress the main characteristics of the clinical picture (stepwise deteriorating course with patchy distribution of deficits; focal neurological signs and symptoms), even if they leave the examiner to judge as to cause-effect relationships between dementia symptoms and evidence (from history, physical-instrumental tests) of "significant" cerebrovascular disease.

The course of MID, in contrast to that of AD, is described as "erratic", and in fact there is no agreement about whether MID is a reversible, a stationary or a progressive disease [6, 11, 12]. Thus, the main concept underlying MID as a nosological entity is that mental deterioration "is determined" by the cumulative effects of (multiple, bilateral, at different times) cerebral infarcts. The total volume of damaged cerebral tissue has been claimed to be the most important factor by several authors [6]. However, isolated lacunar infarcts and minor strokes in discrete subcortical areas (thalamus, hippocampus) have also been described as the only CT finding in patients described as having MID, even if, as a general rule, single strokes are thought not to cause dementia but rather relatively circumscribed changes in mental functions [1, 6].

A tentative approach to the definition and classification of behavioural abnormalities and intellectual decline occurring in (ischaemic) cerebrovascular disease (ICVD) should therefore distinguish between:
a) circumscribed memory disorder (vascular amnestic syndromes from one or more infarctions in appropriate areas);
b) other circumscribed cognitive disorders (such as aphasia and visuo-spatial deficits, as above; and
c) vascular dementia, also MID, including patients with dementia symptoms according to DSM-III, of different severity (from questionable/probable to severe, according to current clinical ratings) presenting with Hachinski ischaemic scores ≥ 7 [9, 13].

Besides clinical criteria, CT, nuclear magnetic resonance (NMR) and other neuroimaging techniques are of particular importance for their role in differential diagnosis against other conditions also causing dementia, but more precise correlations are still required between neuroradiological findings and clinical, neuropsychologic and neuropathologic data in order to define possible subgroups of MID with different pathogenesis and prognosis and also potentially suitable for appropriate treatment [6].

Methods

The present study was aimed at answering some of the open questions about MID, with particular reference to the correlations between clinical picture and neuroradiological findings.

The population examined included 265 cases (206 men, 59 women; mean age 68.2 ± 8.9 SD) of consecutive observation presenting with signs/symptoms of pathological aging of the brain suggesting vascular or degenerative dementia. A preliminary patient selection was therefore made in order to rule out cases of probable or true dementia due to pathological conditions other than those above.

The clinical definition of our patients was based upon the following procedures:
1. Comprehensive interview with the participant and with a reliable informant plus neurological examination.
2. DSM-III criteria for dementia and Hughes' clinical dementia rating (CDR), determined according to published rules [1, 13].
3. Hachinski ischaemic score [9].
4. Mini-Mental Status examination [8].
5. Guidelines for the diagnosis of AD [17].

White matter low attenuation, also leuko-araiosis (LA [10]), seen on the CT was considered when bilateral, symmetrical and diffuse; subcortical infarcts were diagnosed according to Steingart's criteria [20], atrophic changes were considered only when severe degrees of cortical atrophy were encountered (subjective criteria) [5, 21].

Results

A preliminary evaluation of our case series was performed considering the ischaemic scores and the clinical staging of dementia symptoms (Table 1); cases scoring 0.5–1 (questionable/mild dementia) on the CDR were considered altogether. The mean duration of the disease (4.5 ± 2.1 years) may account for the case distribution within the three CDR subgroups: 13.9% with questionable/mild, 34.3% moderate and 51.6% severe dementia. Considering the distribution by ischaemic score, 52.4% of the patients fell in the "vascular" group (score ≥ 7); within this group, the number of cases with questionable/mild dementia was significantly lower than in subgroups with moderate to severe mental deterioration (Table 1).

Table 1. Main clinical characteristics of total population ($n = 265$)

	Hachinski 0–4 ($n = 39$)	ischaemic 5–6 ($n = 87$)	score ≥ 7 ($n = 139$)	Total
Degree of dementia				
Questionable/mild ($n = 37$)	20	11	6	14.0%
Moderate ($n = 91$)	11	28	52	34.3%
Severe ($n = 137$)	8	48	81	51.6%
Total	14.7%	32.8%	52.5%	100.0%

[a] $p < 0.0001$ (χ^2 test between groups)

Table 2. Main neuroradiological (CT) findings ($n = 265$)

CT finding	Hachinski 0–4 ($n = 39$)	ischaemic 5–6 ($n = 87$)	score $\geqslant 7$ ($n = 139$)	Total
Normal ($n = 23$)	12	5	6	8.7%
Severe atrophy ($n = 30$)	8	13	9	11.3%
Leuko-araiosis ($n = 65$)	12	26	27	24.5%
Infarcts ($n = 60$)	4	15	41	22.6%
Combinations ($n = 87$)	3	28	56	32.8%

LA versus Infarcts and respective groups versus combinations, $p < 0.001$; LA versus Infarcts, $p < 0.01$ (χ^2 test between groups)

Table 2 shows the main CT findings of our series, grouped according to presence of severe cortical atrophy, LA, cortical/subcortical infarcts, and combinations of these conditions. Normal CT scans (i. e. absence of density alterations; cortical atrophy in the normal range for age) were found in 8.7% of the total population, 50% of which belonged to the "degenerative" (ischaemic score, 0–4) and 20% to the "vascular" (ischaemic score $\geqslant 7$) subgroup. Findings of severe cortical atrophy (alone) were almost equally distributed in the three diagnostic subgroups (AD, mixed, MID). LA was found in 24.5% of cases, the frequency of this type of alteration (alone) showing an inverse relationship to the ischaemic score (12/39 AD; 26/87 mixed; 27/139 MID). An opposite trend was noted for the CT evidence of cortical/subcortical infarcts (increasing number with the ischaemic scores) as well as for the subgroup "combination of lesions" (56/139 MID versus 3/39 AD). This distribution seems to indicate that the accumulation of CT lesions is significantly correlated with elevated ($\geqslant 7$) ischaemic scores.

In order to evaluate the contribution given by the different CT lesions (infarcts/LA) to the severity of dementia we proceeded by excluding MID cases with either normal CT or isolated cortical atrophy (15 cases); the clinical-neuroradiological correlations in the resulting MID population (124 cases) are reported in Table 3.

Table 3. Clinical-neuroradiological (CT) Findings and degree of dementia in a population with MID ($n = 124$)

CT findings	Degree of dementia Questionable/ mild ($n = 4$)	Moderate ($n = 46$)	Severe ($n = 74$)	Total %
Cortical infarcts ($n = 13$)	–	3	10	10.5%
Subcortical infarcts ($n = 23$)	1	13	9	18.5%
Combinations ($n = 5$)	–	–	5	4.0%
Leuko-araiosis				
Alone ($n = 27$)	3	14	10	21.7%
Plus cortical infarcts ($n = 25$)	–	6	19	20.2%
Plus subcortical infarcts ($n = 31$)	–	10	21	25.0
Total %	3.2	37.1	59.7	100

Cortical versus subcortical infarcts, $p < 0.05$ (χ^2 test between groups)

The frequency of occurrence of multiple cortical infarcts (without concomitant subcortical infarcts and/or LA) that we observed (10.5%, was lower than that reported in MID series by other authors [6]. A significant correlation, instead, existed between severity of dementia and frequency of either cortical or subcortical infarctions. Less severe degrees of dementia, however, were observed in patients presenting with LA plus subcortical infarcts than in those with LA plus cortical infarctions.

The same differences in the distributions of focal lesions by severity of symptoms were found, with a lower degree of significance ($p < 0.02$, x^2 test), when the total number of subcortical infarcts (isolated or combined with LA) was compared to the total number of focal cortical lesions.

Based on presence/absence of cortical versus subcortical infarctions on the CT, correlations were also attempted among the main clinical characteristics of the patients (history, neurological examination, risk factors)."Cortical" subjects (43 cases) were characterized by higher frequency of concomitant coronary heart disease but less severe and less long-lasting arterial hypertension ($p < 0.05$ and $p < 0.01$, respectively) as opposed to subcortical ones. On the other hand, "subcortical" subjects (54 cases) showed more frequent extrapyramidal signs ($p < 0.05$) and a lower number ($p < 0.05$) of clinically relevant cerebrovascular episodes.

Conclusions

From the analysis of our results the following conclusions can be drawn. The Hachinski ischaemic score, despite criticism by some authors [6], can be considered the best suited clinical tool for a preliminary separation between AD and vascular dementia: only 10% of our patients with scores ≥ 7, in fact, do not present ischaemic lesions on the CT. The contribution of isolated LA to the different diagnostic subgroups of dementia, remains controversial. LA may in fact be encountered, even with varying distribution, in normal-aged subjects as well as among patients with either vascular or degenerative dementia [3, 10], its frequency of observation being also a function of the different resolution powers of the methods used (CT/MRI). The frequency of isolated LA among AD patients, however, demonstrates a direct correlation with age, it being more frequent among senile than among presenile groups due to the increasing number and relevance of cardiovascular and metabolic risk factors for cerebral ischaemia [3]. On the other hand, as seen in our series, an overall increase in LA parallels the increase in ischaemic score, even if the role played by LA looks less important when compared to that of cerebral infarcts, either cortical or subcortical.

Moreover, the CT correlates in our MID group bring to our attention the possible existence of three major varieties of findings, in agreement with the definition proposed by Rogers [19]: type I, cortical forms with major infarcts (10% in our series); type II, subcortical forms with multiple (lacunar) infarctions (18%); type III, LA, isolated or combined with pericapsular (lacunar) infarcts (65%). Different pathophysiological mechanisms probably contribute to the three subtypes of MID: thromboembolic events from large-artery disease or chronic ischaemia (poor perfusion) in type I; lacunar strokes from occlusion of penetrating branches of large cerebral arteries in type II; bilateral and diffuse demyelination of subcortical white matter from alterations of the small perforating medullary arteries in type III. Due to common neuropathological characteristics, types II and III most often occur in combination (so-called Binswanger's disease [2]).

Attempts to differentiate between type I and types II–III (cortical versus subcortical MID) based on neuropsychological criteria have so far been inconclusive [6]. From our results, however, type II seems to be characterized by less severe dementia than type III.

The main question to answer, however, concerns the mechanisms underlying the development of mental deterioration among MID patients [15]. It is well known, in fact, that different series of patients with superimposable CT findings may present with different degrees of mental deterioration or may even be non-demented. Large series of patients with type II CT lesions, in particular, should be investigated for a more precise evaluation of their mental functioning. In fact, among patients with pseudobulbar palsy, which is considered the clinical counterpart of the lacunar state, symptoms of dementia have been found only in 15% of cases [14]. The same holds true for type III. As reported elsewhere [3, 16], only 65% of patients with cerebrovascular disease and CT findings of Binswanger's encephalopathy are affected with mild to severe mental deterioration; there are no significant differences in age and risk factors between demented and non-demented subjects.

References

1. American Psychiatric Association Committee on Nomenclature and Statistics (1980) Diagnostic and statistical manual of mental disorders (DSM-III), 3rd edn. American Psychiatric Association, Washington DC
2. Babikian V, Ropper AH (1987) Binswanger's disease: a review. Stroke 18: 2–12
3. Bono G, Martelli A, Merlo P, Trucco M, Sinforiani E, Covelli V, Nappi G (1988) Binswanger's disease: a term in need of revision? New trends in clinical neuropharmacology, 2: 263–268
4. Cummings JL, Miller B, Hill MA, Neshkes R (1987) Neuropsychiatric aspects of multi-infarct dementia and dementia of the Alzheimer type. Arch Neurol 44: 389–393
5. Drayer BP, Heyman A, Wilkinson W, Barret L, Weinberg T (1985) Early-onset Alzheimer's disease: an analysis of CT findings. Ann Neurol 17: 407–410
6. Erkinjuntti T (1988) Dementia. Clinical diagnosis and differential diagnosis, with special reference to multi-infarct dementia. Medical Faculty of the University of Helsinki, Helsinki
7. Fisher CM (1960) Dementia in cerebrovascular disease. Trans Am Neurol Assoc 85: 147–152
8. Folstein MF, Folstein SE, McHugh PR (1975) "Mini Mental State". A practical method for grading the cognitive state of patients for the clinician. J Psychiatr Res 12: 189–198
9. Hachinski VC, Iliff LD, Zilka E, DuBoulay GH, McAllister VL, Marshall J, Russel RWR, Symon L (1975) Cerebral blood flow in dementia. Arch Neurol 32: 632–637
10. Hachinski VC, Potter P, Merskey H (1987) Leuko-araiosis. Arch Neurol 44: 21–23
11. Harrison MJG, Thomas DJ, DuBoulay GH, Marshall J (1979) Multi-infarct dementia. J Neurol Sci 40: 97–103
12. Hershey LA, Modic MT, Jaffe DF, Greenough PG (1986) Natural history of the vascular dementias: a prospective study of seven cases. Can J Neurol Sci 13: 559–565
13. Hughes CP, Berg L, Danziger WL, Coben LA, Martin RL (1982) A new clinical state for the staging of dementia. Br J Psychiatry 140: 566–572
14. Loeb C (1980) Clinical diagnosis of multi-infarct dementia. In: Amaducci L, Davison AN, Antuono P (eds) Aging of the brain and dementia. Raven, New York, pp 251–260
15. Loeb C (1985) Vascular dementias. In: Frederiks JAM (ed) Handbook of clinical neurology neurobehavioural disorders, vol 2. Elsevier Science, Amsterdam, pp 353–369

16. Martelli A, Micieli G, Rodriguez y Baena R, Locatelli D, Bono G, Nappi G (1982) CT abnormalities of deep biemispheric white matter in cerebrovascular disorders. J Neurosurg Sci 26: 95–97
17. McKhann G, Drachman D, Folstein M, Katzman R, Price D, Stadlan EM (1984) Alzheimer's disease: report of the NINCDS-ADRDA work group under the auspices of Department of Health and Human Service Task Force on Alzheimer's Disease. Neurology 34: 939–944
18. SIR (ed) (1981) Drug and methods in C.V.D. Proceedings of the international Symposium on experimental and clinical methodologies for study of acute and chronic cerebrovascular diseases, 24–26 March 1980, Paris, SIR (ed) Pergamon, pp 3–14
19. Rogers RL, Meyer JS, Mortel KF, Mahurin RK, Judd BW (1986) Decreased cerebral blood flow procedes multi-infarct dementia but follow senile dementia of Alzheimer type. Neurology 36: 1–6
20. Steingart A, Hachinski VC, Lau C, Fox AJ, Fox H, Lee D, Inzitari D, Merskey H (1987) Cognitive and neurologic findings in demented patients with diffuse white matter lucencies on computed tomographic scan (leuko-araiosis). Arch Neurol 44: 36–39
21. Valentine AR, Mosely IF, Kendall BE (1980) White matter abnormality in cerebral atrophy: clinico-radiological correlation. J Neurol Neurosurg Psychiatry 43: 139–142
22. Whitehouse PJ, Price DL, Struble RG, Clark AW, Coyle JT, De Long MR (1982) Alzheimer's disease and senile dementia – loss of neurons in the basal forebrain. Science 215: 1237–1239

Affective Disorders in Elderly and Dementing Patients

M. A. JENIKE

Overview

Depression is a common and potentially life-threatening disorder with a community prevalence as high as 13% (Gurland 1976). As many as 20%–35% of elderly patients with concurrent medical illness are depressed (Anonymous 1979; Moffie and Paykel 1975), and those over age 65 account for about 11% of the United States population but commit about 25% of all suicides (Sendbuehler and Goldstein 1977). Depressed elderly patients are often malnourished and agitated for months or even years (Jefferson and Marshall 1981), and untreated major depression lowers life expectancy and is associated with a greater risk for cardiac disease (Kay and Bergman 1966; Avery and Winokur 1976, Tsuang et al. 1980). Depression in the context of a dementing illness can present special challenges.

Psychiatric Symptoms Associated with Dementing Illnesses

Many patients with neurological illnesses suffer from affective symptoms as well as cognitive difficulties (Jenike 1986a, b). Even though the underlying neurological illness may not be treatable, the resolution of concomitant psychiatric symptoms often improves the quality of both the patient's and the caregiver's lives.

Alzheimer's Disease

Some dementing patients suffer from treatable depressive symptoms; estimates of the prevalence of clinical depression among such patients have been reported from 0% to 57% (Kral 1983; Ron et al. 1979; Liston 1978; Cummings et al. 1987, Knesevich et al. 1983); our experience would indicate that major depression seems to be relatively uncommon in patients with Alzheimer's disease. Cummings et al. (1987) found that only 17% of 30 Alzheimer's patients manifested depressive symptoms, and none had major depression. Knesevich and coworkers (1983) found no evidence of depression in a group of Alzheimer's patients when first seen or even when reexamined 1 year later.

Bergener, Reisberg (Eds.)
Diagnosis and Treatment
of Senile Dementia
© Springer-Verlag Berlin Heidelberg 1989

Psychosis (Caine and Shoulson 1983; Cummings et al. 1987) with delusions of persecution, infidelity, and theft occur at some time in the course of the illness in 50% of patients (Cummings et al. 1987). Psychosis may occur alone or in the context of a depressive illness.

Personality changes in Alzheimer's patients, a cortical dementia, occur but are usually not as troubling as those observed in patients with subcortical dementias (Cummings and Benson 1988). Alzheimer's patients tend to maintain a facade of acceptable social behaviors despite intellectual deterioration and occasional emotional indifference.

One problem with using scales such as the Hamilton Depression Rating Scale (Hamilton 1960) in an attempt to diagnose depression versus dementia is that some items assess impairment in work and daily activities as well as psychomotor retardation, weight loss, fatigue, decreased libido, and insomnia – items that may be secondary to dementia alone. This overlap of symptoms in dementia and depression may account for elevated depression rating scale scores in patients with primary degenerative dementia (Alzheimer's disease), leading to an overestimation of the prevalence of depression in dementing patients (Miller 1980). Lazarus and associates (1987) studied the frequency and severity of depressive symptoms among elderly patients who had a DSM-III presumptive diagnosis (definitive diagnosis can be made only at autopsy) of primary degenerative dementia as compared with normal, age-matched, community-dwelling control subjects. They attempted to identify specific depressive symptoms in the demented patients to ascertain whether there are specific signs and symptoms that provide a reliable basis for accurately diagnosing concomitant depression. They found that 18 (40%) of the dementing patients, compared with 5 (12%) of the control subjects, exhibited evidence of at least mild depression, and that within the dementia group, there was no relationship between degree of cognitive impairment and extent of depressive symptoms. To determine which symptoms of depression predominate in dementia, they performed an item analysis of the Hamilton scale and found significant differences between patients and controls on 11 of the 24 items. Significant elevations in the depressed patients with dementia were found on the Hamilton items that assess signs and symptoms reflecting inner feeling states of depression and despair, rather than somatic or vegetative symptoms of depression. For example, depressed mood, anxiety, and feelings of helplessness, hopelessness, and worthlessness were significantly greater in the depressed patients than in the control subjects. In contrast, the dementing patients did not score significantly higher than control subjects on the majority of items assessing vegetative symptoms, such as sleep disturbance, weight loss, and insomnia. This study demonstrates that the evaluation of possibly depressed demented patients should focus more on symptoms reflective of an intrapsychic state of depression, such as depressed mood, anxiety, and feelings of helplessness, hopelessness, and worthlessness, rather than on vegetaive signs of depression which may be the result of the dementing process alone.

Stroke

In contrast to Alzheimer's disease, depression occurs commonly in stroke patients, and these depressions can and should be treated aggressively. Each year roughly

440000 people have thromboembolic strokes in the United States (Wolf et al. 1977), and between 30% and 60% become clinically depressed, with the period of high risk lasting for 2 years after the stroke (Robinson 1981; Lipsey et al. 1984). Statistically, patients with left frontal lobe damage are most likely to suffer from severe depression (Robinson et al. 1983). Robinson and colleagues concluded from animal studies that brain catecholamines are depleted in cerebrovascular accidents and suggested that antidepressant medications might be used to treat these conditions (Robinson et al. 1983; Robinson and Szetela 1981).

Information from close friends, family members, or caregivers is helpful in diagnosing depression in the stroke patient. In general, cognitive impairment in stroke patients does not prevent them from giving accurate responses concerning depressive symptoms, although this is not invariably so. Patients with right-sided brain damage (for right-handed and most left-handed individuals) may suffer aprosodias and have impaired ability to receive the emotional meaning of words and situations or may be unable to communicate emotional distress or depression.

Recent evidence indicates that half the depressions occurring in the acute post-stroke period fulfill DSM-III-R diagnostic criteria for major depression (Robinson et al. 1983), and that, untreated, these disorders last more than 6 months (Robinson et al. 1984). Patients with poststroke affective illness and patients with functional major depression have very similar depressive symptoms (Lipsey et al. 1986).

There are case reports that psychostimulants, which may exert their effects by blocking the reuptake of depleted catecholamines, may be useful in stroke-induced depressions (Kaufmann et al. 1984; Robinson 1981; Woods et al. 1986).

In one study, the tricyclic nortriptyline significantly improved poststroke depression when compared in a double-blind manner to placebo (Lipsey et al. 1984), with successfully treated patients having nortriptyline levels in the therapeutic range (50–150 ng/ml). Bacaese the number of patients in this study was small (34), the authors were unable to determine the relationship between lesion location and response to medication. Another control trial demonstrated the safety and efficacy of trazodone in treating depressed stroke patients (Reding et al. 1986).

Stroke patients have many difficulties dealing with rehabilitation and loss of function and should not be forced to suffer concomitant depression when we have the tools at hand to effectively treat such smyptoms.

Parkinson's Disease

Cummings (1988) in a review of 27 studies representing 4336 Parkinson's disease patients found that the prevalence of overt dementia was 39.9%. The studies reporting the highest incidence of intellectual impairment (69.9%) used psychologic assessment techniques, whereas studies identifiying the lowest prevalence of dementia (30.2%) depended on nonstandardized clinical examinations. Neuropsychologic investigations revealed that parkinsonian patients manifested impairment in memory, visuospatial skills, and set aptitude while language function was largely spared. Intellectual deterioration correlated with age, akinesia, duration, and treatment status. Neuropathologic and neurochemical observations demonstrated that Parkinson's disease is a heterogeneous disorder: the classic subcortical pathology with dopamine deficiency may be complicated by atrophy of nucleus basalis and super-imposed cortical cholinergic deficits, with a few patients having the histopathologic hallmarks of Alzheimer's disease. Mild intellectual impairment also occurs with the classic pathology, and the more severe dementia syndromes have cholinergic altera-tions or Alzheimer's disease. Cummings concluded that Parkinson's disease includes several syndromes of intellectual impairment with variable pathologic and neurochemical correlates.

Parkinson's disease is complicated by depression in one-quarter to one-half of the cases (Mayeux 1982). Depressive symptoms have been reported in up to 34% of patients even prior to onset of motor manifestations (Patrick and Levy 1922). Most studies in which severity of symptoms was recorded found depression to be of mild to moderate intensity (Celesia and Wanamaker 1972; Mayeux et al. 1981; Warburton 1967); suicidal thoughts were common, but actual attempts rare (Mjones 1949). Some patients may experience depression as a reaction to the knowledge of the disease or its disability, but others develop affective symptoms prior to obvious indications of the disease. Most investigators concur that neither the presence nor the intensity of depression can be consistently related to any factor such as age, sex, degree of disability, or type of treatment (Mayeux 1982; Horn 1974; Mayeux, et al. 1981).

L-Dopa, the drug most drug most commonly used to treat Parkinson's disease, may also provoke depression, sometimes with suicidal tendencies (Raft et al. 1972). It may also induce other mental symptoms, such as paranoid ideation and psychotic episodes (Adams & Victor, 1981). Patients with a history of depression prior to onset of motor symptoms may be particularly prone to L-dopa-induced depression (Mayeux 1982).

There are a number of reports of favorable responses to tricyclic antidepressants in depressed parkinsonian patients (Anderson et al. 1980; Laitinen 1969; Strang 1965). Imipramine and its major metabolite desipramine have been effective in placebo-controlled trials (Laitinen 1969; Strang 1965) in reducing depression and fatigue. A few reports of improvement in mood (as well as in bradykinesia and rigidity) have been reported following electroconvulsive therapy (Asnis 1977; Lebensohn and Jen-kins 1975; Yudofsky 1979), which is a reasonable option in depressed parkinsonian patients who fail medication trials.

Psychosis, even in the setting of depression, is uncommon in untreated idiopathic Parkinson's diesease (Cummings and Benson 1988). When the clinician is faced with a parkinsonian patient, it is likely that cognitive and/or psychiatric symptoms will complicate the clinical picture.

Huntington's Disease

Personality changes may occur early in the course of Huntington's chorea and may be of two general types (McHugh and Folstein 1975). In one, the patient becomes generally apathetic, may appear depressed, and tends to neglect himself or herself, his or her job, and his or her former interests. In the other, the patient becomes increasingly irritable and oversensitive, with a tendency toward angry outbursts and violence.

Psychiatric symptoms occur commonly in patients with Huntington's chorea. Episodes of depression can last from weeks to months and may persist for several years. When Huntington patients with disease-related affective symptomatology were examined with the Schedule for Affective Disorders and Schizophrenia (SADS; Endicott and Spitzer 1978), 20% received a diagnosis of dysthymic syndrome, and 17% were diagnosed with a major depressive syndrome. Caine and Shoulson (1983) found that approximately 50% of patients with Huntington's disease exhibited significant affective disturbances (major depressive episodes or dysthymic disorders). If the mood disorders precede the motor disturbance or dementia, it may be impossible to differentiate them from functional disorders without the family history of Huntington's chorea.

The depression occasionally can reverse into a manic state (which can last for weeks and may resolve spontaneously) in which the patient is elated, expansive, grandiose, and may overeat and talk incessantly. Schizophrenia-like symptoms may also precede motor abnormalities and may consist of feelings of unreality, delusions of influence and control, and hallucinations and illusions. Patients typically are convinced of the reality of these hallucinations and delusions and may act upon them.

Depression in Huntington's patients appears to be responsive to antidepressant agents as well as to electroconvulsive therapy (ECT) (McHugh and Folstein 1975; Brothers and Meadows 1955) and may occasionally resolve spontaneously. Suicide rates in at-risk individuals are significantly greater than for the general population (Schoenfeld et al. 1984), and suicide is the cause of death in as many as 7% of nonhospitalized Huntington's patients (Reed and Chandler 1958).

Psychosis is also common in Huntington's disease (Caine and Shoulson 1983; Cummings et al. 1987).

Treatment Decisions

If there is any doubt whether a patient with a neurologic illness is depressed, he or she should be treated. Many patients are both demented and depressed, and the only way to separate the two is by response to treatment. Depression, even in a patient with an underlying dementing process, can usually be resolved. Cognition may not improve, but patients become less negative and more interested in hobbies, social activities, and sex.

Recognizing Depression

Depression in the elderly may present with various clinical pictures, such as chronic pain, multiple somatic complaints, or even dementia (Pseudodementia). Depression is, in fact, the main cause of a treatable dementia in the elderly (Wells 1963, 1979; Feinberg and Goodman 1984; Cole et al. 1983). Although some elderly depressed individuals present atypically, most can be diagnosed according to the Washington University research criteria, which form the basis for the *Diagnostic and Statistical Manual of Mental Disorders Revised*, third edition (DSM-III-R) criteria (Spar and LaRue 1983). A helpful mnemonic, developed by Gross at Massachusetts General Hospital, outlines the clinical picture of major depression as SIG E CAPS (prescription for energy capsules): sleep, interest, guilt, energy, concentration, appetite, psychomotor, and suicide. Each of these corresponds to one of the DSM-III-R criteria for major depression (Jenike 1988b). To elaborate, depressed patients generally complain of insomnia, typically with early awakening in the morning; occasionally, however, hypersomnia is the problem. They lose interest in usually stimulating activities – job, hobbies, social activities, and sex. Guilty ruminations and feelings of self-reproach are the rule. Depressed patients have no energy and feel fatigued all day. They frequently report an inability to concentrate, with slowed or mixed-up thinking. They usually have a poor appetite, with an associated loss of weight, although occasionally they overeat. Psychomotor retardation is usually observed, but agitated depressions in the elderly are not uncommon. They may have recurrent thoughts of suicide or death and may feel that life is not worth living or wish that they were dead. A patient with at least five of these eight criteria is depressed, and if his dysphoric emotional state has persisted for 2–4 weeks, he needs treatment.

Another clue to recognizing depression is the presence of multiple complaints in several body systems. When a patient's complaints do not fit a recognizable pattern or when chronic pain is a component, depression should be suspected and the SIG E CAPS criteria should be investigated.

Cognitive Changes Associated with Depression

When elderly patients appear demented, special care is required to rule out depression. Initially, family members should be asked whether they have observed any of the SIG E CAPS symptoms in the patient.

Clinically, one may find that depressed patients undergoing cognitive testing with the Mini-Mental State Exam and other cognitive tests actually perform better with time; that is, the depressed patient may remember one or none of three items after 3 min, but remember all three if asked again after 15 min. Such an improvement in memory would be very unlikely with Alzheimer's patients.

The term *pseudodementia* is often used to describe depression-related cognitive deficits that are reversible with adequate treatment of the affective illness. Lack of effort on the part of depressed patients is observed frequently by clinicians, who have noted patients increased dependency, indesiveness, and avoidance of responsibility as part of a general picture of motivational change.

Depressed patients perform poorly on a number of motor performance tasks, including tapping, aiming, and circle tracing (Raskin et al. 1982). When retested after adequate treatment of depression, their performance often improves strikingly (Cohen et al. 1982). Increasing severity of depression is strongly associated with decrements in motor performance (Stromgren et al. 1977, Grayson et al. 1987). Byrne (1977) found a significant negative relationship between severity of depression and performance on a signal detection task suggestion that depressed patients are inattentive, as well.

Patients with depression have also been reported to show deficits in memory (Cronholm and Ottosson 1961; Breslow et al. 1980; Sternberg and Jarvik 1976; Henry et al. 1973; Silberman et al. 1983; Raskin et al. 1982; Caine 1986; Feinberg and Goodman 1984) and conceptualization (Raskin et al. 1982; Caine 1986). However, some aspects of memory ability are reported to be preserved in depressed patients:

recognition of high-imagery words (Silberman et al. 1983), recall of related words that have previously been sorted (Weingartner et al. 1981), paired associate learning (Breslow et al. 1980), and rate of forgetting over time (Cronholm & Ottosson, 1961). This suggests that memory tasks that impose structure on the to-be-remembered items are performed relatively well by depressed patients.

Some authors speculate that it may be unreasonable to hypothesize basic memory deficits in depression, and that the most parsimonious explanation of available data would be one based on a single deficit in the central motivational state (Cohen et al. 1982). That is, general deficits in motivation, drive, and attention may account for the clinical and experimental deficits found in patients suffering from depression. For example, studies have found a correlation between intensity of depression and degree of memory impairment (Stromgren, 1977, Byrne, 1977; Cohen et al, 1982).

A number of authors have attempted to identify clues that would separate depressed from demented patients (Grayson et al. 1987). Wells (1979) emphasized the importance of getting a careful history of the disorder. Depressed patients usually develop the symptoms of depression before the onset of cognitive decline. In addition, the cognitive impairments frequently fluctutate along with fluctuations in depression. However, reports that demented patients are invariably unaware of their cognitive deficits, thus differentiating them from depressed patients, appear to be untrue. Many patients with a progressive dementia are clearly aware of their inpairments and the progression of their deficits.

Miller (1980) has discussed the difficulties in distinguishing depressive symptoms from a clinically recognizable depressive syndrome in an organically impaired population and has called particular attention to problems in the interpretation of vegetative indicators common to both dementia and depression. The rates of depression reported in demented patients vary considerably from study to study and probably reflect differences in the definition of both depression and dementia in each study.

In a careful study in which behavioral data was obtained from a structured interview of caregivers who knew patients well, rather than directly from patient – interviewer interaction, Merriam and associates (1988) found that fully 86% of their sample of 175 cognitively impaired patients met full DSM-III criteria for a major depressive episode. With this finding in mind, they questioned the appropriateness of using DSM-III criteria in this population and noted the frequent clinical dilemma that many of the symptoms of depression are present in demented patients who are clearly not depressed. They found that the overwhelming majority of their "depressed" patients were consistently able to be cheered up or distracted, even when most despondent; thus, diagnostic criteria that ignore the capacity for depressed demented patients to be distracted or cheered up may yield false-positive diagnoses of depression. Some researchers are trying to modify standard structured interviews, such as the SADS, so that there is less diagnostic overlap between symptoms of depression and those of dementia (Albert, Jenike, Falk and Keller, unpublished data).

It has recently been suggested that depression in an elderly patient is a red flag warning of an underlying, early dementing illness (Reding et al. 1985). Of 225 patients referred to a dementia clinic over a 3-year period, 57% of those initially felt to be depressed and nondemented went on to develop frank dementia. Many of them had some sign, often subtle, of neurological disease. Depressed elderly patients were found to be at high risk of developing dementia if any of the following were present:

presence of cerebrovascular, extrapyramidal, or spinocerebellar disease; a modified Hachinski ischemic score of 4 or greater; a Mental Status Questionnaire score under 8; or confusion on low doses of tricyclic antidepressants. Numerous patients suffer from both depression and structurally based intellectual impairment. Vigorous therapeutic intervention may benefit the affective state even when there is no rebound in neuropsychological functioning. This may improve the functional status of the patient. It has been reported that depression occurs less frequently as the dementing disease progresses (Reifler et al. 1982), but others (Shuttleworth et al. 1987) have found that the magnitude of depression did not differ as a function of disease severity, and they recommended the use of appropriate antidepressant therapy at any stage of disease in these patients.

Ideally, the uncertain clinician should initially consider the depressed, dementing patients to be suffering from pseudodementia, for which there is hope for recovery, and begin antidepressant therapy (Jenike 1988a, c). The dangers of assuming that cognitive deficits are secondary to neurological disease have been outlined by several authors (Kiloh 1961; Shamoian 1985; Jenike 1988b, c). It is important to guard against fatalistically assuming the cognitively impaired depressed individual as irretrievably demented and withholding treatment as a result. Therapeutic interventions should be based on the presence of responsive target symptoms, and although diagnosis is important, it may not be essential for initiating effective treatment measures. The distinction between a psychiatric and a neurological disorder may not be necessary as long as one establishes that the course is nonprogressive or has completed a work-up to rule out other treatable etiologies.

Cholinergic Alterations in Alzheimer's Disease

When treating affective illness in patients with Alzheimer's disease and probably many other dementing illnesses, abnormalities of the cholinergic system must be considered. Involvement of the cholinergic system with memory impairment is based on a number of findings:
a) anticholinergic drugs, such as scopolamine, induce memory deficits in healthy young subjects similar to those observed in nondemented elderly subjects;
b) these deficits are reversed by physostigmine, a cholinerigic agent that potentiates synaptic acetylcholine;
c) cholinergic drugs such as tetrahydroaminoacridine (THA), arecholine, and physostigmine improve aspects of learning and memory in normal subjects;
d) cholinergic neurons (in nucleus basalis of Meynert) are found to be selectively destroyed early in the course of the illness in the brains of Alzheimer's patients; and
e) the activity of choline acetyltransferase, which catalyzes the synthesis of acetylcholine, is reduced in brain tissue obtained from patients with Alzheimer's disease (Bartus et al. 1982).

In normal subjects, experimental manipulations of the cholinergic system have supported the idea that it is involved in memory. Drachman and Leavit (1975) used an anticholinergic agent, scopolamine, to produce measurable memory deficits in young normal subjects and demonstrated that these deficits could be reversed by intravenous physiostigmine, a cholinomimetic agent, but not by the nonspecific activation of amphetamine. Drachman and Sahakian (1980) later demonstrated that a single subcutaneous injection of physostigmine improved memory and other cognitive functions in normal elderly subjects. Also, Davis et al. (1987) demonstrated improvement after physostigmine in long-term memory processes in normal humans. Agnoli et al. (1983) demonstrated a correlation among the degree of memory loss, intellectual impairment, the quanty of senile plaques, and a decrease in choline acethyltransferase and acetylcholinesterase activity in patients affected by Alzheimer's disease. In this study, patients were subjected to a series of computerized EEG recordings and neuropsychological evaluations after acute administration of a number of cholinergic drugs, including physostigmine, and anticholinergic drugs (scopolamine and orphenadrine). Their results showed that the acute administration of some cholinergic drugs improved memory and also attention performances, whereas anticholinergic drugs induced opposite effects. In addition, the cholinergic drugs exhibited a tendency to shift the EEG spectrum analysis into more normal patterns compatible with the patient's age. This study further supports the view that the cholinergic system plays an important role in memory and attention disturbances found in Alzheimer's disease.

Francis et al. (1985) studied acetylcholine synthesis by measuring the incorporation or radiolabeled glucose into the transmitter in temporal-cortex specimens obtained at diagnostic craniotomy in 17 young patients (mean age, 59; SD, 5) with Alzheimer's disease. They found that synthesis of acetylcholine was significantly negatively correlated with cognitive impairment, and they felt that these results were consistent with the view that the deficit in the presynaptic cholinergic system is a relatively early change in the development of clinical features of the disease.

The loss of cholinergic markers is consistently found in Alzheimer's disease patients, whereas other neurochemical markers are usually decreased to a lesser extent and not as consistently (Terry and Davis, 1980; Davies 1979; Cross et al. 1981), especially early in the course of the illness. In addition, quantitative measurements of cholinergic cell loss correlate with an increase in the number of senile plaques and a reduction in memory function (Perry et al. 1978).

DST, Depression, and Dementia

The dexamethasone suppression test (DST) has often been used to assist clinicians in identifiying patients with depression or in following the resolution of depressive symptoms (Jenike 1985a); the DST is abnormal in about half of patients suffering from major depression. The DST may be of some use in identifying depressive illness in patients with early Alzheimer's disease, but the test in invalidated in the presence of severe dementia where most of the apparently nondepressed patients have abnormal DST (Jenike and Albert 1984).

Treatment of Affective Illness

Psychotherapy

Considerable evidence indicates that medication is more effective when used in combination with some type of psychotherapy.

The elderly are underrepresented in the utilization of outpatient psychiatric facilities in the United States (Steuer 1982). In 1968, only 2% of patients attending outpatient psychiatric facilities or treated by psychiatrists in private practice were over age 65. This situation has changed only slightly over the past decades. One more recent estimate is that only 2.7% of all clinical services provided by psychologists go to older adults (Vandenbos et al. 1981), and that the portion of community mental health center services rendered to this group has remained relatively stable at around 4% over the past decade (General Accounting Office 1982).

This underutilization of services may be the result of many factors. It may reflect a cultural bias; where professionals might believe that resources should go to younger clients who have more years of life ahead of them, and who are economically more productive. Clinicians may view the elderly as inflexible or consider their decline as inevitable. Others may feel that special knowledge is required to help the aged. Countertransference issues may surface. Some elderly patients may view therapists as their children (Grotjahn 1955), and unresolved conflicts with the therapist's own parents may interfere with objective observation and therapy. It has also been argued, however, that mental health system factors – such as reimbursement system inequities, lack of cooperation among community mental health centers and physicians, discrepant perceptions of the help that is needed, and the lack of referrals from other physicians who have contact with older patients who need mental health services – are the most important explanations of why so few older adults are seen by mental health professionals (Kahn 1975).

There are many types of psychotherapeutic approaches that can be used with the elderly, and, unfortunately, no good studies addressing outcome of psychotherapy have been conducted. It has been suggested that four common principles underlie the process of all psychotherapeutic approaches in the elderly:
1. fostering a sense of control, self-efficacy, and hope;
2. establishing a relationship with the caregiver;
3. providing or elucidating a sense of meaning; and
4. establishing constructive contingencies in the environment (Butler, 1975).

Butler (1960, 1968, 1975) pointed out themes common in old age, such as dysfunctioning of one's body, independence and dependence, concerns with time, and stereotypes of the young. Lack of meaningfulness and feelings of uselessness are also common, and therapists may help the aging patient resolve existential crises through reminiscence and self-evaluation.

Busse and Pfeiffer (1977) recommend that the therapist be active in mapping and clarifying the patient's problems and suggest the establishment of limited goals such as symptom relief, support for adaptation to changing life circumstances, acceptance of greater dependency as a normal aspect of the aging process, and renewed or continued involvement in useful activity. They also encourage social conversation during part of each session to enhance the patient's thoughts of being part of a meaningful relationship. Blume and Tross (1980) point out the importance of regularly scheduled sessions as a source of constancy in what may be a life filled with change.

As a means of increasing a patient's of self-worth, Burnside (1978) recommended that the therapist consider touching geriatric patients to express caring and gain the patient's attention. Linden (1975) stressed the importance of optimism in the therapist and emphasized that the personality of the therapist is a main consideration in psychotherapy outcome.

Since the problems of old people are likely to be social as well as intrapsychic, practical interventions are important, and the therapist should have a knowledge of community social agencies and referral sources. A number of agencies and groups are particularly useful in the management of particular types of patients and their families. Support groups and programs involving home visits to frail elderly with the purpose of reducing social isolation have been demonstrated to reduce psychiatric symptoms (Mulligan and Bennet 1977–1978). Programs that enlist elderly persons as teachers, advisors, and consultants benefit both helpers and the helped (Sherman 1981). Foster grandparent programs place older adults in positions to help children in various school or hospital settings (Saltz 1977; Hirschowitz 1973). Pet therapy is reported to diminish feelings of isolation, loneliness, and uselessness (Lago et al. 1983); pets may afford companionship, demand responsibility in terms of caring for them, and provide physical contact.

Tricyclic and Heterocyclic Agents

Pharmacologic strategy for the treatment of depression begins with a choice of antidepressant medication, a decision based upon previous treatment response and anticipation of which side effects may pose the greatest problems or produce therapeutic benefits for the patient. Since the introduction of imipramine about 30 years ago, tricyclics have been the mainstay of pharmacologic treatment for depression. Since these agents are generally considered to be equally effective, the choice of drug should be based on side effects. Tertiary amines such as amitriptyline and imipramine are much more likely to cause hypotension than secondary amines such as desipramine, protriptyline, and nortriptyline (Table 1; Salzman 1982). However, doxepin, a tertiary amine, is safe in elderly patients in terms of orthostatic changes (Neshkes et al. 1985). Tertiary amines also tend to produce more sedation, presumably by blocking synaptic serotonin reuptake or by affecting histamine receptors (Richelson 1982).

Anticholinergic and noradrenergic side effects are also particularly troublesome both in the nondementing and in the dementing elderly patient. Anticholinergic symptoms may be prominent both centrally (delirium, confusion, cognitive impairment) and peripherally (tachycardia, urinary retention, constipation, blurred vision, dry mouth, and exacerbation of narrow angle glaucoma). If desipramine (Norpramin) is assigned an anticholinergic potency of 1, amitriptyline (Elavil) would be eight times more anticholinergic. The other tricyclics lie somewhere in between, with a relative potency of about 2 (Table 1). Clinically, amitriptyline is generally regarded as the tricyclic most likely to cause a clinically hazardous tachycardia (Cassem 1982). The

Table 1. Characteristics of tricyclic and heterocyclic agents in treatment of depression

Generic name	Trade name	Relative anticholinergic effect	Sedative effect
Tricyclic tertiary amines			
Amitriptyline	Elavil and others	8	High
Imipramine	Tofranil and others	2	Moderate
Doxepin	Sinequan, Adapin	2	High
Tricyclic secondary amines			
Desipramine	Norpramin	1	Low
Protriptyline	Vivactil, Triptil	2	Low
Nortriptyline	Aventyl, Pamelor	2	Moderate
Others			
Amoxapine	Asendin	2	Moderate
Maprotiline	Ludiomil	2	Moderate
Trazodone	Desyrel	0	High

[1] Reproduced with (From Jenike 1988 b)

combination of pronounced anticholinergic activity and danger of orthostatic hypotension make amitriptyline the least desirable of all the available tricyclics used to treat depression (Jenike 1985 a, 1988 b). Based on in vitro comparisons of anti-cholinergic potency, amitriptyline is about $\frac{1}{20}$ as active as atropine at central and peripheral muscarinic cholinergic receptors, so that a daily dose of 150 mg amitripty-line corresponds to approximately 7.5 mg atropine, a dose which would almost never be given (Cassem 1982). Because of the well-documented abnormalities in the cholinergic system in dementing patients and the effects of anticholinergic drugs on memory even in normal subjects, any anticholinergic medication given to a dementing patient will worsen cognitive functioning even if it improves affective state.

If a patient has had a prior positive response, or if he has a relative who had a good outcome from a particular drug, it may be best to begin treatment with this drug. In general, tertiary amine tricyclics (except doxepin) and agents with high anticholiner-gic potency should be avoided in the elderly, especially in the context of a dementing illness. Low doses of secondary amine tricyclics with relatively low anticholinergic activity, such as desipramine and nortriptyline, or newer agents, such as trazodone, maprotiline, or fluoxetine, should be the drugs of first choice. If a depressed patient is not sleeping well, trazodone or nortriptyline or maprotiline, given at bedtime, may improve insomnia during the early stages of treatment. In hypersomnic or lethargic patients, daytime doses of desipramine, protriptyline, or fluoxetine may help activate the patient (Jenike 1985 a, 1988 b). These so-called "activating agents" may sedate some patients and should then be given around bedtime.

Amoxapine (Asendin) is the demethylated derivative of the antipsychotic loxapine and is comparable in efficacy to the standard tricyclic agents (Dominquez 1983). Hypotension is an uncommon side effect, but several cases of seizures have been reported. Amoxapine inhibits both norepinephrine and serotonin reuptake and also blocks dopamine receptors and produces extrapyramidal side effects typical of neuroleptics. It has been reported to cause acute dystonia, parkinsonism, and akathisia (Lydiard and Gelenberg 1981; Barton 1982), and there are reports of tardive dyskinesia associated with amoxapine use (Lapierre and Anderson 1983). Since the elderly are particularly prone to develop tardive dyskinesia, and since the movements associated with it are much less likely to be reversible in older individuals (Jenike 1983a), amoxapine should be avoided in elderly patients suffering from uncomplicated depression.

Maprotiline (Ludiomil), also introduced in 1981, is a tetracyclic that is very similar to standard tricyclics in its action (Dominquez 1983). It is a specific blocker of norepinephrine reuptake, with apparently no effect on serotonin uptake. It has little anticholinergic effect and does not commonly produce orthostatic hypotension. In addition, it appears to have a lower incidence of cardiovascular side effects (Wells and Gelenberg 1981). Seizures have been reported, and skin rashes occur in up to 10% of patients (Dominquez 1983).

Trazodone (Desyrel) has a structure different from other antidepressant agents and is a selective, serotonin uptake blocker. It is similar in efficacy to the standard tricyclics (Murphy and Ankier 1980) but has a very low incidence of anticholinergic side effects, although clinically some patients complain of dry mouth. The lack of anticholinergic side effects with trazodone is probably responsible for the low incidence of therapy dropouts in comparative studies with tricyclics and other agents (Newton 1981). The elderly seem to tolerate trazodone very well. Clinically, trazodone is sedating and is particularly helpful for depressed patients who cannot sleep. Other common side effects include indigestion, nausea, and headaches. Priapism is a rare problem and male patients should be cautioned to discontinue the drug if prolonged or painful erections occur. Trazodone appears to have a more benign cardiac side effect profile compared with the tricyclics (Himmelhoch 1981). Caution is still recommended in using trazodone in patients with preexisting cardiac disease. It appears to be particularly nonmalignant when taken in overdose; at this point, there have been no life-threatening complications after trazodone overdose alone such as those frequently associated with overdose of tricyclic antidepressants. The dosing schedule is different from most of the other heterocyclic antidepressants; approximately 400 mg trazodone is equivalent to 150 mg amitriptyline or imipramine. Clinicians frequently underdose patients with trazodone (Jenike 1985a, 1988b).

A new antidepressant, fluoxetine (Prozac) appears to be relatively free of major side effects and may be a useful drug for elderly patients. It is a highly specific, highly potent blocker of serotonin uptake with essentially no ability to block other neurotransmitters nor does it block postsynaptic receptor sites. Its overall place in the armamentarium of antidepressants awaits further research in elderly patients. It has a dosage range of 20 to 80 mg/day.

Prior to starting any antidepressant medication, an ECG should be performed on all elderly patients. Treatment should begin with a very low dose – a maximum of 25 mg for most drugs (except 5 mg for protriptyline, 20 mg for fluoxetine, and 50 mg for trazodone). The dosage can be increased slowly every few days. Subjective response and heart rate must be monitored, and the clinician must be on the alert for anticholinergic, cardiovascular, or central nervous system side effects. Dosage increase should be slowed if tachycardia, excessive sedation, or orthostatic hypotension develops. Often the patient is the last to know that he is getting better, and family members commonly report that the patient is sleeping and eating better before the

Table 2. Suggested blood levels for some tricyclic agents

Drug	What is measured	Total therapeutic level
Imipramine	Imipramine and desipramine	>200 ng/ml
Desipramine	Desipramine	>125 ng/ml
Amitriptyline	Amitriptyline and nortriptyline	>160 ng/ml[b]
Nortriptyline	Nortriptyline	50–150 ng/ml[a]
Doxepin	Doxepin and desmethyldoxepin	>100 ng/ml[b]

[a] Therapeutic window: Levels above or below the therapeutic range are associated with decreased response
[b] Rough estimates (From Jenike 1988b)

dysphoria resolves. An adequate trial takes at least 4 weeks, and probably 6 weeks at therapeutic levels. Drugs should not be changed until an adequate therapeutic trial is completed; Quitkin and coworkers (1984) reviewing drug trials involving patients on a representative spectrum of antidepressants, found that 40% of patients unresponsive at 4 weeks responded to treatment if the drug trial was extended to 6 weeks.

If these agents are not helpful after a reasonable trial, a blood level determination (when available) will assist the clinician in determining the next step (Table 2). Blood levels are well worked out for imipramine and nortriptyline and less so for desipramine (Task Force 1985). We have rough estimates of therapeutic values for amitriptyline and doxepin. We can get blood levels for other agents such as trazodone, but we have no idea what levels correspond with clinical improvement; such levels are, however, occasionally useful to check on compliance. Blood samples should be drawn in the morning before any morning dose of medication or 10–14 h after the evening dose for patients on a once daily dosing schedule. With the same dose, blood levels can vary from ten to as much as 30 times among individuals. Nortriptyline appears to be unique among these agents in that it has a therapeutic window; that is, levels above as well as below the therapeutic range are associated with a decreased response (Task Force 1985). When the level is not in the appropriate range, dosage should be adjusted.

Monoamine Oxidase Inhibitors

Among the somatic treatments available for treating depressed elderly patients, monoamine oxidase inhibitors (MAOIs) are the least used. Many clinicians avoid the use of MAOIs in elderly patients because of fears of adverse reactions. In fact, many textbooks of geriatrics make no mention of the use of MAOIs for the elderly. It is now known that these agents can be safely used for the elderly when certain precautions are taken (Jenike 1984a). Many patients who do not respond to tricyclics or some of the newer antidepressants improve with MAOIs. Also, MAOIs have been found to be especially effective in treating depression related to dementia (Ashford and Ford 1979; Jenike 1985b). Dementing patients have higher levels of monoamine oxidase (MAO) than age-matched control subjects, and this may account for the improvement in some depressions in dementing patients with MAOIs (Jenike 1985b). The following is an example of a not uncommon case:

Mr. A, a 72-year-old retired laborer, was brought to the psychiatric memory disorders clinic of Massachusetts General Hospital with a year history of worsening memory. In addition, the patient's wife told us that he had become increasingly withdrawn and was losing interest in his hobbies. Previously an avid traveler, he now wanted to just sit at home, often alone and in the dark. He was refusing to drive, had lost his appetite, with a resultant weight loss of 12 lb, and seemed frequently confused and unable to concentrate. He denied any suicidal ideation but admitted to feeling very depressed and hopeless. He had a strong family history of depression, and his mother had received electroconvulsive therapy on one occasion, with good result.

Results from Mr. A's dementia work-up were entirely negative, and neuropsychiatric testing results were consistent with the initial impression that Mr. A was suffering from an affective illness with secondary memory impairment (pseudodementia).

Mr A was started on desipramine, 25 mg at bedtime, and the dose was increased slowly to 200 mg daily. He suffered no side effects but also got no better over the next 8 weeks, despite measured blood levels in the therapeutic range. Desipramine was eventually discontinued and nortriptyline was begun, starting with a low dosage. Once again, he failed to respond despite blood levels in therapeutic range.

Because Mr. A had not improved on two tricyclic antidepressants, and the family feared electroconvulsive therapy. a MAOI was begun After a 10-day drug-free period, tranylcypromine was started at 10 mg twice an day and slowly increased to 20 mg twice a day. After 2 weeks, Mr. A was much improved, and within weeks he was "back to his former self." He has continued on tranylcypromine, and at a return visit to the clinic 3 months later was observed to be doing well. Repeat clinical testing at that time showed that his cognitive disturbances had resolved.

As regards precautions and side effects of MAOIs, it is essential that all patients on MAOIs receive dietary and drug precautions (Tables 3, 4) (Jenike 1984a, 1988b). Elderly patients comply well and rarely complain about such restrictions. A low-tyramine diet is required, necessitating avoidance of foods such as fermented cheese, yogurt, beer, red wine, and excessive amounts of caffaine and chocolate. Patients can safely drink white wine, vodka, gin, and whiskey, and a blanket instruction to avoid all alcohol is not only unwarranted but may also decrease compliance dramatically (Jenike 1983b). Combination cold tablets, nasal decongestants, appetite suppressors,

Table 3. Dietary and drug precautions for patients taking monoamine oxidase inhibitors

Danger of rise in blood pressure	Food and drink	Drugs
Very dangerous	All cheese All foods containing cheese (e. g., pizza, fondue, many Italian dishes, salad dressing) Broad bean pods (English, Chinese pea pods)	Cold medications (e. g., Dristan, Contac) Nasal decongestants, sinus medicine Asthma inhalants Meperidine (Demerol) Amphetamines Indirect-acting sympathomimetic amines (e. g., amphetamines, methylphenidate, phenylpropanolamine, ephedrine, cyclopentamine, pseudoephedrine, tyramine) Direct- and indirect-acting sympathomimetic amines (e. g., metaraminol, phenylephrine) Buspirone (Buspar)

Table 3. continued

Danger of rise in blood pressure	Food and drink	Drugs
Moderately dangerous	Sour cream All fermented or aged foods, especially aged meats or aged fish (e. g., corned beef, salami, fermented sausage [pepperoni, summer sausage], pickled herring) Liver (chicken, beef, or pork) Liverwurst Meat or yeast extracts (e. g., Bovril or Marmite) Spoiled or dry fruit (e. g., spoiled bananas, figs, raisins) Red wine, sherry, vermouth, cognac Beer and ale	Allergy and hay fever medications Antiappetite (diet) medicine Direct-acting sympathomimetic amines (e. g., epinephrine, isoproterenol, methoxamine, norepinephrine) Local anesthetics with epinephrine Levodopa for parkinsonism Dopamine
Minimally dangerous	Chocolate, anchovies, caviar, coffee, colas, sauerkraut, mushrooms, beet root (beets), rhubarb, curry powder, junket, Worcestershire sauce, soy sauce, licorice, snails[a]	
Safe	Fresh cottage cheese, cream cheese, yogurt in moderate amounts Baked products raised with yeast (e. g., bread) Yeast Fresh fruits, except pineapple and avocados Other alcoholic drings (e. g., gin, vodka, whiskey, in true moderation)	Pure steroid asthma inhalants (e. g. beclomethasone diproprionate [Vanceril]) Pure antihistamines (chlorpheniramine, brompheniramine) Other narcotics (e. g. codeine) in lowered doses Local anesthetics without epinephrine (e. g. mepivacaine [Carbocaine]) Diabetics taking insulin may have increased hypoglycemia requiring a decreased dose of insulin, but insulin is otherwise safe Patients on hypotensive agents for high blood pressure may have more hypotension, requiring a decrease or stopping of in the hypotensive agent, which otherwise is safe

[a] These foods rarely have been reported to cause hypertensive reactions with MAOIs. The evidence supporting these claims is weak and often based on a single isolated case. Warnings based on such evidence have been uncritically perpetuated, especially in view of the large number of patients taking MAOIs who have eaten these foods with no problem. In practice, a blanket prohibition of these foods seems unjustified, unless they are clearly spoiled or decayed, except for specific patients in whom they have already caused symptoms. (From Jenike 1988b)

and amphetamines must be avoided. Pure antihistamines, such as chlorpheniramine, however, can safely be used to treat patients who have rhinitis (Jenike 1983 a, 1984).

There is a poorly understood, potentially fatal toxic interaction between MAOIs and meperidine hydrochloride, which was first described in 1955 (Mitchell 1955) and has been reported occasionally since that time (Meyer and Halfin 1981). Clinically, patients appear agitated, disoriented, cyanotic, hyperthermic, hypertensive, and tachycardic. In this event, chlorpromazine has been used as an effective treatment (Papp and Benaim 1958; Jenike 1984). There have been no clinical reports of the same severe toxic interactions with other narcotics, although increased potency has been noted experimentally in animals (Meyer and Halfing 1981). Should narcotics be needed for a patient on a MAOI, a prudent course would be to begin with half the

Table 4. Instructions for patients taking monoamine oxidase inhibitors

Avoid all the food and drugs mentioned on the dietary restrictions list. Be particularly careful to avoid those foods and drugs that are considered moderately and very dangerous

In general, avoid all foods that are decayed, fermented, or aged in some way. Avoid any aged food even if it is not on the list

If you get a cold or flu, you may use aspirin or acetaminophen (Tylenol). For a cough, glycerin cough drops or *plain* Robitussin may be used

All laxatives or stool softeners may be used for constipation

All antibiotics, e.g., penicillin, tetracycline, and erythromycin, may be safely used to treat infections

Do not take other medications without first checking with me. This includes any over-the-counter medicines bought without prescription, e.g., cold tablets, nose drops, cough medicine, diet pills

Eating one of the restricted foods may cause a sudden elevation of your blood pressure. When this occurs, you get an explosive headache, particularly in the back of your head and temples. Your head and face will feel flushed and full, your heart may pound, and you may perspire heavily and feel nauseated

If you need medical or dental care while on this medication, show these restrictions and instructions to the doctor. Have the doctor call my office if he has any questions or need further clarification or information

Side effects such as postural lightheadedness, constipation, delay in urination, delay in ejaculation and orgasm, muscle twitching, sedation, fluid retention, insomnia, and excess sweating are quite common. Many of these side effects lessen considerably after the 3rd week

Lightheadedness may occur following sudden changes in position. This can be avoided by getting up slowly. If tablets are taken with meals, lightheadedness and the other side effects are lessened

The medication is rarely effective in less than 3 weeks

Care should be taken while operating any machinery or while driving, since some patients have episodes of sleepiness in the early phases of treatment with MAO inhibitors

Take the medication precisely as directed. Do not regulate the number of pills without first consulting me

In spite of the side effects and special dietary restrictions, your medication, an MAO inhibitor, is safe and effective when taken as directed

If any special problems arise, call me at my office

(From Jenike 1988b)

usual dosage and titrate the dosage slowly on the basis of symptomatic response, bearing in mind that increased potency will be more pronounced if the narcotic is given close to the time that the MAOI was taken that day (Meyer and Halfin 1981).

Because MAOIs have essentially no anticholinergic effects, they are useful for patients who are sensitive to these side effects, such as patients with dementing illnesses. For example, the elderly patient who has urinary retention with only a 10-mg dosage of desipramine may do very well on a MAOI. Some women taking MAOIs are unable to achieve orgasm. (The Medical Detter, July 11, 1980, p 58). Serious hepatic toxicity, which used to occur frequently with earlier MAOIs, is rare with those currently available.

The side effects of MAOIs that cause the most problems for the elderly are hypotension and insomnia. Insomnia can be minimized by giving the last daily dose no later than 4 P.M. Some patients, however, feel drowsy on these agents, particularly phenelzine, and can be given the drug at bedtime. It is best to start with a daytime dosing schedule and switch to evening only if the patient complains of drowsiness. Orthostatic hypotension is a dangerous side effect for geriatric patients, because they tolerate falls poorly. It had been thought that MAOI-induced orthostatic hypotension occured early in the course of treatment and that if patients could tolerate the first few days of medication, hypotension would rarely necessitate discontinuing the drug (Mielke 1976; Robinson et al. 1978). Recently, however, Kronig and associates (1983) carefully followed a small group of patients ($n = 14$; average age, 52) and reported that the mean orthostatic drop increased with time and peaked between 3 and 4 weeks after MAOIs were begun. Their data imply that clinicians should continue to watch for orthostatic changes at least throughout the 1st month of treatment.

The most important adverse effect associated with MAOIs is the uncommon, but frightening, occurrence of a hypertensive crisis caused by a toxic interaction with certain drugs or tyramine-containing foods. Tyramine and other amines can cause hypertension by a mechanism that is not completely understood. Normally, ingested tyramine is inactivated by monoamine oxidase in the gastrointestinal tract and liver; when this is prevented by MAOIs, palpitations, severe headaches and hypertensive crises can result (The Medical Letter, July 11, 1980, p. 58). The elderly patient who has fragile atherosclerotic blood vessels could easily suffer a stroke during such a crisis. Intravenous phentolamine, an alpha-adrenergic blocker, is recommended for treatment of severe hypertensive reactions. Alternatively, chlorpromazine which also has alpha-adrenergic blocking activity, can be given intramuscularly. A recent report suggests that intravenous labetalol (20 mg given over 5 min) may also be effective in treating tyramine-induced hypertensive crises (Abrams et al. 1985).

One systematic study of dietary noncompliance showed that although nearly 40% of 98 patients taking tranylcypromine acknowledged "cheating" on their restrictions, no serious complications ensued (Neil et al. 1979).

Little is gained by measuring platelet MAO activity while patients are on these agents. The assay is generally not readily available, and some researchers have found no significant relationships between clinical response and platelet MAO inhibition (Davidson and White 1983). Also, White and colleagues found that MAO inhibition levels were not consistent and could vary with assay methodology, laboratory technique, and gender unmatched comparison groups (White et al. 1983).

At the Massachusetts General Hospital we have for a number of years routinely used MAOIs as maintenance therapy for patients who have received electroconvulsive therapy for severe depressive disorders. Most of these patients are over the age of 60 years. To my knowledge, we have not had a single patient develop a hypertensive episode; the overwhelming majority tolerate these agents very well. Tranylcypromine is our preferred MAOI for elderly patients because it is shorter acting and, when discontinued, is out of the patient's system within 24 h. In contradistinction, phenelzine's effects may persist for over a week when discontinued (Goodman and Gilman 1975). Our usual starting dose of tranylcypromine is 10 mg twice daily and most elderly patients can be treated effectively on this dose, but some may require gradual increase to as much as 60 mg daily. Phenelzine should be started at 15 mg once daily and may need to be increased slowly to as high as 75 mg for some patients. There are no known long-term adverse effects of MAOIs, such as the tardive dyskinesia that occurs with chronic use of neuroleptics.

Clinicians frequently find that positive antidepressant effects of MAOIs begin to decrease over a few weeks on MAOIs. Full antidepressant effect can usually be regained by increasing the dose or, if the patient is already at the maximum dose, by stopping the medication completely for 1–2 weeks and then restarting it.

The following conclusions may be drawn with regard to MAOIs:
1. MAOIs are safe and effective for the elderly when certain simple precautions are taken.
2. Give patients a list of foods to avoid (Table 3) and an instruction sheet (Table 4); advise them not to take any medications that are not listed as safe on the instruction sheet unless they check with a physician.
3. To lessen chances of insomnia, give the last dose of medication before 4 P. M.
4. Reasonable starting doses are 10 mg twice daily for tranylcypromine or 15 mg once daily for phenelzine; maintain elderly patients on this dose for at least 1 week and increase the dose slowly.
5. Monitor blood pressure for orthostatic changes for at least 1 month, as recent evidence indicates that such changes may not be present initially.
6. If a hypertensive crisis develops, phentolamine, chlorpromazine, or labetalol can be used for rapid blood pressure control.
7. Do not administer meperidine for pain relief to patients taking MAOIs; other narcotics can be used safely but should be started at a lower than usual dosage.

Lithium

Therapeutic Uses

Lithium is occasionally used in the elderly. It is unusual for mania to occur initially past the age of 65 years, and most elderly patients who present in a manic state have a history of prior manic episodes (Jefferson 1983). Only about 5% of patients admitted to psychogeriatric wards suffer from manic episodes. Of those elderly patients admitted for affective disorders, Roth (1955) found that 13% were suffering predominantly from manic symptoms.

The median age at onset for bipolar illness is 30 years; the risk of illness remains fairly high until age 50 and then decreases sharply. Almost 90% of all cases have onset before age 50 years (Angst et al. 1973). Early-onset bipolar disorder is an illness that usually continues into later life; so even though the initial onset of bipolar disorder may be rare after age 65, the bipolar population that eventually reaches old age is substantial. The New York State Psychiatric Institute Lithium Clinic reported that about 20% of 200 active patients were over 65 years of age (Dunner et al. 1979). The proportion of patients suffering from dementia was not specified.

As in younger patients, the primary uses of lithium in the elderly are to treat mania and prevent recurrent episodes in bipolar patients. Lithium has also been used with some success in schizoaffective disorder and recurrent unipolar depression (Jefferson 1983). The utility of lithium in treating acute depression is not well established although occasional lithium-responsive bipolar and unipolar depressives are reported (Jefferson 1983). Lithium is not the drug of first choice for depression in elderly patients but may be a useful adjuvant in tricyclic antidepressant-resistant unipolar depressed patients (see below). DeMontigny and associates (1981) reported that eight such patients (aged 33–64 years) responded within 48 h when lithium was added to the tricyclic regimen.

Based on little data, it appears that lithium is just as effective in the elderly as it is in younger patients. In patients with coexisting dementia, however, lithium is reportedly less effective and is associated with increased risk (Jefferson 1983).

Special Precautions in the Elderly

The glomerular filtration rate (GFR) decreases with advancing age (Rowe et al. 1976), and since lithium is almost exclusively excreted by the kidneys, dosage modification is routinely required, and in patients with renal disease, drastic reductions in dose are needed.

Elderly patients tend to have more diseases than younger patients. These acute and chronic illnesses can complicate lithium use in the elderly. For example, superimposed renal disease not only impairs lithium excretion but also may increase chances of lithium-induced nephrotoxicity. Dementing illnesses may sensitize a patient to lithium-induced neurotoxicity and also decrease ability to comply with dosing schedules (Himmelhoch et al. 1980). Cardiovascular disease may make patients vulnerable to fluid and electrolyte alterations and may increase risk of cardiotoxicity (Jefferson 1983).

Elderly patients with more disease will be on multiple medications. Not only is there then an increased incidence of side effects, but it is harder to establish which drug is responsible for which side effect. Also, compliance problems increase and there is an increased likelihood of adverse drug interactions.

Common Drug Interactions with Lithium

Because many elderly patients suffer from idiopathic hypertension, thiazide diuretics are frequently taken in combination with lithium. They consistently cause decreased renal clearance of lithium and raise serum lithium levels. Whenever a thiazide is added to ongoing lithium therapy, dosage must generally be lowered. Conversely, to avoid subtherapeutic levels, dosage may have to be increased when a thiazide is discontinued.

Nonsteroidal anti-inflammatory drugs, such as indomethacin and phenylbutazone, have been reported to reduce lithium clearance and raise serum lithium levels by 25%–60% (Jefferson and Marshall 1981; Reimann and Frolich 1981). It is unknown whether other prostaglandin synthesis inhibitors cause a similar action.

Case reports of rare and probably idisoyncratic interactions have been reported with neuroleptics, neuromuscular blocking agents, antibiotics, methyldopa, and digitalis (Jefferson and Marshall 1981). Definite recommendations await further data.

Before Starting Lithium

It is important to consider causes of secondary mania. Onset at a late age and the absence of a family history of affective illness should make one suspicious of a medical cause for mania. Medical causes which have been reported to produce the picture of mania include drugs (including levodopa and steroids), metabolic abnormalities, infection, neoplasm, and temporal lobe epilepsy (Krauthammer and Klerman 1978).

Mania is also occasionally seen in previously depressed individuals being treated with tricyclic antidepressants or MAOIs. Some researchers feel that this represents the uncovering of an underlying bipolar disorder while others suggest that it is simply a true drug-induced mania.

To rule out secondary mania, a detailed medical history should be supplemented by a physical examination and appropriate laboratory testing. Because of the potential pitfalls involved in treating the manic elderly patient, hospitalization for evaluation and treatment should be strongly considered – particularly if the patient lives alone or has concurrent medical illnesses.

Renal function must be evaluated prior to initiating lithium treatment. Because of the insensitivity of the serum creatinine in the elderly, a 24-h creatinine clearance is a better test for evaluating GFR.

Thyroid function should be evaluated by measuring serum thyroxine (T_4), L-triiodothyronine (T_3), and thyroid-stimulating hormone (TSH). A baseline ECG is mandatory in all elderly patients. Without focal neurologic signs, there is no need to perform a prior EEG or computed tomography (CT) scan (Jefferson 1983).

Starting lithium

In the elderly it is important to initiate lithium carbonate therapy with a low dose and to increase dosage slowly. Liptzin (1984) recommends beginning with a dose of 75–300 mg per day, while Dunner et al. (1979) begin with a 300-mg daily dose of lithium carbonate in all their healthy elderly manics. Doses of 75 mg can be obtained using lithium citrate and doses of 150 mg by breaking a 300-mg tablet in half. Since the elimination half-life of lithium is prolonged in the elderly to as long as 36 h or more, it may take more than a week to reach steady-state serum levels following either initiation of therapy or a change in dose (Jefferson 1983).

In elderly manics, more frequent sampling of serum levels are generally indicated to minimize the likelihood of toxicity. To interpret serum lithium levels appropriately, samples should be drawn 12 h after the last dose. Unlike most other medications used in psychiatry, the oral dose of lithium is not an adequate guideline, and blood levels are crucial for proper management. Therapeutic levels are still not clearly defined in the elderly. In general, they may respond to lower levels than those generally effective in younger patients. Foster and Rosenthal seek blood levels in the range of 0.4–0.7 mmol/l and do not exceed 0.7 mmol/l unless a very classic manic picture is present clinically (Foster and Rosenthal 1980).

Maintenance of Lithium

Serum lithium levels and clinical evaluations should be performed more frequently in the elderly than in a younger population. If the patient is compliant or is closely watched, he or she can be evaluated on a monthly basis for the 1st year of therapy. It is important that the patient and family be aware of the proper use and toxic side effects, and that they be encouraged to contact the physician whenever questions arise. Psychiatrists should have a good working relationship with the patient's internist or general physician.

Side Effects and toxicity

Patients with therapeutic levels may complain of tremor, urinary frequency, mild nausea, and a subjective feeling of "being medicated". Early signs of intoxication include increasing tremor, ataxia, weakness, slurred speech, blurred vision, tinnitus, and drowsiness or excitement. Severe intoxication produces increased deep-tendon reflexes, nystagmus, confusion, lethargy, and stupor. This may progress to seizures and coma.

Bradyarrhythmia secondary to sinus node dysfunction occurs uncommonly with lithium therapy (Cassem 1982). Routine measurement of pulse and asking about typical symptoms such as dizziness or fainting are necessary.

Extrapyramidal effects, particularly parkinsonian movements, have been reported with lithium use, and the elderly may be more sensitive to such complications (Jefferson 1983).

Lithium produces subtle cognitive changes in healthy young volunteers, and these may be more marked in the elderly. These can progress to the point that early senile dementia may be suspected (Judd et al. 1977).

There are reports of acute worsening of eye lens opacification after lithium was started (Makeeva et al. 1974). The number of cases is small, and this does not seem to be a common effect. Jefferson (1983) states that, at present, lithium use in the elderly is not generally considered reason for periodic eye evaluation.

The elderly are prone to develop lithium intoxication. They are particularly vulnerable because of reduced lithium clearance secondary to reduced renal function and because of increased sensitivity to the drug, more associated illnesses, multiple medications, poor compliance, decreased food and fluid intake, and lack of social supports. The presence of coexisting neurologic illness is the most critical predisposing factor, according to Himmelhoch and colleagues (1980).

Polyuria and polydipsia are so common that they can be considered routine. Thiazide diuretics can be used to decrease these symptoms when they are severe, but the mechanism of this paradoxical response to diuretics remains unclear.

Propranolol hydrochloride in small doses (10–30 mg/day) may be used to treat lithium-induced tremor. Because propranolol may produce worsening of cardiovascular status and induce depression, it should be used at the lowest possible dose (Liptzin 1984).

Psychostimulants

Psychostimulants were used briefly as antidepressants until the advent of the tricyclics, at which time the latter became the first line drugs in the treatment of depression (Myerson 1936). Nonetheless, recent studies advocating their use in medically ill depressed patients (Kayton and Raskind 1980; Hackett 1978; Kaufmann et al. 1984; Woods et al. 1986), as adjuvants to morphine in the treatment of postoperative pain (Forest 1977), and for adjustment reactions in patients recovering from chronic illnesses or surgical procedures (Hackett 1978) have rekindled interest in the investigation of these agents. Silberman (1981), in a double-blind study of 18 endogenously depressed patients, demonstrated superiority of amphetamine over placebo in improving mood and psychomotor activity. Two studies have shown the effectiveness of methylphenidate hydrochloride in treating depressive symptoms in patients with concurrent dementia. In the first study (Holliday and Joffe 1965), depressed patients with dementia responded better to methylphenidate than to the tricyclic antidepressant protriptyline. In the second (Kaplitz 1975), methylphenidate was clearly superior to placebo in a double-blind 8-week study, and the methylphenidate group was free of significant side effects. Kaufmann and colleagues (Kaufmann et al. 1982, 1984; Kaufmann 1982) have reported a number of patients with neurologic or medical disease who responded to psychostimulants.

At our hospital, stimulants such as methylphenidate or dextroamphetamine are frequently used to treat medically ill or postoperative elderly patients who are apathetic, withdrawn, or depressed.

Stimulants are also helpful for patients with abulia secondary to frontal lobe disease or in demented patients with coexistent retarded-depressive features. Alternatives to tricyclic antidepressants may be necessary in the treatment of depression in medically ill patients. The development of confusional states secondary to anticholinergic side effects and excessive sedation of some antidepressants have been discussed. As noted above, depressed patients with structurally compromised brain function who are undergoing treatment with tricyclic antidepressants may have a deficit of acetylcholine and therefore may be especially vulnerable to these adverse reactions (Crook and Cohen 1981).

Hackett has described the usefulness of psychostimulants in diagnosing and effectively treating medically ill, apathetic, weakened patients in whom depression might be easily masked by their concomitant illness (Hacket 1978). The rapid improvement in the physical and psychological symptomatology speeds up the recovery, in some cases dramatically. This rapid response to treatment, usually within 24–48 h, is of additional benefit for this type of patient, since concurrent medical illness makes it more of a hazard to wait 10–14 days for the tricyclic antidepressants to become clinically effective.

The therapeutic use of amphetamine and methylphenidate for depression may not be legal in some jurisdictions, and not considered acceptable in others. It is tempting to speculate from previous studies, however, (Forest 1977; Holliday and Joffe 1965; Kaplitz 1975; Myerson 1936; Kayton and Raskind 1980) that there is a wide margin of safety between therapeutic and toxic doses where unwanted physical and psychological side effects may appear. Further well-designed clinical studies are warranted to confirm these observations.

Dextroamphetamine is roughly twice as potent as methylphenidate. Therapeutic effects are usually achieved with daily doses of 20–40 mg methylphenidate or 10–20 mg dextroamphetamine given orally in two divided doses, preferably 30 min before meals (Kaufmann 1982). It is best to administer the last dose before 4 P. M. in order to avoid insomnia. If there is no therapeutic response in 48–72 h, the medication should be discontinued. Occasionally, patients may develop some emotional lability, at which point the dose may be reduced.

The duration of treatment is usually empirical and individualized to the clinical situation (Kaufmann 1982; Kaufmann et al. 1984). For example, if the onset of depressive symptoms is recent, of moderate intensity, and associated with a concurrent medial illness, the stimulant might be needed for only 1–2 weeks. In other cases, if the symptoms are progressing in severity, or if there has been a relapse, treatment may be necessary for a few months.

Although no clinically significant alterations in blood, serum, or urinary parameters occur at therapeutic dosages, during prolonged therapy it is recommended that routine laboratory tests be performed on a regular basis. Vital signs, especially blood pressure, should be monitored in hypertensive patients (Kaufmann 1982).

Psychostimulants may exert their antidepressant effects by blocking reuptake of catecholamines, thus prolonging the effects of synaptically released dopamine and norepinephrine (Brown 1977).

The response to methylphenidate in many patients illustrates three important issues:
a) the quick remission of symptoms following a small dose of stimulant;
b) the lack of toxic side effects and;
c) no recurrence of symptoms after stimulant was discontinued.

Although stimulants are not a panacea, there are specific indications for their short-term use.

Potentiation by Lithium or Thyroid Hormone

As noted earlier, lithium may be a useful adjuvant in tricyclic antidepressant-resistant unipolar depression. DeMontigny and associates (1981) reported that eight such patients (aged 33–64) responded within 48 h after low-dose lithium was added to the tricyclic regimen. In addition, Louie and Meltzer (1984) reported on nine patients who were unresponsive to antidepressants alone who were given lithium carbonate to potentiate the antidepressant. Two of their patients showed sustained improvement, two showed transient improvement but then relapsed, two other cases with bipolar histories became manic, and three did not respond. In their study, the time between lithium addition and improvement of depressive symptoms was frequently longer than that reported by deMontigny et al. and ranged from 2 to 12 days. Kushnir (1986) reported successful lithium augmentation of an antidepressant in five elderly patients (mean age, 81 years; range, 65–93). No significant complications were noted.

L-Triiodothyronine (T_3) has also been reported to potentiate the effect of the tricyclics. Goodwin et al. (1982) reported six women and six men who were treated in a double-blind fashion for major depressive illness which did not respond to imipramine or amitriptyline, 150–300 mg/day during periods ranging from 26 to 112 days. After the addition of T_3, 25 µg/day (ten patients) or 50 µg/day (two patients), nine patients showed statistically significant improvement in depression scores; in eight the response was marked. Improvement generally began within 1–3 days and was noted in all aspects of the depressive syndrome. Side effects were minimal, and T_3 did not change plasma levels of imipramine or desipramine or their ratio but did suppress thyroxine. The work of Goodwin el al. followed earlier uncontrolled reports of T_3 acceleration of response to tricyclic antidepressants; five studies suggested that some depressed patients who were not responsive to tricyclics became responders when T_3 was added (Earle 1970; Ogura et al. 1974; Banki 1975, 1977; Tsutsui et al. 1979).

These adjuvants may be particularly helpful in treatment-resistant patients. Despite the well-established efficacy of tricyclic antidepressant agents (Baldessarini 1977), controlled studies indicate that the rate of nonresponse or partial response is in the range of 20%–35% (Goodwin et al. 1982; Klein and Davis 1969). Goodwin and colleagues went so far in their report as to suggest that a trial of a tricyclic antidepressant in a depressed patient should not be considered a failure until T_3 potentation has been tried.

Cardiac Patients

Physicians probably allow many moderately severe depressions to go untreated because of unwarranted fears about the cardiac side effects of antidepressants. Cassem (1982) reviewed the relevant issues in detail and concluded that when certain precautions are taken, antidepressants can generally be safely used even in very ill cardiac patients. There are four main side effects that are of particular concern in using antidepressant in cardiac patients:
a) orthostatic hypotension,
b) anticholinergic effects,
c) cardiac conduction effects, and
d) decreased cardiac contractility. These will be reviewed individually.

Orthostatic Hypotension. Postural changes in blood pressure occur commonly with antidepressant agents. Tertiary amine tricyclics (amitriptyline, imipramine), with the exception of doxepin (Neshkes et al. 1985), tend to cause more severe hypotensive effects than secondary amines (nortriptyline, desipramine). With tricyclics, the best clinical predictor of drug-induced postural hypotension is the predrug orthostatic fall in blood pressure. Cassem (1982) estimates that in patients with a mean predrug fall in systolic blood pressure of 10 mmHg between lying and standing, the mean orthostatic change on imipramine is about 25 mmHg. It is not known whether such predrug conclusions can be drawn for the newer nontricyclic antidepressants or for the MAOIs. The newer agents such as amoxapine, maprotiline, and trazodone appear to offer no advantage in avoiding orthostatic hypotension (Cassem 1982).

Orthostatic hypotension is one of the primary side effects of MAOIs. It is not felt to be dose dependent and has usually been described as an early side effect, although, as noted earlier, recent data indicate that this may be incorrect. Kronig and associates (1983) studied 14 patients with a mean age of 52 years who were treated with phenelzine and found that the mean orthostatic drop increased with time in a generally linear fashion, with a maximum mean orthostatic drop of 12 mmHg which occurred at week 4. It appears, from their data, that the elderly were no more likely to have severe orthostatic changes than were younger patients; the consequences, however, of a fall in blood pressure in an old person are much more likely to be serious. Lithium therapy is not associated with orthostatic hypotension.

Anticholinergic Effects. For elderly patients, anticholinergic effects are particularly toxic (Snyder and Yamamura 1977; Richelson 1982). The cardiac effect of most concern is tachycardia. In general, tertiary amines are more potent anticholinergic agents than scondary amines, with amitriptyline significantly exceeding all other tricyclics (Cassem 1982). Those cardiac patients with ischemic disease are least able to tolerate an increase in heart rate. Amoxapine and maprotiline offer little improvement over earlier tricyclics in terms of anticholinergic properties. Trazodone, however, has no anticholinergic effects and may be useful in patients at risk from tachycardia. One great advantage of the MAOIs is their essential lack of anticholinergic side effects (Jenike 1984a). No regular changes in cardiac rhythm have been associated with the MAOIs, even in cases of overdose. Lithium also has no anticholinergic effects and does not produce tachycardia (Cassem 1982).

Decreased Contractility. It is a frequent fear that tricyclics may induce congestive heart failure because of their negative ionotropic effect. In reviewing the data, Cassem (1982) noted that most studies employed indirect measurements of cardiac function, such as systolic time intervals, which could have reflected slowing of H-V conduction commonly produced by tricyclics rather than decreased contractility. Veith et al. (1982), using radionuclide ventriculograms to measure ejection fractions before and during maximum exercise in depressed patients with heart disease on therapeutic doses of imipramine and doxepin, demonstrated no adverse effects on left ventricular function. Glassman and colleagues (1983) also studied a group of depressed patients with clinically significant preexisting left ventricular dysfunction by means of radionuclide angiography. Of 15 patients in their study, 13 had ejection fraction values that were more than two standard deviations below normal controls. They found that therapeutic levels of imipramine did not further impair left ventricular performance, and that ejection fraction was unchanged during treatment. There is also no evidence that the newer nontricyclic agents, lithium, or the MAOIs affect cardiac contractility.

Cardiac Conduction Effects. Tricyclics slow conduction in the His bundle and Purkinje fibers, with ECG manifestations including increased PR, QRS, and QTc intervals as well as a decrease in T-wave amplitude (Cassem 1982). This effect appears to be correlated with anticholinergic activity, with trazodone causing the least slowing (Gomoll and Byrne 1979; Hayes et al. 1983). This can exacerbate preexisting ventricular conduction deficits (Rudorfer and Young 1980).

The risk of worsening cardiac arrhythmias with antidepressant therapy has been overemphasized in the past, since imipramine and probably the other tricyclic antidepressants are actually effective antiarrhythmic agents, similar in action to group I agents such as quinidine and procainamide (Giardina et al. 1979). In fact, patients on quinidine or procainamide should be followed carefully, and their antiarrhythmic medication may need to be reduced when a tricyclic antidepressant is added. Studies documenting the antiarrhythmic efficacy of imipramine (Raskind et al. 1982) and nortriptyline (Giardina et al. 1981) can be shared with colleagues who may be reluctant to use antidepressants in patients with arrhythmias.

At one time, it was felt that there was no relationship between the initial PR and QRS intervals and drug-related change after starting imipramine (Giardina et al. 1979). That is, patients with preexisting prolonged PR or QRS interval did not have any greater changes than those with an initially short PR or QRS interval. Recent studies, however, indicate that there may be a slightly increased risk, and that these patients should be followed carefully with serial ECGs (Roose et al. 1987).

Clinical problems associated with slowed conduction are rare. Giardina et al. (1979) found that none of 14 patients with conduction abnormalities developed second-degree heart block. Of the 14 patients, five had first-degree heart block, and five had right bundle-branch block. Of those patients who overdose on tricyclics, only 6%–20% develop significant clinical problems with conduction abnormalities (Biggs et al. 1977; Callahan 1979).

It has been demonstrated that increases in PR and QRS intervals are directly related to tricyclic plasma levels (Giardina et al. 1979), and ECGs can provide a reliable guide to the cardiac effects of the tricyclic as dose is increased. In cases of severe conduction abnormalities, such as sick sinus syndrome, Cassem (1982) recommends pacemaker protection from complete heart block.

There are case reports that both amoxapine and maprotiline have been associated with arrhythmias (Cassem 1982; Zavodnick 1981). Trazodone is generally free of clinical conduction problems in healthy individuals but has been associated with arrhythmias in patients with preexisting cardiac illness. There are no consistent changes in cardiac rhythm associated with the MAOIs, even in cases of overdosage (Cassem 1982).

Lithium regularly produces T-wave flattening in the ECGs of about 50% of patients with drug levels over 0.5 mmol/l (Jefferson and Greist 1977). These changes may be secondary to altered ionic equilibrium with intracellular hypokalemia; serum potassium is normal in these cases. Toxic cardiac effects are uncommon, but reversible sinus node abnormalities and other conduction disturbances have been reported (Wellens et al. 1975; Wilson et al. 1976; Jaffe 1977). Cassem (1982) recommends that patients with preexisting cardiac conduction abnormalities be given continuous cardiac monitoring during the initiation of lithium therapy.

Patients with heart disease can generally be managed on antidepressant medication. All elderly patients with heart disease should be followed with occasional ECGs. Inquiry about cardiac symptoms such as ankle edema, dyspnea on exertion, orthopnea, and paroxysmal nocturnal dyspnea should be done at each visit. The patients should be examined for rales and the presence of changing heart sounds.

Electroconvulsive Therapy

Electroconvulsive therapy (ECT) is a commonly used and effective modality for treating depressed elderly patients who are refractory to medication, or who require rapid resolution of depressive symptoms. ECT, as practiced today, is the electrical induction of a series of grand mal seizures, usually from six to ten, in patients with susceptible psychiatric disorders, primarily severe depression. The seizure itself, rather than the electrical stimulus, is the therapeutic agent. The technique of ECT has been refined over the past few decades, and today the use of anticholinergic premedication, short-acting barbiturates for anesthesia, muscle relaxants, oxygenation, low-energy stimulus wave forms, and unilateral stimulus electrode placement have all acted to decrease the risks and side effects without diminishing its therapeutic efficacy (Jenike 1984b; Weiner 1982).

ECT may be the only choice of treatment in the elderly depressed patient whose illness is accompanied by self-destructive behavior, such as suicide attempts or refusal to eat. In these cases, a drug trial lasting 4–6 weeks may be associated with significant risk. In these patients, ECT, which characteristically begins to exert beneficial effects within the 1st week, may be life saving.

Depression is common in all age groups, but ECT is used to a greater extent in the elderly since depression is more likely to be severe in the older patient, and also because the elderly are more likely to suffer from concurrent chronic diseases for which antidepressant drugs may be less desirable due to their anticholinergic, cardiotoxic, and hypotensive effects (Weiner 1982).

ECT is both more effective and faster acting than drugs in the treatment of depression, and many depressed elderly patients, especially those with psychotic symptoms, who do not respond to drugs do respond to ECT. In one study, for example, remission occurred in 80%–85% of drug nonresponders (Scovern and Kilmann 1980). ECT has consistently outperformed tricyclic antidepressants and MAOIs, with 10%–20% more patients showing improvement. Not only is ECT more effective than pharmacologic agents, but it may be safer for those patients with serious illness, particularly that involving cardiac dysfunction.

The mortality rate with the use of ECT has been estimated at around one in 10 000 patients, which is probably considerably less than that associated with any of the drugs indicated in the treatment of depression (Fink 1979; Weiner 1982). Clinically, ECT is commonly associated with confusion and temporary amnesia, and physiologically, by slowing on EEG. Even though some patients complain of mild memory loss for months or even years after receiving ECT, objective memory testing in such cases does not appear to bear out the presence of an organic defect. No studies have documented any significant pathologic changes in the brain (Weiner 1982). Most ECT patients do not consider themselves affected by persistent memory deficits, and they tend to view their treatments as no more upsetting than a visit to the dentist (Hughes et al. 1981).

In ECT therapy, it is the electrical stimulus, not the seizure itself, that is the component most responsible for the side effects of confusion and transient loss of memory. A recent study involving 29 patients (mean age, 73 years) showed that electrical stimuli given only over the nondominant hemisphere produced therapeutic results comparable to bilateral stimulation (Fraser and Glass 1978, 1980). The degree of postictal confusion, however, was much greater for those receiving bilateral ECT, indicating that the acute cerebral impairment was less in those patients who received unilateral, nondominant stimulation.

Even though there are really no absolute contraindications to ECT, there are certain conditions in which a marked increase in associated morbidity and mortality may be seen (American Psychiatric Association Task Force 1978; Fink 1979). These include recent myocardial infarction or stroke, severe hypertension, and the presence of an intracerebral mass. In these patients, ECT should generally be delayed until effective medical management has been initiated, or until adequate recovery time has elapsed. If ECT is urgently indicated, however, appropriate premedication and close monitoring can help to minimize the risk.

Summary

Depression is a common debilitating and often life-threatening illness in the elderly and dementing patient. Diagnosis and medical asessment have been reviewed. Tertiary amines, such as imipramine and amitriptyline (with the exception of doxepin), cause significant orthostatic hypotension and probably should be avoided as agents of first choice in the elderly. Amitriptyline is also extremely anticholinergic and is best avoided. Amoxapine is essentially a neuroleptic with antidepressant properties and may induce neurologic sequelae, including tardive dyskinesia.

If a patient has had a prior positive response, or if he has a relative who had a good outcome from a particular drug, it may be best to begin treatment with this drug. The initial choice of antidepressant can be based largely on the clinical picture. For example, if a depressed patient is sleeping much more than usual and requires an activating agent, desipramine, fluoxetine, or protriptyline are good drugs to try initially. If, on the other hand, the patient is unable to sleep, a more sedating agent such as nortriptyline or trazodone should be given. Risks and side effects, as well as use in cardiac patients, are reviewed in detail.

Many clinicians avoid the use of MAOIs in the elderly patient because of fears of adverse reactions. Precautions, side effects, and specific recommendations are outlined.

Using lithium in the elderly requires special precautions because of decreased GFR and potential interactions with concomitantly used drugs. Side effects and toxicity are discussed.

The use of psychostimulants, such as methylphenidate and amphetamine, to treat medically ill depressed patients is reviewed. These agents are also sometimes useful in demented individuals or in patients with abulic frontal lobe syndromes.

Poststroke depressions are common and recent evidence indicates that they can be adequately treated. Stroke patients have many difficulties dealing with issues of rehabilitation and should not be forced to suffer concomitant depression when we have the tools at hand to treat such symptoms effectively.

Recent data on the potentiation of antidepressant effects by lithium or T_3 indicate that they may possibly be useful in some heterocyclic-resistant patients.

Risks, side effects, and recent procedural advances in the use of ECT are reviewed. ECT is both more effective and faster acting than drugs in the treatment of depression, and many depressed elderly patients, especially those with psychotic symptoms, do not respond to drugs but improve dramatically with ECT.

References

Abrams JH, Schulman P, White WB (1985) Successful treatment of a monoamine oxidase inhibitor – tyramine hypertensive emergency with intravenous labetalol. N Engl J Med 313: 52

Adams RD, Victor M (eds) (1981) Principles of neurology. McGraw-Hill, New York

Agnoli A, Martucci N, Manna L et al. (1983) Effect of cholinergic and anticholinergic drugs on short-term memory in Alzheimer's dementia: a neuropsychological and computerized electroencephalographic study. Clin Neuropharmacol 6: 311–323

Andersen J, Aabro E, Gulmann N et al. (1980) Antidepressive treatment of Parkinson's disease. Acta Neurol Scand 62: 210–219

Angst J, Baastrup P, Grof P et al. (1973) The course of monopolar depression and bipolar psychoses. Psychiatr Neurol Neurochir 76: 489–500

Anonymous (1979) Psychiatric illness among medical patients. Lancet 1: 479

American Psychiatric Association Task Force (1978) Electroconvulsive therapy. American Psychiatric Association Task Force on ECT. Task force report no 14. American Psychiatric Association, Washington DC

Ashford W, Ford CV (1979) Use of MAO inhibitors in elderly patients. Am J Psychiatry 136: 1466

Asnis G (1977) Parkinson's disease, depression and ECT: a review and case study. Am J Psychiatry 134: 191–195

Avery D, Winokur G (1976) Mortality in depressed patients treated with electroconvulsive therapy and antidepressants. Arch Gen Psychiatry 33: 1029–1937

Baldessarini RJ (1977) Chemotherapy in psychiatry. Harvard University Press, Cambridge MA

Banki CM (1975) Triiodothyronine in the treatment of depression. Orv Hetil 116: 2543–2546

Barton JL (1982) Amoxapine-induced agitation among bipolar depressed patients. Am J Psychiatry 139: 387

Bartus RT, Dean RL, Beer R et al. (1982) The cholinergic hypothesis of geriatric memory dysfunction. Science 217: 408–416

Biggs JT, Spiker DG, Petit JM et al. (1977) Tricyclic antidepressant overdose. JAMA 238: 135–138

Blume JE, Tross S (1980) Psychodynamic treatment of the elderly: a review of issues in theory and practice. In: Eisdorfer D (ed) Annual Review of Gerontology and Geriatrics, Vol 1, Springer Publishing, New York

Breslow R, Kocsis J, Belkin B (1980) Memory deficits in depression: evidence using the Wechsler Memory Scale. Percept Mot Skills 51: 541–542

Brothers CRD, Meadows AW (1955) An investigation of Huntington's chorea in Victoria. Ment Sci 101: 548–563

Brown WA (1977) Psychologic and neuroendocrine responses to methylphenidate. Arch Gen Psychiatry 34: 1103–1108

Burnside IM (1978) Principles from Yalom. In: Burnside IM (ed) Working with the Elderly: Group Process and Techniques. Duxbury Press, North Scituate MA

Busse EW, Pfeiffer E (1977) Behavior and adaptation in late life, 2nd edn. Little Brown, Boston

Butler RN (1960) Intensive psychotherapy for the hospitalized aged. Geriatrics 15: 644

Butler RN (1968) Toward a psychiatry of the life-cycle: implications of sociopsychologic studies of the aging process for the psychotherapeutic situation. Psychiatr Res Reports 23: 233

Butler RN (1975) Psychotherapy in old age: In: Arieti S (ed) American handbook of psychiatry, 2nd edn, vol 5. Basic Books, New York

Byrne DC (1977) Affect and vigilance performance in depressive illness. J Psychiatr Res 13: 185–191

Caine ED (1986) The neuropsychology of depression: The pseudodementia syndrome. In: Grant I, Adams KM (eds) Neuropsychological assessment of neuropsychiatric disorders. Oxford, New York, pp 221–243

Caine ED, Shoulson I (1983) Psychiatric syndromes in Huntington's disease. Am J Psychiatry 140: 728–733

Callahan M (1979) Tricyclic antidepressant overdose. JACEP 8: 413–425

Cassem NH (1982) Cardiovascular effects of antidepressants. J Clin Psychiatry 43: (11/2): 22–28

Celesia GG, Wanamaker WM (1972) Psychiatric disturbances in Parkinson's disease. Dis Nerv Syst 33: 577–583

Cohen RM, Weingartner H, Smallberg SA et al. (1982) Effort and cognition in depression. Arch Gen Psychiatry 39: 593–597

Cole JO, Branconnier R, Solomon M et al. (1983) Tricyclic use in the cognitively impaired elderly. J Clin Psychiatry Sept (sec 2): 14–19

Cronholm G, Ottosson J (1961) Memory functions in endogenous depression. Arch Gen Psychiatry 5: 193–197

Crook T, Cohen GD (eds) (1981) Physicians' handbook on psychotherapeutic drug use in the aged. Powley, New Canaan CT

Cross AJ, Crow TJ, Perry EK et al. (1981) Reduced dopamine beta-hydroxylase activity in Alzheimer's disease. Br Med J 282: 93–94

Cummings JL (1988) Intellectual impairment in Parkinson's disease: clinical, pathologic, and biochemical correlates. J Geriatr Psychiatry Neurol 1: 24–36

Cummings JL, Benson DR (1988) Psychological dysfunction accompanying subcortical dementias. Annu Rev Med 39: 53–61

Cummings JL, Miller BL, Hill M et al. (1987) Neuropsychiatric aspects of multi-infarct dementia and dementia of the Alzheimer type. Arch Neurol 44: 389–393

Davidson J, White H (1983) The effect of isocarboxazid on platelet MAO activity. Biol Psychiatry 18: 1075–1079

Davies P (1979) Neurotransmitter-related enzymes in senile dementia of the Alzheimer type. Brain Res 171: 319–327

Davis KL, Mohs RC, Tinklenberg JR et al. (1978) Physostigmine: improvement of long-term memory processes in normal humans. Sciene 201: 272–274

deMontigny C, Grunberg F, Mayer A et al. (1981) Lithium induces rapid relief of depression in tricyclic antidepressant drug non-responders. Br J Psychiatry 138: 252–256

Dominquez RA (1983) Evaluating the effectiveness of the new antidepressants. Hosp Community Psychiatry 34: 405–407

Drachman DA, Leavitt J (1974) Human memory and the cholinergic system. Arch Neurol 30: 113–121

Drachman DA, Sahakian BJ (1980) Memory and cognitive function in the elderly: a preliminary trial of physostigmine. Arch Neurol 37: 674–675

Dunner DL, Roose SP, Bone S (1979) Complications of lithium treatment in older patients. In: Gershon S, Kline NS, Shou M (eds) Lithium controversies and unresolved issues. Excerpta Medica, Amsterdam, pp 427–431

Earle BV (1970) Thyroid hormone and tricyclic antidepressants in resistant depressions. Am J Psychiatry 126: 1667–1669

Endicott J, Spitzer RL (1978) A diagnostic interview: the schedule for affective disorders and schizophrenia. Arch Gen Psychiatry 35: 837–844

Feinberg T, Goodman B (1984) Affective illness, dementia, and pseudodementia. J Clin Psychiatry 45: 99–103

Fink M (1979) Convulsive therapy: theory and practice. Raven, New York

Forest WH (1977) Dextroamphetamine with morphine for the treatment of postoperative pain. N Engl J Med 296: 712–715

Foster JR, Rosenthal JS (1980) Lithium treatment of the elderly. In: Johnson FN (ed) Handbook of lithium therapy. MTP Press, Lancaster England, pp 414–420

Francis PT, Palmer AM, Sims NR et al. (1985) Neurochemical studies of early-onset Alzheimer's disease: possible influence of treatment. N Engl J Med 313: 7–11

Fraser RM, Glass IB (1978) Recovery from ECT in elderly patients. Br J Psychiatry 33: 524

Fraser RM, Glass IB (1980) Unilateral and bilateral ECT in elderly patients. Acta Psychiatr Scand 62: 13

Giardina E-GV, Bigger JT, Glassman AH et al. (1979) The electrocardiographic and antiarrhythmic effects of imipramine hydrochloride at therapeutic plasma concentrations. Circulation 60: 1045–1052

Giardina EGV, Bigger JT, Johnson LL (1981) The effect of imipramine and nortriptyline on ventricular premature depolarizations and left ventricular function. Circulation 64: 316

Glassman AH, Johnson LL, Giardina EGV et al. (1983) The use of imipramine in depressed patients with congestive heart failure. JAMA 250: 1997–2001

Gomoll AW, Byrne JE (1979) Trazodone and imipramine: comparative effects on canine cardiac conduction. Eur J Pharmacol 57: 335–342

Goodman LS, Gilman A (eds) (1975) The pharmacological basis of therapeutics. MacMillan, Publishing Co, New York

Goodwin FK, Prange AJ, Post RM et al. (1982) Potentiation of antidepressant effects of L-triiodothyronine in tricyclic nonresponders. Am J Psychiatry 139: 34–38

Grayson DA, Henderson AS, Kay DWK (1987) Diagnoses of dementia and depression: a latent trait analysis of their performance. Psychol Med 17: 667–675

Grotjahn M (1955) Analytic psychotherapy with the elderly. Psychoanal Rev 42: 419

Gurland BJ (1976) The comparative frequency of depression in various adult age groups. J Gerontol 31: 283–292

Hackett TP (1978) The use of stimulant drugs in general hospital psychiatry. tape, vol 7 (12). Audio-Digest Foundation, Glendale CA

Hamilton M (1960) A rating scale for depression. J Neurol Neurosurg Psychiatry 23: 56–62

Hayes RL, Gerner RH, Fairbanks L et al. (1983) EKG findings in geriatric depressives given trazodone, placebo or imipramine. J Clin Psychiatry 44: 180–183

Henry A, Weingartner H, Murphy DL (1973) Influence of affective states and psychoactive drugs on verbal learning and memory. Am J Psychiatry 130: 966–971

Himmelhoch JM (1981) Cardiovascular effects of trazodone in humans. J Clin Psychopharmacol 1(65): 765–815

Himmelhoch JM, Neil JF, May SJ et al. (1980) Age, dementia, dyskinesias, and lithium response. Am J Psychiatry 137: 941–945

Hirschowitz RG (1973) Foster grandparents program: preventive intervention with the elderly poor. Hosp Comm Psychiatry 24: 418–420

Holliday AR, Joffe JR (1965) A controlled evaluation of protriptyline compared to placebo and to methylphenidate hydrochloride. J New Drugs 5: 257

Horn (1974) The psychological factors in parkinsonism. J Neurol Neurosurg Psychiatry 37: 27–31

Hughes J, Barraclough BM, Reeve W (1981) Are patients shocked by ECT? JR Soc Med 74: 283

Jaffe CM (1977) First-degree atrioventricular block during lithium carbonate treatment. Am J Psychiatry 134: 88–89

Jefferson JW (1983) Lithium and affective disorder in the elderly. Compr Psychiatry 24: 166–178

Jefferson JW, Greist JH (1977) Primer of lithium therapy. Williams and Wilkins, Baltimore

Jefferson JW, Marshall JR (1981) Neuropsychiatric features of medical disorders. Plenum, New York

Jenike MA (1983a) Tardive dyskinesia: special risk in the elderly. J Am Geriatr Soc 31: 71–73

Jenike MA (1983b) Alcohol and antihistamines not contraindicated with MAOIs? Am J Psychiatry 140: 1107

Jenike MA (1984a) The use of monoamine oxidase inhibitors in elderly depressed patients. J Am Geriatr Soc 32: 571–575

Jenike MA (1984b) Electroconvulsive therapy: what are the facts? Geriatrics 38: 33–38

Jenike MA (1985a) Handbook of geriatric psychopharmacology. PSG, Littleton MA

Jenike MA (1985b) MAO inhibitors as treatment for depressed patients with primary degenerative dementia (Alzheimer's disease) Am J Psychiatry 142: 763–764

Jenike MA (1986a) Alzheimer's disease: clinical management. Psychosomatics 27: 407–416

Jenike MA (1986b) Alzheimer's disease. Sci Am Med 9: 1–4

Jenike MA (1988a) Alzheimer's disease – what the practicing clinician needs to know. J Geriatr Psychiatry Neurol 1: 37–46

Jenike MA (1988b) Assessment and treatment of affective illness in the elderly. J Geriatr Psychiatry Neurol 1: 89–107

Jenike MA (1988c) Depression and other psychiatric disorders. In: Albert MS, Moss M (eds) Geriatric neuropsychology. Guildford, New York, pp 115–144

Jenike MA, Albert MS (1984) The dexamethasone suppression test in patients with presenile and senile dementia of the Alzheimer's type. J Am Geriatr Soc 32: 441–444

Judd LL, Hubbard B, Janowsky DS et al. (1977) The effect of lithium carbonate on the cognitive functions of normal subjects. Arch Gen Psychiatry 34: 355–357

Kahn RL (1975) The mental health system and the future aged. Gerontologist 15(1/II): 24–31

Kaplitz SE (1975) Withdrawn, apathetic geriatric patients responsive to methylphenidate. J Am Geriatr Soc 23: 271–276

Kaufmann MW (1982) Use of methylphenidate in the elderly. Top Geriatr 1: 3–4

Kaufmann MW, Murray GB, Cassem NH (1982) Use of psychostimulants in medically ill depressed patients. Psychosomatics 23: 817–819

Kaufmann MW, Cassem NH, Murray GB et al. (1984) Use of psychostimulants in medically ill patients with neurological disease and major depression. Can J Psychiatry 29: 46–49

Kay DWK, Bergman K (1966) Physical disability and mental health in old age. J Psychosom Res 10: 3–12

Kayton W, Raskind M (1980) Treatment of depression in the medically ill elderly with methylphenidate. Am J Psychiatry 137: 963–965

Klein DF, Davis JM (1969) Diagnosis and drug treatment of psychiatric disorders. Williams and Wilkins, Baltimore

Knesevich JW, Martin RL, Berg L et al. (1983) Preliminary report on affective symptoms in the early stages of senile dementia of the Alzheimer type. Am J Psychiatry 140: 233–235

Kral VA (1983) The relationship between senile dementia (Alzheimer type) and depression. Can J Psychiatry 28: 304–306

Krauthammer C, Klerman GL (1978) Secondary mania. Arch Gen Psychiatry 35: 1333–1339

Kronig MH, Roose SP, Walsh BT et al. (1983) Blood pressure effects of phenelzine. J Clin Psychopharmacol 3: 307

Kushnir SL (1986) Lithium-antidepressant combinations in the treatment of depressed, physically ill geriatric patients. Am J Psychiatry 143: 378–379

Lago D, Connell CM, Knight B (1983) Initial evaluation of PACT (People and Animals Coming Together): a companion animal program for community-dwelling older persons: In: Smyer M, Gatz M (eds) Mental health and aging: programs and evaluations. Sage, Beverly Hills CA

Laitinen L (1969) Desipramine in treatment of Parkinson's disease. Acta Neurol Scand 45: 109–113

Lapierre YD, Anderson K (1983) Dyskinesia associated with amoxapine antidepressant therapy: a case report. Am J Psychiatry 140: 493–494

Lazarus LW, Newton N, Cohle RB et al. (1987) Frequency and presentation of depressive symptoms in patients with primary degenerative dementia. Am J Psychiatry 144: 41–45

Lebensohn Z, Jenkins RB (1975) Improvement of parkinsonism in depressed patients treated with ECT. Am J Psychiatry 132: 283–285

Linden ME (1957) The promise of therapy in the emotional problems of aging. Paper presented at the fourth congress of the International Association of Gerontology, July, Merano, Italy

Lipsey JR, Pearlson GD, Robinson RG et al. (1984) Nortriptyline treatment of poststroke depression: a double-blind study. Lancet 1: 297–300

Lipsey JR, Spencer WC, Rabins PV et al. (1986) Phenomenological comparison of poststroke depression and functional depression. Am J Psychiatry 143: 527–529

Liptzin B (1984) Treatment of mania. In: Salzman C (ed) Clinical geriatric psychopharmacology. McGraw-Hill, New York, pp 116–13

Liston EH (1978) Diagnostic delay in presenile dementia. J Clin Psychiatry 39: 599–603

Louie AK, Meltzer HY (1984) Lithium potentiation of antidepressant treatment. J Clin Psychopharmacol 4: 316–321

Lydiard RB, Gelenberg AJ (1981) Amoxapine: an antidepressant with some neuroleptic properties? Pharmacotherapy 1: 163–175

Makeeva VL, Gol'davskach IL, Pozdnyakova SL (1974) Somatic changes and side effects from the use of lithium salts in the prevention of affective disorders. Zh Nevropatol Psikhiatr 74: 602–607

Mayeux R (1982) Depression and dementia in Parkinson's disease. In: Marsden CC, Fahn S (eds) Movement disorders. Butterworth, London, pp 75–95

Mayeux R, Stern Y, Rosen J et al. (1981) Depression, intellectual impairment, and Parkinson's disease. Neurology 31: 645–650

McHugh PR, Folstein MF (1975) Psychiatric syndromes of Huntington's chorea: a clinical and phenomenologic study. In: Benson DF, Blumer D (eds) Psychiatric aspects of neurologic disease. Grune and Stratton, New York, pp 267–286

Merriam AE, Aronson MK, Gaston P et al. (1988) The psychiatric symptoms of Alzheimer's disease. J Am Geriatr Soc 36: 7–12

Meyer D, Halfin V (1981) Toxicity secondary to meperidine in patients on monoamine oxidase inhibitors: a case report and critical review. J Clin Psychopharmacol 1: 319

Mielke DH (1976) Adverse reactions to thymoleptics. In: Gallant DM, Simpson GM (eds) Depression: behavioral, biochemical, diagnostic and treatment concepts. Spectrum, Holliswood NY

Miller NE (1980) The measurement of mood in senile brain disease: examiner ratings and self reports. In: Cole JO, Barrett JE (eds) Psychopathology in the aged. Raven, New York

Mitchell RS (1955) Fatal toxic encephalitis occurring during iproniazid therapy and pulmonary tuberculosis. Ann Intern Med 42: 417

Mjones H (1949) Paralysis agitans. Acta Psychiatr Neurol 54 (Supp 1): 1–195

Moffie HS, Paykel ES (1975) Depression in medical inpatients. Br J Psychiatry 126: 346–353

Mulligan MA, Bennett R (1977–1978) Assessment of mental health and social problems during multiple friendly visits: the development and evaluation of a friendly visiting program for the isolated elderly. Int J Aging Hum Dev 8: 43–65

Murphy JE, Ankier SI (1980) An evaluation of trazodone in the treatment of depression. Neuropharmacology 19: 1217–1218

Myerson A (1936) The effect of benzadrine on fatigue in normal and neurotic persons. AMA Arch Neurol Psychiatry 36: 816–822

Neil JF, Licata SM, May SJ et al. (1979) Dietary noncompliance during treatment with tranylcypromine. J Clin Psychiatry 40: 33–37

Neshkes RE, Gerner R, Jarvik LE et al. (1985) Orthostatic effect of imipramine and doxepin in depressed geriatric outpatients. J Clin Psychopharmacol 5: 102–106

Newton R (1981) The side effect profile of trazodone in comparison to an active control and placebo. J Clin Psychopharmacol 1(65): 895–935

Ogura C, Okuma T, Uchida Y et al. (1974) Combined thyroid (triiodothyronine) tricyclic antidepressant treatment in depressive states. Folia Psychiatr Neurol Jpn 28: 179–186

Papp C, Benaim S (1958) Toxic effects of iproniazid in a patient with angina. Br Med J 2: 1070

Patrick HT, Levy DM (1922) Parkinson's disease: a clinical study of 146 cases. Arch Neurol Psychiatry 7: 711–720

Perry EK, Tomlinson BE, Blessed G et al. (1978) Correlation of cholinergic abnormalities with senile plaques and mental test scores in senile dementia. Br Med J 2: 1457–1459

Quitkin FM, Rabkin JG, Ross D et al. (1984) Duration of antidepressant drug treatment. Arch Gen Psychiatry 41: 238–245

Raft D, Newman M, Spencer R (1972) Suicide on L-dopa. South Med J 65: 312

Raskin A, Friedman AS, DiMascio A (1982) Cognitive and performance deficits in depression. Psychopharmacol Bull 18: 196–202

Raskind M, Veith R, Barnes R et al. (1982) Cardiovascular and antidepressant effects of imipramine in the treatment of secondary depression in patients with ischemic heart disease. Am J Psychiatry 139: 1114–1117

Reding M, Haycox J, Blass J (1985) Depression in patients referred to a dementia clinic: a three-year prospective study. Arch Neurol 42: 894–896

Reding MJ, Orto LA, Winter SW et al. (1986) Antidepressant therapy after stroke: a double-blind trial. Arch Neurol 43: 763–765

Reed E, Chandler JR (1958) Huntington's chorea in Michigan. I. Demography and genetics. Am J Hum Genet 10: 201–225

Reimann IW, Frolich JC (1981) Effects of diclofenac on lithium kinetics. Clin Pharmacol Ther 30: 348–352

Richelson E (1982) Pharmacology of antidepressants in use in the United States. J Clin Psychiatry 43(11/2): 4–11

Robinson DS, Nies A, Revaris CL et al. (1978) Clinical pharmacology of phenelzine. Arch Gen Psychiatry 35: 629

Robinson RG (1981) Depression in aphasic patients: frequency, severity, and clinicopathological correlations. Brain Lang 14: 282–291

Robinson RG, Szetela B (1981) Mood change following left hemisphere brain injury. Ann Neurol 9: 447–453

Robinson RG, Kubos KL, Starr LB et al. (1983) Mood changes in stroke patients: relationship to lesion location. Compr Psychiatry 24: 555–566

Robinson RG, Starr LB, Price TR (1984) A two year longitudinal study of mood disorders following stroke: prevalence and duration at six months follow-up. Br J Psychiatry 144: 256–262

Ron MA, Toone BK, Garraida ME et al. (1979) Diagnostic accuracy in presenile dementia. Br J Psychiatry 134: 161–168

Roose SP, Glassman AG, Giardina EGV et al. (1987) Tricyclic antidepressants in depressed patients with cardiac conduction disease. Arch Gen Psychiatry 44: 273–275

Roth M (1955) The natural history of mental disorder in old age. J Ment Sci 101: 281–301

Rowe JW, Andres R, Tobin JD et al. (1976) The effect of age on creatinine clearancc in mcn: a cross-sectional and longitudinal study. J Gerontol 31: 155–163

Rudorfer MV, Young RC (1980) Desipramine: cardiovascular effects and plasma levels. Am J Psychiatry 137: 984–986

Saltz R (1977) Foster grandparenting: a unique child-care service. In: Troll LE, Israel J, Israel K (eds) Looking adhead: a woman's guide to the problems and joys of growing older. Prentice-Hall, Englewood Cliffs

Salzman C (1982) A primer on geriatric psychopharmacology. Am J Psychiatry 139: 67–76

Schoenfeld M, Myers RG, Cupples LA et al. (1984) Increased rate of suicide among patients with Huntington's disease. J Neurol Neurosurg Psychiatry 47: 1283–1287

Scovern AW, Kilmann PR (1980) Status of ECT: a review of the outcome literature. Psychol Bull 87: 260

Sendbuehler J, Goldstein S (1977) Attempted suicide among the aged. J Am Geriatr Soc 25: 245–248

Shamoian CA (ed) (1985) Treatment of affective disorders in the elderly. American Psychiatric Association, Washington DC

Sherman E (1981) Counseling the aging: an integrative approach. Free Press, New York

Shuttleworth EC, Huber SJ, Paulson GW (1987) Depression in patients with dementia of Alzheimer type. J Nat Med Assoc 79: 733–736

Silberman EK (1981) Heterogeneity of amphetamine response in depressed patients. Am J Psychiatry 138: 1302–1306

Silberman EK, Weingartner H, Post RM (1983) Thinking disorder in depression. Arch Gen Psychiatry 40: 775–780

Snyder SH, Yamamura HI (1977) Antidepressants and the muscarinic acetylcholine receptor. Arch Gen Psychiatry 34: 236–239

Spar JE, LaRue A (1983) Major depression in the elderly: DSM III criteria and the dexamethasone suppression test as predictors of treatment response. Am J Psychiatry 140: 844–847

Sternberg DE, Jarvik ME (1976) Memory functions in depression. Arch Gen Psychiatry 33: 219–224

Steuer J (1982) Psychotherapy for depressed elders. In: Blazer DG (ed) Depression in late life. Mosby, St Louis

Strang RR (1965) Imipramine in treatment of parkinsonism: a double-blind placebo study. Br J Med 2: 33–34

Task Force (1985) Task Force on the Use of laboratory Test in Psychiatry. Tricyclic antidepressants – blood level measurements and clinical outcome. Am J Psychiatry 142: 142–149

Terry RD, Davies P (1980) Dementia of the Alzheimer type. Annu Rev Neurosci 3: 77–95

Tsuang MT, Woolson RF, Fleming JA (1980) Premature deaths in schizophrenia and affective disorders. Arch Gen Psychiatry 37: 979–983

Tsutsui S, Yamazaki Y, Namba T et al. (1979) Combined therapy of T and antidepressants in depression. J Intern Med Res 7: 138–146

Vandenbos GR, Stapp J, Kilburg RR (1981) Health service providers in psychology: results of the 1978 APA Human Resources Survey. Am Psychol 36: 1395–1418

Veith RC, Raskind MA, Caldwell JH et al. (1982) Cardiovascular effects of tricyclic antidepressants. N Engl J Med 306: 954–959

Warburton JW (1967) Depressive symptoms in parkinsonian patients referred for thalamotomy. J Neurol Neurosurg Psychiatry 30: 368–370

Weiner RD (1982) The role of electroconvulsive therapy in the treatment of depression in the elderly. J Am Geriatr Soc 30: 710–712

Weingartner H, Cohen RM, Murphy DL et al. (1981) Cognitive processes in depression. Arch Gen Psychiatry 38: 42–47

Wellens H, Cats B, Durren D (1975) Symptomatic sinus node abnormalities following lithium carbonate therapy. Am J Med 59: 285–287

Wells BG, Gelenberg AJ (1981) Chemistry, pharmacology, pharmacokinetics, adverse effects and efficacy of the antidepressant maprotiline hydrochloride. Pharmacotherapy 1: 121–139

Wells CE (1963) Pseudodementia. Am J Psychiatry 120: 244–249

Wells CE (1979) Pseudodementia. Am J Psychiatry 136: 895–900

White K, MacDonald N, Razani J et al. (1983) Platelet MAO activity in depression. Compr Psychiatry 24: 453–458

Wilson J, Kraus E, Bailas M et al. (1976) Reversible sinus node abnormalities due to lithium carbonate therapy. N Engl J Med 294: 1223–1224

Wolf PA, Dawber TR, Thomas HE et al. (1977) Epidemiology of stroke. In: Thompson RA, Green JR (eds) Advances in neurology. Raven, New York, pp 5–19

Woods SW, Tesar GE, Murray GB et al. (1986) Psychostimulant treatment of depressive disorders secondary to medical illness. J Clin Psychiatry 47: 12–15

Yudofsky SC (1979) Parkinson's disease, depression, and electroconvulsive therapy: a clinical and neurobiologic synthesis. Compr Psychiatry 20: 579–581

Zavodnick S (1981) Atrial flutter with amoxapine: a case report. Am J Psychiatry 138: 1503–1504

*Psychological Assessment
of Aging and Dementia*

Psychological and Cognitive Factors in Psychogeriatric Memory Assessment

L. W. Poon

Introduction

Decline in intellectual and cognitive functioning is the hallmark of senile dementia. Most notably, memory decline has been identified as the most prominent deficit and could be the only apparent cognitive deficit in the early stages of senile dementia (DSM III, American Psychiatric Association, 1980).

Although there are numerous standardized memory test batteries in the market place, there is unfortunately no general concensus among researchers and clinicians on which battery is most appropriate in diagnosing memory and cognitive dysfunction with the elderly (Erickson et al. 1980). For example, the often used Wechsler Memory Scale has been criticized for having limited predictive power for detecting specific deficits; it has been criticized for lacking a measure for long-term retention, for not differentiating modality-specific memory funcitons, and for not being validated for the elderly population (Erickson and Scott 1977; Erickson et al. 1980). The Randt Memory Test (Randt et al. 1980) was found lacking in the measurement of nonverbal memory, and the Guild Memory Test (Gilbert et al. 1971) was found by some clinicians to be too complex for people with more than a mild deficit. The problem of test sensitivity and specificity is illustrated by the common complaints among clinicians that the results of some memory tests bear no resemblance to the everyday memory functioning and complaints of the patients.

Given the litany of criticisms and complaints of existing tests and confusion in test selection and data interpretation, this chapter reviews current findings in memory changes in normal aging and provides answers to three sets of frequently asked questions:
1. Why is memory so difficult to assess in early stages of dysfunction for elderly patients?
2. What are the basic ingredients pertinent to memory assessment that could be used as criteria for test selection?
3. Are some tests better than others? How many tests are sufficient to evaluate all of the basic factors in cognition and memory? Is there an easily administered and efficient test that can provide a comprehensive test of memory and cognition?

Bergener, Reisberg (Eds.)
Diagnosis and Treatment
of Senile Dementia
© Springer-Verlag Berlin Heidelberg 1989

Table 1. Evidence for age-related declines in memory capacity

Type of study and type of evidence	Memory store				
	Sensory	Primary	Secondary	Working	Tertiary
Cross-Sectional studies					
Anecdotal	–	Positive	Positive	Positive	Positive
Psychometric	–	Negative	Positive	–	Negative
Experimental	Positive	Negative	Positive	Positive	Negative
Longitudinal studies					
Anecdotal	–	–	–	–	–
Psychometric	–	Negative	Positive	–	Negative
Experimental	–	–	Positive	–	–

From Fozard (1980) and Poon (1985)

Why Is Memory so Difficult To Assess in Early States of Dysfunction?

Memory and Aging Research

The study of memory and aging has a long and distinguished tradition. Surveys of published literature in psychological sections of gerontological journals have shown that 68% of the papers published in the period 1963–1968 were on memory and aging, 72% in 1964–1974, and 58% in 1979–1980 (Poon 1985). Research on memory and

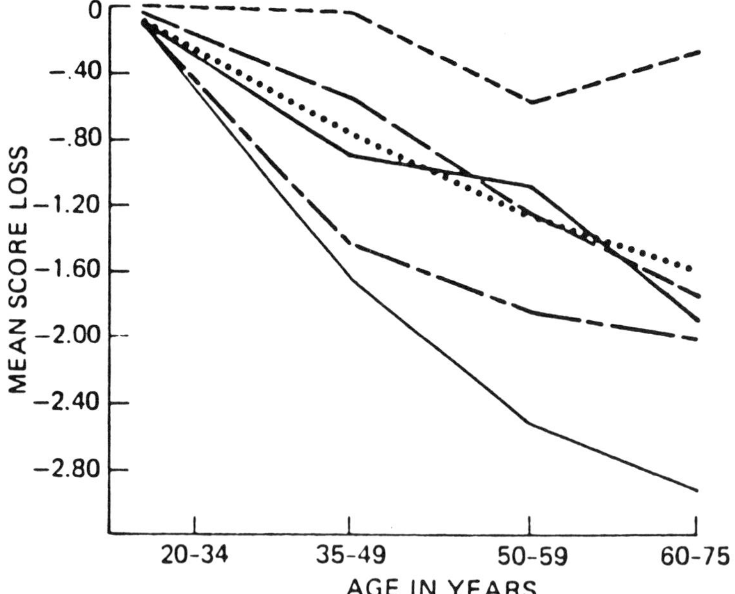

Fig. 1. Differential decline on memory tests throughout maturity. (Adapted from Gilbert and Levee 1971 and Poon 1985)
— – — – Paragraphs 182; ⋯⋯ Paired Associates; – – – – – Digits; — — — Designs; ———— Retention of Paragraphs 182; ———— Retention of Paired Associates

aging has dominated the psychological literature, and investigators have proposed a variety of models postulating mechanisms and causes of memory changes with normal aging (see Craik 1977, Salthouse 1982, and Poon 1985 for selective reviews).

Investigations on age differences in memory performances have produced surprisingly reliable results. Table 1 produces a summary of findings by Fozard (1980). In general, the locus of memory deficits can be isolated in secondary or long-term memory and in the acquisition and retrieval of new information. These findings are representative of the performance differences in six subtests of the Guild Memory Test reported by Gilbert and Levee in 1971. Figure 1 shows minimal age difference in tests of primary or short-term memory (e. g., digit span); substantial age difference is found in secondary memory (retention of paragraphs).

While findings on group differences across the adult age range have been reliable, findings on memory performances across individuals of the same age show a substantial amount of variability (Poon 1985). The vast individual difference in memory performance presents substantial difficulty to clinical diagnosis. Why is memory so difficult to assess in early stages of dysfunction? There are three primary reasons:

Table 2. Some components found to influence observed memory performance

Memory processes	Dynamic processes
	  Encoding
	  Storage
	  Retrieval
	
	Memory capacity
	  Iconic memory
	  Primary memory
	  Secondary memory
	  Working memory
	  Tertiary memory

Information characteristics	Verbal Spatial Tactile Olfactory Visual
Individual differences	Health Affect Education Intelligence Experiences Personality Cognitive styles
Environmental influences	Stresses Environmental support
Task characteristics	Familiarity Difficulty Pacing Practice

a) Memory is a multifaceted phenomenon involving a multitude of dependent processes.
b) There are a number of peripheral and environment factors that are known to affect memory functioning.
c) The range of memory functioning that can be considered normal is large.

To comprehend the sources of individual and age-related variabilities in memory performanes, it is important to understand the mechanisms of memory and the many factors that have been found to influence memory performance. Table 2 provides a list of pertinent variables that have been found to interact with each other to influence the observed memory performance. First of all, remembering involves encoding, storage, and retrieval. Memory failure could be due to inadequate encoding or acquisition or to failure in the storage or retrieval of acquired information. An example of failure to retrieve stored information is the tip-of-the-tongue phenomenon (Bowles et al., in press). It should be noted that encoding, storage, and retrieval are dependent processes, and that it is difficult to separate these components.

A theoretical division into primary and secondary memory is usually employed to describe the acquisition and retention of new information. Primary memory is conceptualized as a limited-capacity store in which information is still "in mind," as it is being used. If the information is stored, it enters secondary memory, which is conceptualized as an unlimited, permanent store of newly acquired information. If the information in primary memory is not rehearsed or acquired in a deeper level, the information is then lost and will not be registered in secondary memory. Tertiary memory is hypothesized as a repository of remote of very well-learned information, such as the name of one's spouse. All lines of research show that primary and tertiary memory are preserved, and that significant age-related decline is observed in secondary memory in normal aging.

Memory performances have been shown to be influences by a number of factors (Poon 1985). Day-to-day fluctuation could be caused by changes in mood, affect, interest, motivation, and level of attention/concentration which could affect encoding, storage, and retrieval of information. Person-to-person differences could be due to differenes in education, intelligence, skills, and familiarity with the task, as well as biological and motivational factors. The many factors that have been found to influence the level of memory functioning make it clear why the level of functional memory is fluid and subject to a large range of intra- and interpersonal variability.

The following quotation from Talland (1968 p. 24) provides one way of viewing memory disorders:

Occasional failure in recall or a temporary difficulty in learning need not be taken as symptomatic of a disorder in a function. All our functions are exercised within limits and, with such heterogeneous and often complex functions as remembering and learning, the limits are wide. Every so often one's performance can exceed as well as fall short of those mean values that correspond to the bulk of one's efforts and achivments. We infer a disorder from a permanent or extensive disability in comparison with previous performance or in comparison with a suitably defined control group.

Age-Associated Memory Impairment

When there is a memory dysfunction, especially in the early stages and prior to the full expression of the impairment, the variable and fluid nature of normal memory functioning makes it difficult to estimate the probability of dysfunction and to isolate the locus of its disorder. The variability of normal memory functioning provides the background for a current controversy surrounding the discussion regarding a possible diagnostic category of age-associated memory impairment (AAMI; Crook et al. 1986). Some pertinent questions surrounding the definition of AAMI are: What critical components are affected in AAMI in normal aging, and should they be labeled impairments? What is the appropriate control group from which to measure and compare symptoms of AAMI? Are the tests proposed for criterion measures appropriate or sensitive enough to define AAMI? One possible impact of an AAMI diagnosis is the opportunity for remediation. Owing to the variable nature of memory and the different possible causes of lower performance *at any given time,* how would one define and differentiate transient and stable biological, psychological, and environmental antecedents of AAMI to recommend a specific course for remediation for an individual?

The current discussion on AAMI is beneficial and adds to our sensitivity of cognitive assessment issues for older individuals. To illustrate the variable nature of memory functioning, neither the clinicians nor the elderly individuals could accurately diagnose or define memory complaints at early stages of dysfunction. The cognitive aging research literature shows that community-dwelling older persons themselves cannot articulate their memory complaints accurately. In this population, memory complaints have been found to relate to level of depression but not objective memory performances (see Gelewski and Zelinski 1986, for a review). In comparison, preofessionals are not immune to misclassifying the degree of cognitive and memory dysfunction in diagnosing cases of possible senile dementia of the Alzheimer type. The percentage of misdiagnoses has been estimated between 10% and 50% (Garcia et al. 1981; Gurland and Toner 1983; Ron et al. 1979). Although memory and cognition is one of several presenting symptoms in the diagnosis of Alzheimer's disease, the level of possible misdiagnosis seems to indicate that there is a genuine need to improve our current understanding of memory assessment.

Basic Precepts for Memory Assessment

What basic precepts should a clinician be cognizant of in selecting or designing a memory battery to meet specific clinical assessment goals? First and foremost, the selection of tests should be guided by the clinical questions that precipitated the assessment. It is clear that no one test could assess the global status of memory abilities for an individual. Tests that are selected or designed to answer specific questions should increase the sensitivity of the assessment.

In addition to issues of test reliability, issues of test validity are important for the interpretation of results. *Face validity* or *ecological validity* pertains to whether the test seems to reflect the everyday memory demands and complaints. *Construct validity* pertains to whether the test actually measures the process that it is thought to be measuring, and *convergent validity* addresses whether a particular test is in agreement with other tests that purport to measure the same process (Cunningham 1986).

While face validity can be independent of construct and convergent validity and is not needed for the prediction of a process, it would be comforting for a patient to know that the memory tests which they are taking seem to assimilate their complaints and relate to everyday memory demands.

High construct validity for a test is mandatory for the accurate interpretation of the result for presence or absence of a particular type of dysfunction. This criterion is often violated in published papers (of experiments evaluating memory functioning of specific patient groups or the efficacy of a treatment on specific memory process) in that the construct validity of a memory test used to measure a process is often assumed or is incorrectly assumed. If that test is used to demonstrate changes of an assumed memory process or the effectiveness of a particular treatment on a particular memory process, an incorrectly assumed construct validity of the test would constitute a fatal flaw in that published study.

Perhaps an example of an attempt to follow sound psychometric practice in memory testing is in order here. Crook and his colleagues (Crook and Larrabee, in press) have attempted to construct or modify existing tests that imitate everyday memory demands or evaluate typical memory complaints of older individuals. Tests that imitate everyday memory demands would satisfy the face validity criterion. A number of the tests were evaluated experimentally to examine component changes in normal aging as well as in dementia and other pathologies. This effort could establish the construct validity of the instruments. Further, factor analysis of data is being carried out to identify the communality of these tests with similar tests that purport to evaluate the same process. From these analyses, convergent validity of the tets could then be indentified. Crook's efforts should be lauded, for few clinical laboratories carry out the test validation process in a systematic way.

In summary, some basic notions about memory functioning should be kept in mind. First, it is important to realize that memory is a consolidation process, and tests of memory must reflect the real-life demands on the individual. That is, tests of rote learning and immediate retrieval of new information do not represent an individual's complete repertoire of memory abilities – unless we are interested specifically in these processes or the effects of treatment on these specific processes. Second, sound psychometric principles of reliability and validity of tests should be practiced in order to produce accurate and meaningful interpretation of observed performance.

Figure 2 presents a diagram used by Jenkins (1979) and adapted by Smith (1980) to describe the contributions and interactions of four major factors that have been found to affect cognitive performances. These factors are equally pertinent to memory assessment and can contribute to the clinician's understanding of individual memory performance differences.

Individual Characteristics

The first factor describes the characteristics of the individual in addition to chonological age. The pioneering work of many investigators have shown the important influences of anatomical, physiological, neurochemical, genetic, and other biomedi-

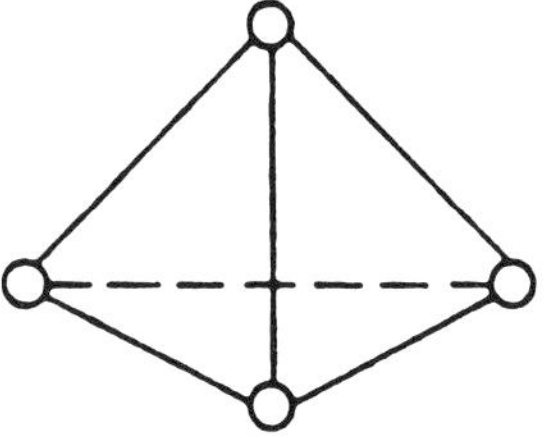

Fig. 2. Basic ingredients in memory assessment. (Adapted from Poon et al. 1985)

cal factors on behavior and cognitive performances (see Finch and Schneider 1985 for a review). Psychologists have also shown that education, intelligence, affect, environmental influences, skills, knowledge and self-rating of memory all could account for significant amounts of age-related variance of the observed memory performance (see Poon 1985 for a review). In general, higher level of education, higher premorbid intelligence, more familiarity with the memory task, less amount of depression and test anxiety, and higher level of motivation all tend to contribute to better performance. Poon et al. (1984) have demonstrated that age differences could be under- or overestimated if these variables are not properly controlled in cognitive aging research. In the case of diagnostic judgment, the magnitude of dysfunction could be similarly under- or overestimated when these individual difference effects are overlooked.

Criterion Task

The criterion task is the actual test, and its dependent measure(s) are used to measure performance. For a particular task, it is important to note that different dependent measures evaluate different aspects of a process and may contain different levels of sensitivity for differentiating processes. In the evaluation of age differences and early SDAT, for example, recognition recall is less sensitive to free recall (Kaszniak et al. 1986). Figure 3 shows the results reported by Perlmuter (1979), who found that the rate of age decline is different for free, cued, and recognition recall. This differential age decline is further affected by incidental and intentional learning of the informa-

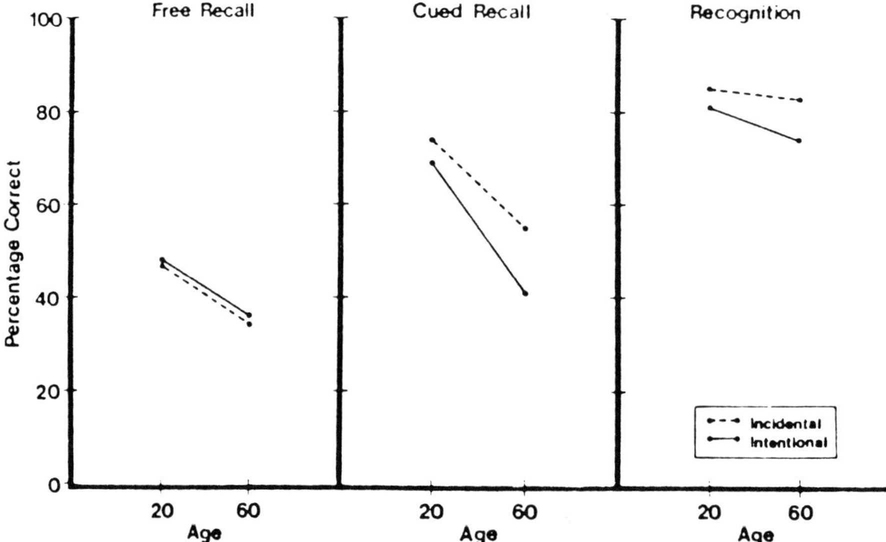

Fig. 3. Intentional and incidental memory measured in three ways as a function of age (From Perlmutter 1979)

tion. When drawing conclusions about differences in memory performance, one must keep the specific dependent measure in mind.

Another crucial aspect of the task factor to consider in interpreting results is the relative difficulty of the task. It has been empirically demonstrated that task difficulty interacts with age as well as with pathology (Poon 1985; Kaszniak et al. 1986). Figure 4 shows the disproportionate decline in performance of older compared to younger adults when the task was made more difficult by increasing the presentation rate of the stimuli. The lesson to be learned in task selction is that the magnitude of memory dysfunction of a process can range from negligible to significant, depending on the relative difficulty of a task or test. To complicate the diagnostic picture further, task difficulty can interact with the severity of dysfunction, an individual difference characteristic.

Nature of Stimuli

The nature of the stimuli, e. g., verbal or nonverbal, dictates the type of processing to be measured. One dimension of the stimuli, the familiarity, is critical to the evaluation of memory functions in older individuals. Figure 5 presents the results of an experiment that measured the speed of correct retrieval from tertiary memory (naming latency) of pictures of objects. The figure shows that the direction of age differences – that is, young perform better than old, or old perform better than young – can be manipulated simply by the selction of test stimuli (Poon and Fozard 1978). Cohort-specific effects have also been shown for memory of words and prose (see Poon 1985 for a review). One lesson to learn is that the use of neutral or unfamiliar stimuli may

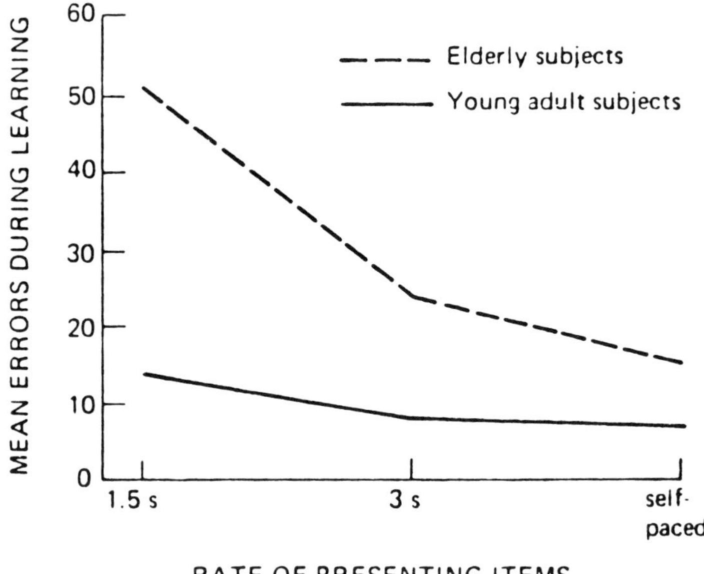

Fig. 4. Age differences in paired-associate learning proficiency as affected by rate of presenting items. (Adapted from Canestrari 1963 and Poon 1985)

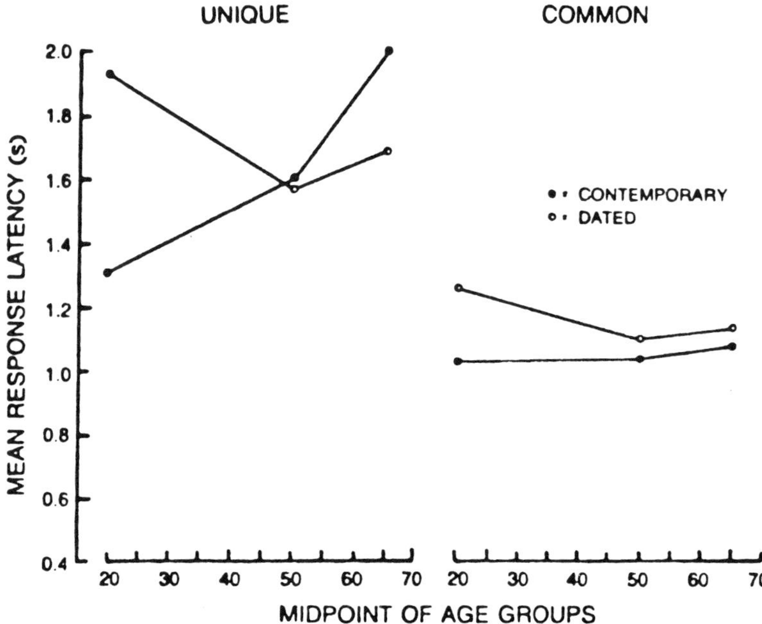

Fig. 5. Mean response latencies for the unique and common versions of contemporary and dated exemplars for the 20-, 50-, and 65-year-old groups. (Adapted from Poon and Fozard 1978 and Poon 1985)

exaggerate the degree of memory difficulty for older people; the observed deficit could, therefore, be the result of the stimuly employed rahter than an indication of a flawed memory process.

Cognitive Strategies

Treat et al. (1981) substantiated the findings that older individuals tend not to use efficient strategies to enhance their memory performance unless they are retaught the strategies. Substantial memory facilitation is observed once a mnemonic, or memory aid, is provided for the elderly (see Poon et al. 1980 for a review). Figure 6 shows the performances of paired-associate memory of young, middle-aged, and elderly adults and their retention of the paired-associate information over a 16-month period. Older adults could acquire 30% less information compared to the young adults at initial learning, and their retrieval rate was substantially lower than that in the middle-aged and young adults over the 16-months period. However, when an imagery mnemonic or a cartoon mnemonic was taught to all the subjects during acquisition, the performance of the older adults improved so that there was no difference in the rate of initial acquisition among the three age groups, and the retention performance of old subjects equaled that of middle-age subjects. It is therefore important to monitor the acquisition and retrieval strategies of the subjects. Tests that may reflect the strategies of the subject could provide cues on reasons for superior or poor performance.

Informed Decision Making in Test Selection

The preceding sections of this chapter have shown that there are different models of memory as well as approaches to the study of memory. Memory performances are shown to depend on the memory process measured, stimuli employed, cognitive strategies used by the person, as well as the individual's biomedical and psychological status. It is perhaps judicious to state that there is no one test or battery that is suitable to evaluae the different aspects of memory.

Because memory tests are used to confirm clinical hypotheses, a number of tests may be appropriate if they are suitable for the milieu of the individual and provide a qualitative profile of underlying mechanisms that are the basis of the clinical hypothesis. The selection of a test or a set of tests should therefore be guided by the prototypical behavioral symptoms of the disease, the hypotheses of the clinician, and the previously demonstrated sensitivity and specificity of a test, as well as the psychometric properties of the test. This process necessitates informed decision making on the part of the clinician. A standardized memory test may be completely appropriate for one individual but provide incomplete data for another individual. This philosophy argues against the relative appropriateness or usefulness of one standardized memory battery (or task) against another, and it places the responsibility for selecting an effective assessment instrument squarely on the clinician.

In order to select the most cost-effective memory assessment instruments to test or evaluate a specific set of clinical questions or hypotheses, a clinician needs a wide range of information on:

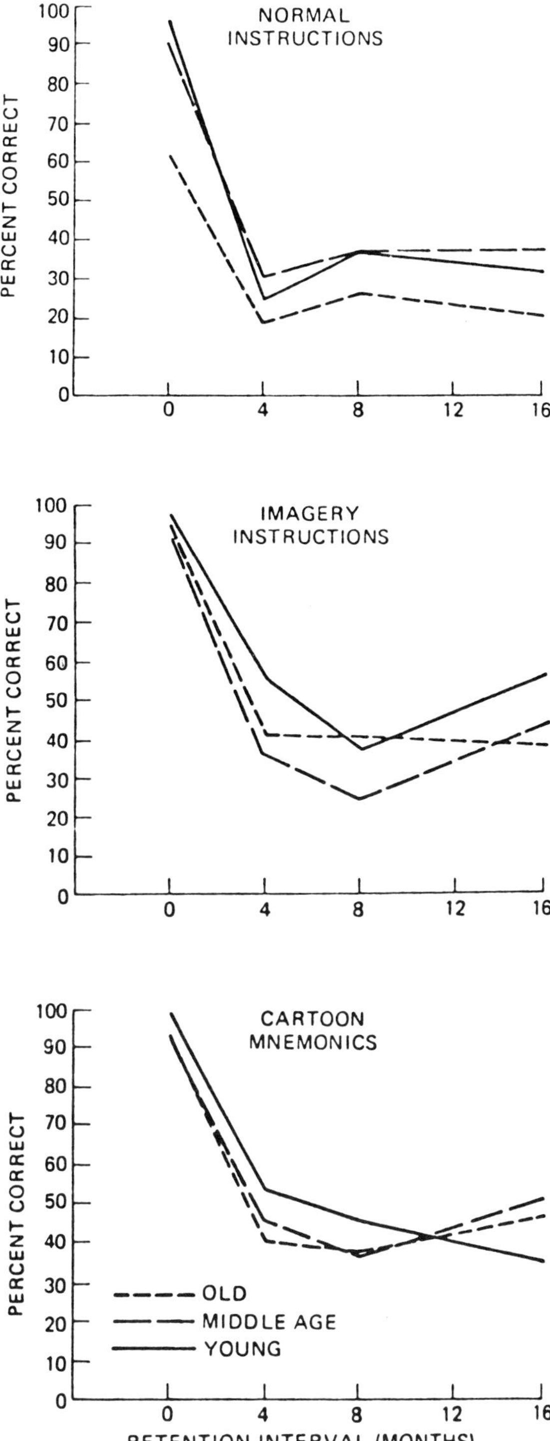

Fig. 6. Paired-associate retrieval performances of young, middle-aged, and elderly subjects over a 16-months span. (Adapted from Thomas and Ruben 1973 and Poon 1985)

a) memory function, including the four basic ingredients of memory assessment,
b) available instruments or paradigms for different assessment purposes, and
c) demonstrated sensitivity of specific tests in evaluating change and clinical diagnosis.

Summary and Conclusion

With the current knowledge on experimental and clinical aspects of memory and aging, we can take comfort in knowing that when diagnostic instruments are judiciously selected, it is possible to obtain a great deal of sophistication in identifying and differentiating patterns of performance between control and patient groups, over time, with different clinical presentation across patient groups, and with some reliable degree of association to other anatomical, physiological, and biochemical correlates. This level of sophistication can only be obtained with close collaboration among biomedical and behavioral scientists and among researchers and clinicians. I hope this chapter provides further communication between cognitive psychologists and psychogeriatric researchers and practitioners and facilitates cross-fertilization of ideas and concepts in memory functioning in normal aging and disease.

References

American Psychiatric Association (1980) Diagnostic and statistical manual of mental disorders (3rd edn). American Psachiatric Association, Washington DC

Bowles N, Obler L, Poon LW (in press) Aging and word retrieval: naturalistic, clinical, and laboratory data. In: Poon LW, Rubin D, Wilson B (eds) Everyday cognition in adulthood and late life. Cambridge University Press, New York

Canestrari REJ (1963) Paced and self-paced learning in young and elderly adults. J Gerontol 18: 165–168

Craik FIM (1977) Age differences in human memory. In: Birren J, Schaie KW (eds) Handbook of the psychology of aging. Van Nostrand Rhinehold, New York

Crook T, Larrabee G (in press) Interrelationship among everyday memory tests: stabiolity for factor structure with age. Neuropsychology

Crook T, Bartus R, Ferris S, Whitehouse P, Cohen G, Gershon S (1986) Age-associated memory impairment: proposed diagnostic criteria and measures of clinical change. Report of a National Institute of Mental Health Work Group. Dev Neuropsychol 2: 261–276

Cunningham W (1986) Psychometric perspectives: validity and reliability. In: Poon LW, Gurland B, Eisdorfer C et al. (eds) Handbook for memory assessment of older adults. American Psychological Association, Washington DC

Erickson R, Scott M (1977) Clinical memory assessment: a review. Psychol Bull 84: 1130–1149

Erickson R, Poon LW, Walsh-Sweeney L (1980) Clinical memory testing of the elderly. In Poon LW, Fozard JL, Cermak LS et al. (eds) New directions in memory and aging: proceedings of the George Talland memorial conference. Erlbaum, Hillsdale

Finch C, Schneider E (1985) Handbook of the biology of aging. Van Norstrand Reinhold, New York

Fozard J (1980) Time for remembering. In: Poon LW (ed) Aging in the 1980's: psychological issues. American Psychological Association, Washington DC

Garcia D, Reding M, Blass J (1981) Overdiagnosis of dementia. J Am Geriatr Soc 29: 407–410

Gilbert J, Levee R (1971) Patterns of declining memory. J Gerontol 26: 70–75

Gilewski M, Zelinski E (1986) Questionnaire assessment of memory complaints. In: Poon LW, Gurland B, Eisdorfer C et al. (eds) Handbook for memory assessment of older adults. American Psychological Association, Washington DC

Gurland B, Toner J (1983) Differentiating dementia from nondementing conditions. In: Mayeux R, Prosen W (eds) The dementias. Raven, New York

Jenkins J (1979) Four points to remember: a tetrahedral model of memory experiments. In: Cermak L, Craik FIM (eds) Levels of processing in human memory. Erlbaum, Hillsdale NJ

Kaszniak A, Poon LW, Reige W (1986) Assessing memory deficits: an information processing approach. In: Poon LW, Gurland B, Eisdorfer C et al. (eds) Handbook for memory assessment of older adults. American Psychological Association, Washington DC

Perlmutter M (1979) Age difference in adults' free recall, cued recall, and recognition. J Gerontol 34: 533–539

Poon LW (1980) Aging in the 1980's. Psychological Issues. American Psychological Association, Washington DC

Poon LW (1985) Differences in human memory with aging: nature, causes and clinical implications. In: Birren J, Schaie KW (eds) Handbook of the psychology of aging. Van Nostrand Rhinehold, New York

Poon LW, Fozard J (1978) Speed of retrieval from long-term memory in relation to age, familiarity and datedness of information. J Gerontol 5: 711–717

Poon LW, Walsh-Sweeney L, Fozard J (1980) Memory skill training for the elderly: salient issues on the use of imagery mnemonics. In: Poon LW, Fozard IL, Cermak LS et al. (eds) New directions in memory and aging: proceedings of the George Talland memorial conference. Erlbaum, Hillsdale

Poon LW, Krauss E, Bowles NL (1984) On subject selection in cognitive aging research. Exp Aging Res 10: 43–49

Randt C, Brown R, Osborne D (1980) A memory test for longitudinal measurement of mild to moderate deficits. Clin Neuropsychol 2: 184–194

Ron M, Toone B, Garralda M, Lishman W (1979) Diagnostic accuracy in presenile dementia. Br J Psychiatry 134: 161–168

Salthouse TA (1982) Adult cognition. An experimental psychology of human aging. Springer, Berlin Heidelberg New York (Springer series in coignitive development)

Smith AD (1980) Cognitive issues: advances in cognitive psychology of aging. In: Poon LW (ed) Aging in the 1980's: psychological issues. Amercian Psychological Association, Washington DC

Talland G (1968) Disorders of memory and learning. Penguin, Harmondsworth, Middlesex

Thomas JC, Reuben H (1983) Age and Mneumonic Techniques in Paired Associate Learning. Miami

Treat N, Poon LW, Fozard J (1981) Age, imagery and practice in paired associate learning. Exp Aging Res 7: 337–342

Essentials of Psychological Assessment
of the Mentally Ill Elderly:
Mild Cognitive Impairment and the Issue of Plasticity

E. U. Kranzhoff

General Propositions

Though the present book is concerned with diagnosis and treatment of senile
dementia, the title of this chapter deliberately avoids the term senile dementia. The
psychiatrically oriented reader deserves a brief explanation. Dementia refers to a
clinical syndrome of alterations in cognitive functions, motor function, affect, and
personality. Any combination of these symptoms may appear in an individual
dementing disorder; none of these could be regarded as pathognomonic. While in
pariticular, the determination of presence or absence of cognitive impairments –
unanimously regarded as central inclusion criteria by currently favored diagnostic
systems (Diagnostic and Statistical Manual of Mental Disorders, DSM III, ADRDA/
NINCDS, National Institute of Aging/American Medical Association) – is one of the
domains of clinical psychology, determining the presence or absence of the various
exclusion criteria is the responsibility of various experts. The final clinical diagnosis of
senile dementia or of any of its subtypes thus constitutes a "joint venture" of different
specialities and has to be considered a multidisciplinary task. The present argument
leads to the first proposition concerning essentials of psychological assessment of the
mentally ill elderly. *Proposition 1: The outcome of psychological assessment procedures never can be a clinical psychiatric diagnosis.*

It is the clinical gerontologist's conviction that the determination of deficits is only
one side of the coin, however important. Of no less importance are the ways an
individual copes with "objective" alterations in abilities and possibilities, i. e., the
"subjective" dimension. Thus the gerontologist at least ought to be constantly on the
look-out for potential resources in the patient to compensate for his/her cognitive
impairments and which may be undiscovered and consequently unrealized hitherto;
this objective introduces the issue of plasticity which is discussed more extensively
below. *Proposition 2: Concerning the diagnostic efforts of the clinical geropsycholog-
ist, deficit measurement is frequently widely overemphasized.*

When the deficit side of the coin is considered, the psychological diagnosis of
presence of advanced cognitive impairments rarely presents difficulties; even clinical
judgement is highly accurate in these cases. The issue at stake here is not so much
diagnosis but adequate staging, particularly for judging course and possible outcome
of treatment, and the respective literature has presented hopeful models in recent
years (see Reisberg's Global Deterioration Scale or Copeland's AGECAT in the
present volume). Challenging and intriguing, however, remains the determination of

Bergener, Reisberg (Eds.)
Diagnosis and Treatment
of Senile Dementia
© Springer-Verlag Berlin Heidelberg 1989

mild cognitive impairments as an indication of possible early signs of a dementing process. When trying to detect mild cognitive impairments, it is vital to bear in mind the tripartite question: What is normal in a particular age group for a particular individual? Norm-oriented psychodiagnostic procedures in principle try to resolve this problem by establishing central tendencies/average scores, i. e., norms, on tests for certain age groups with which the individual score is compared; "normal" in this tradition usually is defined statistically, e. g., central tendency ± one standard deviation. Criterion-oriented procedures differ from this approach in that they determine a certain standard of behavior or performance which, if complex, is subdivided into small hierachically ordered steps. Normal in this perspective is the attainment of the target criterion; age-group standards may influence the criterion definition, but are irrelevant with respect to the judgement of an individual's performance as being normal or impaired. Quite a number of assessment instruments developed following the first mentioned procedure supply useful age norms even for the higher age groups. The data base in these cases, however, is cross-sectional, giving an unduly simplified picture of cognitive decline in some areas and relative stability in others, at the same time neglecting intraindividual variability and cohort differences. The criterion-oriented approach, on the other side, up to now has not produced any significant number of assessment tools for clinical settings. *Proposition 3: The complexities of notions such als "normality" and "variability" require proceeding from status-oriented to process-oriented approaches in particular in the assessment of cognition in the mentally impaired elderly.*

Average Performance Versus Potential

In particular the assessment of mild cognitive impairments as early signs of dementia has by and large arrived at a dead end using status-oriented diagnostic instruments. When it comes to looking for potential conceptual alternatives, one obvious candidate is life-span developmental psychology, a field in which the elderly have been the main focus of attention for several decades. Within this research tradition, when dealing with psychometric intelligence in old age, a distinction between average performance and plasticitiy is offered (e. g., Willis and Baltes 1980) which could prove potentially helpful especially in the assessment of mild cognitive impairments in the elderly. The former term – average performance – conceives of intelligence as a rather stable and invariant property, much resembling a "trait" in the traditional meaning of the term in personality psychology. "This general trait approach is reflected in the usual observational scheme associated with psychometric intelligence, which involves an average performance per individual based on a static, single-occasion measurement of intellectual performance in a variety of tasks. Note that averaging is based on averaging of tasks given on one occasion, rather than on consideration of a developmental (longitudinal) time continuum or the individual's adaptive capacity to different life situations (Willis and Baltes 1980, p 265)". While even in this tradition attention has been drawn to the fact that there is decline along with stability in certain differential aspects of psychometric intelligence – a major example is the distinction between fluid and cristallized intelligence and its differential development in old age (e. g., Horn 1970, 1982) – obviously, such an average performance- and trait-oriented approach does not lead to information on the range (limits) of behavior (Baltes and Baltes 1980; Baltes et al. 1984).

Most, if not all norm-oriented psychological testing procedures can be subsumed among this cross-sectionally oriented focus on average performance.

The counterpart term – plasticity (potential) – becomes central as soon as one is interested no longer in what aged persons do "if they live in the context of the current social ecology, if they are not exposed to varying biological and environmental conditions (whether construed as facilitative or interfering) before assessment begins, and if they are asked to participate in one mode of assessment, one dictated by procedures and models developed in the life context of the young adult" (Willis and Baltes 1980, p 265), but instead what they could do; in other words if one is no longer interested in performance, but in potential. The literature on gerontological intelligence abounds with references to how large an extent the aged person's performance on intelligence tests is influenced by so-called performance factors, e. g., fatigue, test familiarity, lack of performance-enhancing motivational conditions, psychotropic drugs, unfamiliar surroundings (Baltes and Labouvie 1973; Goulet 1973; Botwinick 1977). Consequently, any given performance is a potentially biased sample from an unspecified universe of potentials.

In psychodiagnostics the traditional, but largely neglected technique of testing the limits has been developed exactly for this purpose of obtaining information reflecting the extent of realizable potentials. The implications of focusing on potential rather than on performance for the assessment of mild cognitive impairments in mentally ill elderly people are obvious. While cross-sectionally comparing healthy elderly with mentally ill elderly, persons' average performances either may leave unnoticed subtle impairments or may lead one to interpret noted deficits alternatively as being determined by some kind of performance factor, usually drug intake or hospital atmosphere conditions. The application of testing-the-limits procedures (for possible strategies see Baltes and Kindermann 1985 and Kühl and Baltes 1988) might, while counteracting the possible effects of performance factors, at the same time give evidence of absence or presence of cognitive plasticity. Inherent in this argument is the expectation that absent or significantly reduced plasticity – particularly on tests of fluid intelligence – should turn out to be indications of early dementing processes (Kühl and Baltes 1988).

Preliminary Empirical Evidence

Proceeding from the hypothesis that elderly persons without even mild cognitive impairments, though gaining relatively low subnormal pretest performance scores, should exhibit cognitive plasticity in testing-the-limits procedures, while cognitively impaired elderly should not substantially gain from repeated testing (Baltes & Kindermann 1985), we performed two studies to obtain preliminary empirical evidence on the efficiency of the lacking-plasticity approach in the differential diagnosis of early dementing processes.

Study I

In an initial retrospective study we selected 24 psychogeriatric patients for whom three diagnostic procedures had identified early dementing processes:
a) the psychiatrist's judgement of presence of symptoms indicative of early dementia,
b) Mini Mental Status score below 26 points, and
c) a raw score of 11 or 12 points on the Sandoz Clinical Assessment Scale in Geriatric (SCAG) cognitive impairment factor.

These patients were coached during five sessions on tasks of fluid intelligence, following the suggestions from a paper by Baltes (1984). The three tasks each covered one of the main aspects of fluid intelligence, i.e., figural reasoning (RAVEN type matrices), inductive thinking (numbers and letters series), and associative memory (picture number test). Figure 1 shows that the data gathered thus far – the study is still in progress – in part seem to support the hypothesis derived from the lacking-plasticity assumption. On the task we think most indicative of fluid intelligence, i.e., matrices of rising difficulty and complexity, our subjects as a group exhibited no statistically significant increase in the number of correct solutions. Even in this rather small and homogeneous group there is, however, an impressingly high interindividual variability which casts doubt on the utility of the procedure in the assessment of individual patients at the present time. Also, at present there is no evidence that an unimpaired comparison group will show an increase in correct solutions on that very task. In this respect we have thus far only the evidence from the Baltes (1984) investigations, and task-specific influences will have to be ruled out. With respect to the inductive thinking task and the associative memory task there was a substantial increase in

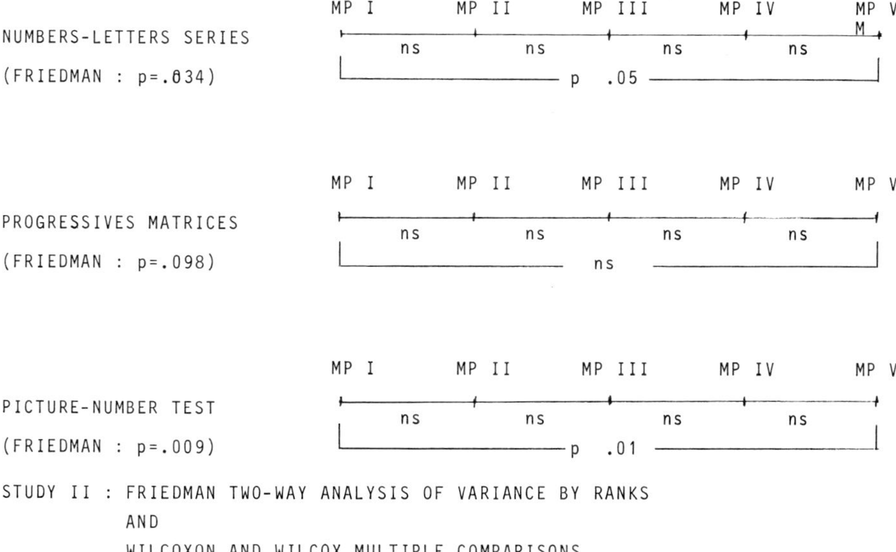

Fig. 1. Results of tests of fluid intelligence using Friedman two-way analysis of variance by ranks and Wilcoxon and Wilcox multiple comparisons. *MP*, NS, not significant

performance on both, particularly on the latter. This finding, however, only discredits the lacking-plasticity assumption if it should turn out that an unimpaired comparison group shows an equal and not a substantially higher increase in performance. Methodologically, of course, issues of reliability and validity are tapped when interpreting the results. What do we know about the reliability of our often imaginative and creative experimental tasks? And if instead we apply established tests, and if there is – rarely enough – general information about retest reliability, are we justified in transferring this information to samples of elderly psychiatric inpatients? And, more basically, how should we tackle the fundamental problem inherent in classical test theory that the higher the reliability, the better assessment procedures are, while only instruments of moderate reliability are able to demonstrate change over time?

Study II

The second study draws upon the argument that if there is a certain range of performance of cognitive abilities the unimpaired elderly person can demonstrate under favorable circumstances he should gain substantially on learning tests. Lack of plasticity then should show up in an impaired ability to access new information i. e., first signs of early dementing processes might be reflected in subtle learning disabilities. To follow this line of reasoning further we analyzed the picture-learning test scores of 65 unselected psychogeriatric inpatients. The impaired group in this study was defined via an extended battery of performance tests as well as by an expert psychiatric evaluation. The testing-the-limits procedure applied consisted in repeatedly presenting a table of 12 common, colored objects to the patient – at a maximum five times. Learning was considered to be reflected in the number of correctly reproduced items per presentation. As Fig. 2 shows, both groups learned. The increase was significantly greater, however, in the unimpaired group. The result thus seems to support the assumption of defective plasticity in mentally impaired elderly persons. As none of the impaired group raised their performances to 12 or at least 11 reproduced items after the fifth presentation and only two subjects reproduced 10 items, and while only 6 out of 37 subjects in the unimpaired group had a score lower than 10 after the last presentation, this procedure holds some promise for the assessment of individual patients.

Conclusions

Efforts to reliably and validly assess mild cognitive impairments in psychogeriatric populations by means of either screening tests or elaborated neuropsychological procedures have been widely unsatisfactory. As we pointed out in our theoretical considerations, at least one reason for the low diagnostic accuracy of traditional one-measurement-point assessment strategies is the large overlap of mental test scores between mentally unimpaired and mentally impaired elderly people. Only testing-the-limits procedures are believed to have the potential to substantially reduce the region of overlap such that by mobilizing baseling reserve capacities the two groups of people approach their current maximum performance. Preliminary empirical evi-

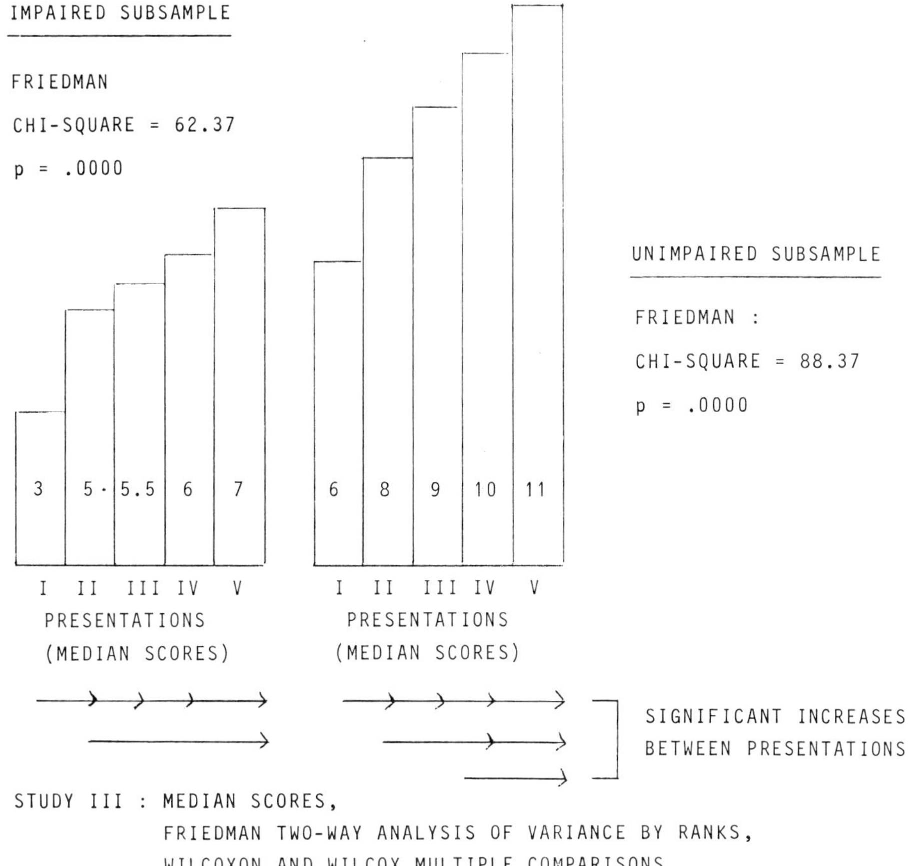

Fig. 2. Median Scores of picture-learning test using Friedman two-way analysis of variance by ranks and Wilcoxon and Wilcos multiple comparisons. *Left*, Impaired subsample, Friedman: Chi-square = 62.37; *P* = 0.0000; *right*, Unimpaired subsample, Friedman: Chi-square = 88.37, *P* = 0.0000. *Arrows* represent significant increases between presentations

dence seems to support this view. The development of standardized testing-the-limits strategies is thus highly recommended as they may substantially widen our very rudimentary knowledge about the early stages of dementia. Also, the meaning of the growing preoccupation with age-associated memory impairments (AAMI; see the respective chapters in this volume) could be judged from this perspective.

References

Baltes PB (1984) Intelligenz im Alter. Spektr Wiss 5: 46–60
Baltes PB, Baltes MM (1980) Plasticity and variability in psychological aging: methodological and theoretical issues. In: Gurski G (ed) Determining the effects of aging on the central nervous system. Schering, Berlin

Baltes MM, Kindermann T (1985) Die Bedeutung der Plastizität für die klinische Beurteilung des Leistungsverhaltens im Alter. In Bente D, Coper H, Kanowski S (eds) Hirnorganische Psychosyndrome im Alter II. Springer, Berlin Heidelberg New York

Baltes PB, Labouvie GV (1973) Adult development of intellectual performance: description, explanation, and modification. In: Eisdorfer C, Lawton MP (eds) The psychology of adult development and aging. American Psychological Association, Washington DC

Baltes PB, Dittmann-Kohli F, Dixon RA (1984) New perspectives on the development of intelligence in adulthood: toward a dual-process conception and a model of selective optimization with compensation. Life-Span Dev Behav 6: 33–76

Botwinick J (1977) Aging and intelligence. In: Birren JE, Schaie KW (eds) Handbook of the psychology of aging. Van Nostrand Reinhold, New York

Goulet L (1973) The interfaces of acquisition: models and methods for studying the active, developing organism. In: Nesselroade JR, Reese HW (eds) Life-span developmentel psychology: methodological issues. Academic, New York

Horn JL (1970) Organization of data on life-span development of human abilities. In: Goulet LR, Baltes PB (eds) Life-span developmental psychology: research and theory. Academic, New York

Horn JL (1982) The aging of human abilities. In: Wolman BB (ed) Handbook of developmental psychology. Prentice-Hall, Englewood Cliffs

Willis SL, Baltes PB (1980) Intelligence in adulthood and aging. In: Poon LW (ed) Aging in the 1980s. American Psychological Association, Washington DC

Psychological Methods for the Assessment
of Performance and Emotionality in Elderly Patients

W. JANKE, and M. HÜPPE

Introduction

A broad repertoire of measures have been developed in psychology for measuring performance and, to a lesser degree, emotionality. In order to evaluate the usefulness of these in gerontology it is helpful to consider their respective goals.

As Table 1 shows, the measures may refer to experience, behavior, expression, or somatic (physiological, biochemical) variables. Thus, the measures may refer to *different kinds of organismic activity*.

Most measures in old persons refer to behavior and experience. In patients, however, the level of experience is generally omitted because of the difficulty in obtaining valid self-reports. However, it must be emphasized that other data sources should be used to assess aspects of experience. Somatic variables for the assessment of emotions always involve many difficulties because the most relevant autonomic indicators change their meaning in old age (e.g., electrodermal activity). Somatic variables for the assessment of cognitive deficits will probably be used more and more if the promising field of brain imaging and the specific extensions of the variables fulfill the hope that there is good covariation between performance and electrophysiological data. In particular, interesting results have been reported on the topographical electrophysiology of the brain in Alzheimer's dementia (see Maurer and Dierks 1987). This method clearly has an advantage in comparison to computed tomography because of the possibility to measure brain changes during tasks, and in comparison to positron emission tomography because of its being much less invasive

Table 1. Types of organismic activity measured by different methods

Type of activity	Specific aspect
Experience	Self
	Mood
Expression	Mimic
	Gestures
	Posture
Behavior	Activities
	Actions
Somatic activity	CNS activity (e.g., EEG, evoked potentials, contingent negative variation)
	ANS activity (e.g., heart rate, electrodermal activity)
	Chemical activity (e.g., hormones, transmitters)

Bergener, Reisberg (Eds.)
Diagnosis and Treatment
of Senile Dementia
© Springer-Verlag Berlin Heidelberg 1989

Table 2. Different methodological approaches used in measurement

Methodological approach	Recorded feature
Judgment	Self
	Others
Observation	Molar and molecular behavior
Testing	Performance tests
	Personality tests
Reactivity in experimental settings	Response to emotional stimuli/situations
	Response to stressors during performance tests

and much cheaper. At the present time, however, each method should be used when possible in order to get information about advantages and disadvanges. Thus, interesting results on the relationship between neuropsychological testing and computed tomography were obtained by Albert and Stafford (1986).

The measurement of behavior will, in any event, maintain its dominant role in providing information on the integrative work of the brain.

Each level of organismic activity may be approached by *different methodological approaches.* As presented in Table 2, data may be obtained by judgment (rating), by observation, by tests, or by measurements of reactivity in experimental settings. The methodological aspect is particularly important with respect to objectivity and reliability. Moreover, some age-related and disease-related behavioral changes determine the type of methodological approach which is to be used; the utility of self-report, for example, is limited in persons with dementia or states of confusion.

Finally, the measures to be used may refer to different *kinds of psychic functions.* Table 3 lists the most important functions which may be approached by diagnostic methods in gerontology. The functions which have been investigated in old age are frequently those of information processing and psychomotor behavior; a number of tests are available here. To a lesser degree, language has been investigated outside the

Table 3. Functions measured by different methods

Area	Specific aspects (examples)
Information processing	Perception (e. g., recognition speed)
	Thinking (e. g., problem solving)
Information storage	Learning
	Memory
Psychomotor	Speed, accuracy, and strength of motor behavior
	produced spontaneously or elicited by stimuli
Language (speaking and understanding)	Naming of words
	Recognition of words
Behavior	Social
Emotion	General tension
	Specific emotions (e. g., anxiety, anger, joy, sadness)
Motivation	General activity
	Specific motivations
	Biological motives (e. g., hunger, thirst, sex, sleep)
	Personal motives (e. g., need for success)
	Social motives (e. g., need for social contacts)

contexts of intelligence tests and specific tests for measuring language changes in brain-damaged patients. It seems necessary, however, to develop new or better tests in this area for the testing of dementia, because language disturbances seem to be very early indicators of cortical dementias (e.g., Bayles 1982; summary, Benson 1979). Very neglected areas are those which relate to personality, emotion and motivation, and social behavior. There are only a few well-established measures which can be used with old persons. This has been observed earlier (Janke and Baltissen 1979), and the situation has not improved much since (summary, Janke and Hüppe, in press).

The outcome with old and ill persons is dramatic. The reason for this is not evident since the anatomical changes which have been found in cortical and subcortical-frontal dementia according to the classification of Cummings and coworkers (Cummings 1986; Cummings and Benson 1983, 1984) are very pronounced in those brain structures which are also responsible for emotional behavior, e.g., hippocampus. Moreover, alterations in emotions seem to be very early signs in diseases with dementia (e.g., Kazniak 1986; Orsini et al. 1988). In addition, it is important to note that changes in performance are often caused by specific and nonspecific emotional factors. In some cases nonspecific arousal or emotions might increase performance scores. Usually, however, motivational and emotional changes reduce performance. Changes which occur rather frequently in old patients are overarousal, anxiety, dysphoria, and anger.

As is well-known, the influence of motivational and emotional conditions is particularly dramatic in so-called pseudodementia, in which certain depressive patients have severe cognitive deficits that are not due to brain dysfunctions. As has been shown, the differentiation of elderly patients with major depression from those with the Alzheimer type of dementia is not an easy task. La Rue et al. (1986) found that patients with major depression and those with Alzheimer's dementia could be differentiated only in a test for selective reminding. In many other cognitive tests both groups deviated equally from a healthy aged group. From these results and others, it must be concluded that emotion, motivation, and personality are basic characteristics which must be included in test batteries, not only in their own right but also as control variables to explain performance variables.

Approaches to the Assessment of Performance and Emotionality

Judgment Measures

The first group of measures involves a rater who judges the presence or absence, the degree, or the quality of a behavior pattern, of expressive behavior, or of traits or states. The rater may be the subject himself, who judges his own characteristics; such methods are usually called self-ratings or self-reports. More commonly, however, the rater is a psychologist or psychiatrist who judges the subject with respect to the above-mentioned individual characteristics. The basis of this judgment may be a more or less structured interview, nonsystematic or systematic observation, and statements by the subject himself or those about him by relatives or other persons who know him. Judgment or rating scales are the most commonly used techniques in geriatrics; reviews have been made by Goga and Hambacher (1977), Hamilton (1986),

Kochansky (1979), and Salzman et al. (1972). The measures available differ according to:
a) number of items,
b) number and type of functions measured,
c) psychometric properties (reliability, validity),
d) norms and data for reference populations, and
e) use in distinguishing among different disorders.

Observer Rating Methods. Numerous scales are used in gerontopsychology and gerontopsychiatry. Frequently these are not constructed according to the principles of test construction but are ad hoc scales for which no data about reliability, validity, and norms exist. Lehmann (1984) reported that with only 5 of 13 scales used in 67 studies for the measurement of drug effects in organic psychosyndromes sufficient data on reliability were available. Tables 4 and 5 list rating scales for which such data are known. All scales are multidimensional and refer to performance as well as to emotionality. The rating methods listed are directed towards:
a) measurement of momentary mood (e.g., Adjective Checklist),
b) assessment of the severeness of dementia (e.g., CDR, DRS), or
c) differentiation of Alzheimer's dementia from other forms (e.g., DAT).

Some rating methods are mixtures of data from judgments derived from impressions during a clinical interview and from the evaluation of structured observations or tasks (e.g., repetition of words, enumerations of objects, or arithmetic tasks).

Rating scales differ considerably with respect to the type of factors that lead to the final judgment. Some scales are very well operationalized (e.g., FAST, SCAG, DAT). The sensitivity of observer-rating methods seems to vary according to the context and aim of a study. Regarding sensitivity in therapeutic trials, there is evidence that expert ratings indicate improvement earlier than self-ratings (e.g., Debus et al. 1978). In respect to sensitivity in the differentiation of patient populations, observer-based ratings seem to distinguish quite well the different populations of patients (e.g., Cummings and Benson 1986).

On the other hand, many problems are involved in all observer ratings (see Janke and Baltissen 1979):
1. Observer ratings are basically only indirect with respect to the experience of a subject.

Table 4. Psychogeriatric observer-rating methods for the assessment of aspects of performance and emotionality: *mental state*

Methods	Rater	No. of items	No. of alternatives to respond	Recorded features	Authors
Dementia of the Alzheimer Type Inventory (DAT)	Physician/ psychologist	10	3	5 Mental functions: memory, visuospatial, cognition, personality, language; 5 motor functions: speech, psychomotor speed, posture, gait, movements	Cummings and Benson (1986)

Table 4. continued

Methods	Rater	No. of items	No. of alternatives to respond	Recorded features	Authors
Mini-Mental State Examination (MMSE)	Nursing staff	11	3–9	Mental state: orientation, registration, attention and calculation, recall, language	Folstein et al. (1975)
SHORT-CARE	Physician/ psychologist	143		6 Scales: depression/demoralization, dementia, subjective memory impairment, sleep disorders, somatic symptoms, disability	Gurland et al. (1984)
Extended Scale	Physician/ psychologist	23		Dementiating, movements, graphomotor, block design, similarities, differences, identities, sentences, orientation, information, count, simple arithmethic, association learning, verbal recognition and memory, design recognition and memory	Hersch (1979)
London Psychogeriatric Rating Scale (LPRS)	Nursing staff	36	3	4 Scales and total score: mental disability, physical disability, socially irritating behavior, disengagement	Hersch et al. (1978)
Clinical Dementia Rating (CDR)	Physician/ psychologist and reference person	60	4	6 Scales: memory, orientation, judgment/problem solving, community affairs, home/hobbies, personal care	Hughes et al. (1982)
Orientation-Memory-Concentration Test	Physician/ psychologist	6/26	2	Orientation, memory, concentration	Katzman et al. (1983)
Dementia Rating Scale (DRS)	Physician/ psychologist	27	2	4 Factors and total score: orientation, emotional control, motor ability, communication	Lawson et al. (1977)
Brief Cognitive Rating Scale (BCRS)	Physician/ psychologist	10	7	10 Functions: concentration, memory (recent/post), orientation, functioning/ self care, speech, psychomotor, mood/ behavior, praxis, calculation ability	Reisberg et al. (1985)
Functional Assessment Staging Test (FAST)	Physician/ psychologist	1	7	Cognitive state	Reisberg et al. (1985)
Global Deterioration Scale (GDS)	Physician/ psychologist	1	7	Cognitive state	Reisberg et al. (1982)
Alzheimer's Disease Assessment Scale (ADAS)	Physician/ psychologist	21	6/2	Cognitive functions: memory, language, praxis; noncognitive functions: mood, behavioral disorders, total scores	Rosen et al. (1984)

Table 5. Psychogeriatric observer-rating methods for the assessment of aspects of performance and emotionality: *emotional state*

Methods	Rater	No. of items	No. of alternatives to respond	Recorded features	Authors
Adjective Checklist (EWL 60-F)	Physician/ psychologist/ reference person	60	4	15 Emotional aspects related to 6 factors: performance-orientated activation, general disactivation, extraversion/introversion, general well-being, emotional irritation, anxiety/depression	Janke et al. (1987)
Nuremberg Geriatric Rating (NAR)	Psychologist	9	7	3 Factors: activity, mood, anxiety	Oswald (1979)
Brief Psychiatric Rating Scale (BPRS)	Physician/ psychologist	18	7	Anxiety/depression, mental impairment, activity, hostility	Overall and Gorham (1962)
Plutchik Geriatric Rating Scale (PLUT)	Nursing staff	31	3	Social behavior, aggressiveness, self-care, sleep disorders, working performance	Plutchik et al. (1970)
Sandoz Clinical Assessment Geriatric Scale (SCAG)	Physician/ psychologist	18	7	18 Scales related to 5 factors and overall impression: cognitive dysfunction, interpersonal relationships, affective disorders, apathy, somatic functioning	Shader et al. (1974)

2. Most observer ratings show rather low interrater reliability. Reliability may be improved by standardization, but this is not possible for all areas measured, in particular not for mood areas such as anxiety or sadness.
3. The validity of an instrument is not fixed but differs with different judges.
4. In therapeutic trials with several repeated measurements the correlations between subtests or scales vary. Correlations generally increase, which means that the characteristics measured are losing their relative independence.
5. Sensitivity in the differentiation of states or traits seems to be low. This follows from studies in which intercorrelations have been determined.

Self-Ratings. Self-ratings are usually well constructed according to the principles of test theory. Even in patients, it has been found that subjects maintain their factorial structure in therapeutic trials (Debus et al. 1978). On the other hand, self-report methods have severe limitations:
1. Self-report methods are limited to the evaluation of emotional and motivational states and traits. Usually they are not useful for assessing performance (for summaries in German see Janke 1984; Janke and Hüppe, in press; in English see Oswald and Fleischmann 1985).

Table 6. Self-rating methods for the assessment of immediate (I), medium-term (M) and long-term (L) aspects of emotionality: *multidimensional tests*

Methods	No. of items	No. of alternatives to respond	Time range	Recorded features	Authors
Symptom Check List (Self-Report Symptom Inventory, SCL-90-R)	90	5	I	9 Aspects of mood, e. g., depression, anxiety	Derogatis (1977)
Freiburg Personality Inventory (FPI-R)	138	2	L	10 Dimensions, e. g., life-satisfaction, social orientation, inhibition, irritability, aggressiveness, extraversion, emotionality	Fahrenberg et al. (1984)
Questionnaire of Psychic and Somatic Complaints	46	4	M	8 Aspects: depression, anxiety, cognitive impairment, somatic symptoms, sleep disorders, social problems, psychotic experiences, sexual impairment	Hautzinger (1984)
Adjective Checklist (EWL-K)	123	2	I	15 Aspects related to 6 dimensions (see EWL 60-S)	Janke and Debus (1978)
Adjective Checklist (EWL 60-S)	60	2	I	Performance-oriented activation, general disactivation, extraversion/introversion, general well-being, emotional irritation, anxiety/depression	Janke et al. (1984)
Profile of Mood States (POMS)	35	7	I	4 Aspects: dejection, fatigue, thirst for action, ill-humor	McNair et al. (1971)
Multiple Affect Adjective Checklist (MAACL)	132	2	I	3 Aspects: anxiety, depression, hostility	Zuckerman and Lubin (1965)

2. Self-report methods may lose their validity in old populations because of response sets.
3. In the case of old patients with cognitive deficits the validity of self-report methods is diminished by contamination due to cognitive and emotional factors.
   Tables 6 and 7 list multidimensional and unidimensional self-report measures.

Observation Methods

Methods of observation are, on the one hand, very common methods in pathopsychology and psychiatry. On the other hand, they are rather unusual techniques

Table 7. Self-rating methods for the assessment of immediate (I), medium-term (M) and long-term (L) aspects of emotionality: *unidimensional tests*

Methods	No. of items	No. of alternatives to respond	Time range	Recorded features	Authors
General well-being					
Nuremberg Geriatric Self-Rating Scale (NAS)	12	5	M	Self-rated aging	Oswald and Fleischmann (1986)
Mood Scale (Bf-S)	28	3	I	General well-being	von Zerssen (1976a)
Live satisfaction					
Life Satisfaction Index A (LSI-A)	20	3	M	Happiness	Neugarten et al. (1961)
Life Satisfaction Scale	19(12)	2(3)	M	Satisfaction with past and present life	Wiendieck (1970)
Depression					
Beck Depression Inventory	21	3	M	Depressiveness	Beck et al. (1961)
Depression Scale of the Center for Epidemiology (CES-D)	20	4	M	Depressive mood	Radloff (1977)
Depression Scale (D-S)	16	4	I	Anxious-depressive mood	von Zerssen (1976b)
Self-Rating Depression Scale (SDS)	20	4	M	Depressive mood	Zung (1965)
Anxiety					
State-Trait-Anxiety Inventory (STAI-X1)	20	4	I	State anxiety	Spielberger et al. (1970); Laux et al. (1981)
State-Trait-Anxiety Inventory (STAI-X2)	20	4	L	Trait anxiety	Spielberger et al. (1970); Laux et al. (1981)
Self-Rating Anxiety Scale (SAS)	20	4	M	Clinical anxiety	Zung (1976)

insofar as they are only rarely standardized. Observation methods differ in terms of various factors, including the degree of standardization of conditions, the kind of observation and registration, and the nature of the observation sample.

An important distinction, based on the type of behavior to be observed, is that between macroanalysis and microanalysis. The macroanalytic approach involves the observation and registration of general behavioral aspects. Examples include the Ward Behavior Rating Scale (Burdock et al. 1960) and the Nuremberg Geriatric Observation Scale (NAB) from the Nuremberg Geronto psychological Inventory (NAI; Oswald and Fleischmann 1986). Both methods involve ratings based on non-systematic behavioral observation. In the NAB the rater scores 15 behaviors (e. g., appearance, behavior outside, cultural activities) on a scale with three points. The total score is an indicator for activity level and self-care. Norms for patients with Alzheimer's and multi-infarct dementia are given.

The microanalytic approach involves systematic observation of specific behaviors, usually in a standardized situation, e.g., in a clinical interview. Very often the behavior to be observed is expressive behavior. Behavioral aspects which have frequently been used in clinical psychology or psychiatry are:
a) manumotor behavior (Ekman and Friesen 1972; Freedman 1972; Ulrich 1981);
b) speech behavior (Ellgring 1977; Hoffmann et al. 1985; Klos and Ellgring 1985; Pope et al. 1970; Ulrich 1981); and
c) mimic activity (Ellgring and Ploog 1984).

The clinical population that has been investigated most frequently is that of depressive patients. In gerontopsychology Hüppe (1987) investigated gestures and speech characteristics as indicators of emotions in experimental situations which are thought to induce emotions. The most important feature of this approach is the possibility to obtain information by means of nonobtrusive measures. There are many problems in the observation of expressive behavior:
a) It is questionable whether expressive characteristics have the same meanings in different patients.
b) It is not clear whether expressive behavior indicates states or traits; probably in most cases a mixture of trait and state is involved which cannot be recognized easily.
c) It is not clear whether individual differences are due to emotions or to other factors e.g., illness.

Standardized Tests

Tests that may be useful in healthy and sick old persons are derived from different areas of psychology and have different theoretical backgrounds. At least two types are used that may be applied with other methodological approaches, e.g., with ratings. These are trait/state oriented tests and neuropsychological tests.

Trait/State oriented tests are the common psychological tests to measure behavior indicating traits or states. The test most frequently used in gerontology are performance tests which measure general concentration ability and vigilance, perception, thinking and intelligence, learning and memory, and psychomotor abilities. Most tests are derived from the classical intelligence tests, such as the Wechsler Intelligence Test, which includes several verbal ability tests and tests for visual-spatial orientation. Specific tests such as the Wechsler Memory Scale are used very often as supplements to a general intelligence test. Summaries of tests for measuring age-related cognitive performance are given by Birren and Schaie (1985), Kramer and Jarvik (1979), and Miller (1980). General discussions about intelligence and other performance tests may be found in the German *Enzyklopädie der Psychologie,* specifically the volume *Intelligenz- und Leistungsdiagnostik* (Groffmann und Michel 1983); a survey of tests is given by Brickenkamp (1975).

Neuropsychological tests are methods which are sensitive to alterations of brain functions, and which for this reason are used in testing the behavioral correlatates of brain function alterations induced by diseases of the brain. Contrary to the goals of common psychological tests they do not aim to be indicators of traits and states or to be predictors of behavior or performance in specific settings such as the workplace or hospitals. Numerous tests have been developed in clinical neuropsychology. In part these are the same as those in trait or state testing. Examples for this are psychomotor tests (e. g., for reaction time), memory tests, and perception tests (e. g., the Bender Gestalt Test). Some tests refer to rather specific abilities in the area of sensory and perceptual, motor and language functions. In particular, visual-spatial items are included in batteries for detecting brain changes. The most elaborated batteries which have been used in measuring changes in elderly persons are the Halstead-Reitan Battery and the Luria-Nebraska Neuropsychological Battery (for summaries and critical comments see Goldstein 1984; Porish and Sbordone 1986; Wittling 1983). The essential difference here is that neuropsychological tests try to indicate brain functions and not the underlying traits or states. Summaries of neuropsychological tests are given by Goldstein (1984), Hamsher (1984), Lezak (1983), and Wittling (1983).

Table 8 lists performance tests which are frequently administered in patients with impaired cognitive functioning. The most well-known tests in the Federal Republic of Germany are the Nuremberg Gerontopsychological Inventory (NAI; Oswald and Fleischmann 1986) and the Syndrome Short Test (SKT; Erzigkeit 1977). The NAI is derived from the most well-known intelligence tests and other performance tests. It is specifically adapted to elderly persons and measures a broad spectrum of performance. It consists of 11 subtests, most of which are contructed according to principles of classical test theory and are well suited for old subjects. For some subtests there are parallel forms. For five subtests norms for brain-damaged patients are available. Table 9 shows the principles of the performance tests of the NAI. The SKT, on the other hand, aims at the differentiation of different grades of psychoorganic syndromes. The test contains various assessments of memory and attention. There are five parallel forms, with nine subtests each.

Table 8. Standardized tests for subjects with demential symptoms

Name	Structure	Recorded aspect	Authors
Stimulus Recognition Test (SRT)	Recognition of 10 stimuli	Short-term memory	Brink et al. (1979)
Syndrome Short Test (SKT)	9 Subtests (5 parallel forms)	Organic psychosyndrome	Erzigkeit (1977)
Philadelphia Geriatric Center Mental Status Questionnaire	Answers to 35 questions and visual counting	Dementia	Fishback (1977)
Set Test	Naming of 40 colors, animals, fruits, cities	Dementia	Isaacs and Kennie (1973)
Nuremberg Geronto-psychological Inventory (NAI)	11 Performance tests	Wide range of intellectual performance	Oswald and Fleischmann (1986)
Memory Check	Answers to 15 questions	Mental competence	Tobacyk et al. (1983)

Table 9. Performance tests of the Nuremberg Gerontopsychological Inventory (NAI)

Test	Kind	Task	Norms	Recorded aspect
Modified Trail-Making Test (ZVT)	S	Connecting numerals	55–69 Years 70–79 Years 80–96 Years Organic brain patients (OBP)	General cognitive performance speed
Maze Test G	S	Time-controlled drawing of the way to the center of a labyrinth	(see ZVT)	Visual information process and visual-motor coordination
Digit-Symbol Test G	S	Allocation of symbols to digits	(see ZVT)	Attention, visual-motor coordination
Color-Word Test	S	Reading of colorwords, colors	(see ZVT without OBP)	Interference attention
Digit Span G	M	Repeating numerals forward and backward	55–96 years	Recent memory
Word List	M	Recognition and reproduction of words	(see ZVT)	Short- and long-term remembering
Picture Test	M	Verbal reproduction of visual patterns	(see ZVT without OBP)	Performance in visual remembering
Word Pairs	M	Association of word pairs	(see ZVT without OBP)	Reproduction of associations
Figure Test	M	Recognition of geometric figures	No standard	Visual remembering (without encoding)
Sentence Test	M	Repeating given sentences	56–96 years	Recent memory (with verbal encoding)
Incidental Learning	M	Describing the practiced subtests	(see ZVT)	Attention, memory

S: speed-orientated tests; M: memory-orientated tests

Many other tests have also been proposed which discriminate between normal subjects and persons with dementia (Brouwers et al. 1984; Butters et al. 1983).

Measurements of Reactivity

The approach that aims at the measurement of reactivity examines responses to all kinds of stimuli, in particular to emotional stimuli/situations. These are explained with respect to the following characteristics:
a) elicitation of responses (perceptual, emotional, motivational, social),
b) speed and quality of adaptation processes,
c) speed and degree of habituation processes, and
d) recovery and refractory time.

Examples include the study of performance under stress (e.g., tapping under noise), performance and emotional responses under failure conditions, and emotional response to stressors (e.g., noise, sleep deprivation).

Until now the reactivity approach has been administered mainly in psychophysiology for measuring reactivity in specific physiological systems with the aim to predict susceptibility to illness. Another application is in the diagnosis of emotions. However, even in the psychology of emotions, research is only beginning (Hüppe 1987; Janke 1984; Janke and Baltissen 1979; Janke and Hüppe, in press). Stimuli/situations which have been used in old persons include: symbolic stimuli (pictures, words, sentences with emotional meaning), performance tasks (arithmetic, learning), cold pressor test, pain stimuli, noise, thermal stimuli, and isometric exercise.

The reactivity approach is also of importance outside the research on emotions. The approach may be used, in particular, in performance measurements to assess the vulnerability of the ability to achieve normal performance under nonoptimal internal and external conditions. As shown in many experiments, the vulnerability of performance to internal and external factors/stressors seems to be an important age-related individual characteristic. Reactivity measurement may be directed to all types of organismic activity (experience, expression, behavior, somatic). Thus, the approach allows the recognition of dissociations between the various levels of the organism. Dissociations, however, may be sensitive indicators of age- or illness-related changes.

One important advantage of the reactivity approach is its applicability in all subject populations, in particular in patients with dementia. Regrettably, only very few investigators have used several dependent variables in testing the reactivity to stimuli. Physiological or biochemical variables have been applied in studies with old persons. This means that almost no data on the type of emotions which have been induced are available.

Problems and Conclusions

Many problems in the psychodiagnostics of elderly patients remain unsolved. A first problem is the lack of measures which refer to the different levels of organismic activity (most measures are limited to only one level), to different methodological approaches (most are observer-rating scales), and to the various psychic functions (most refer to performance and ignore personality and emotionality). With the exception of rating scales based on observers, most methods mentioned above have not been used extensively with old persons, and even less so with elderly patients who are ill or have cognitive deficits.

A second problem lies in the kind of inferential conclusions made. It has been stated in the neuropsychological assessment literature that inferences may be based on different rationales (Lezak 1983; Wittling 1983). The usual rationale is the comparison of an individual measure with a reference group. This procedure, however, is burdened with the problem of obtaining reference groups, a problem which frequently cannot be solved. Another rationale, which seems to be a better one, is to use intraindividual comparisons. One possibility is to use premorbid measures; these, however, are rarely available. A promising strategy is the use of pathognomic signs, for example, speech disturbances. Pathognomic signs can be used only for basic functions which are present in every normal person. The disadvantage of this approach is that frequently no quantification of degree is possible.

References

Albert MS, Stefford JL (1986) CT-scan and neuropsychological relationship in age and dementia. In: Goldstein G, Tarter RT (eds) Advances in clinical neuropsychology, vol 3. Plenum, New York, pp 31–53

Bayles KA (1982) Language function in senile dementia. Brain Lang 16: 265

Beck AT, Ward CH, Mendelson M, Mock J, Erbaugh J (1961) An inventory for measuring depression. Arch Gen Psychiatry 4: 561–571

Benson F (1979) Neurologic correlates of anomia. In: Whitaker H, Whitaker HA (eds) Studies in neurolinguistics, vol 4. Academic Press, New York, pp 293–328

Birren JE, Schaie KW (1985) Handbook of psychology of aging, 2nd edn. Van Nostrand Reinhold, New York

Brickenkamp R (1975) Handbuch psychologischer und pädagogischer Tests. Hogrefe, Göttingen

Brink TL, Bryant J, Catalano ML, Janakes C, Oliveira C (1979) Senile confusion: assessment with a new stimulus recognition test. J Am Geriatr Soc 27: 126–129

Brouwers P, Cox C, Martin A, Chase T, Fedio P (1984) Differential perceptual-spatial impairment in Huntington's and Alzheimer's dementias. Archiv Neurol 41: 1073–1076

Burdock EI, Hardesty AS, Hakerem G, Zubin J (1960) A ward behavior rating scale for mental hospital patients. J Clin Psychol 15: 246–247

Butters N, Albert MS, Sax DS, Miliotis P, Nagode J, Sterste A (1983) The effect of verbal mediators on the pictorial memory of brain-damaged patients. Neuropsychologia 21: 307–323

Cummings JL (1986) Subcortical dementia: an analysis of the contributions of subcortical brain structures to human thought and emotion. Br J Psychiatry 149: 682–697

Cummings JL, Benson DF (1983) Dementia. A clinical approach. Butterworth, Boston

Cummings JL, Benson DF (1984) Subcortical dementia: review of an emerging concept. Arch Neurol 41: 874–879

Cummings JL, Benson DF (1986) Dementia of the Alzheimer type. An inventory of diagnostic clinical features. J Am Geriatr Soc 34: 12–19

Debus G, Dietsch P, Janke W (1978) Die Wirkung von Carpipramin – Ergebnisse der Eigenschaftswörterliste, des Strukturierten Interviews und der Zustandsbeurteilung durch den Arzt. In: Boeters U, Ihm P, Janke W (eds) Carpipramin. Eine multizentrische Doppelblindstudie. Aulendorf, Bad Buchau, pp 21–45

Derogatis CR (1977) SCL-90. Administration, scoring & procedures. Manual-I for the R(evised) version and other instruments of the psychopathology rating scale series. John Hopkins University School of Medicine, Baltimore

Ekman P, Friesen WV (1972) Hand movements. J Commun 22: 353–374

Ellgring H (1977) Kommunikatives Verhalten im Verlauf depressiver Erkrankungen. In: Tack WH (ed) Bericht über den 30. Kongreß der Deutschen Gesellschaft für Psychologie in Regensburg 1976, Vol 2. Hogrefe, Göttingen, pp 190–192

Ellgring H, Ploog D (1984) Sozialkommunikatives Verhalten in klinischer Perspektive. In: Bente D, Coper H, Kanowski S (ed) Hirnorganische Psychosyndrome im Alter. Springer, Berlin Heidelberg New York, pp 217–243

Erzigkeit H (1977) Manual zum Syndrom-Kurztest Formen A-E. Vless, Vaterstetten

Fahrenberg J, Selg H, Hampel R (1984). Das Freiburger Persönlichkeitsinventar (FPI-R). Hogrefe, Göttingen

Fishback DB (1977) Mental status questionnaire for organic brain syndrome, with a new visual counting test. J Am Geriatr Soc 25: 167–170

Folstein MF, Folstein SE, McHugh PR (1975) "Mini-Mental State": a practical method for grading the cognitive state of patients for the clinician. J Psychiatr Res 12: 189–198

Freedman N (1972) The analysis of movement behavior during the clinical interview. In: Siegman AW, Pope B (eds) Studies in dyadic communication. Pergamon, New York, pp 153–175

Goga JA, Hambacher WO (1977) Psychologic and behavioral assessment of geriatric patients: a review. J Am Geriatr Soc 25: 232–237

Groffman KJ, Michel L (1983) Enzyklopädie der Psychologie, vol II (2): Intelligenz- und Leistungsdiagnostik. Hogrefe, Göttingen

Goldstein G (1984) Comprehensive neuropsychological assessment batteries. In: Goldstein G, Hersen M (eds) Handbook of psychological assessment. Pergamon, New York, pp 181–210

Gurland B, Golden RR, Teresi JA, Challop J (1984) The SHORT-CARE: an efficient instrument for the assessment of depression, dementia and disability. J Gerontol 39: 166–169
Hamilton M (1986) Psychometric scales for dementia. Gerontology 32: 30–32
Hamsher K deS (1984) Specialized neuropsychological assessment methods. In: Goldstein G, Hersen M (eds) Handbook of psychological assessment. Pergamon, New York, pp 235–256
Hautzinger M (1984) Ein Fragebogen zur Erfassung psychischer und somatischer Beschwerden bei älteren Menschen. Z Gerontol 17: 223–226
Hersch EL (1979) Development and application of the extended scale for dementia. J Am Geriatr Soc 27: 348–354
Hersch EL, Kral VA, Palmer RB (1978) Clinical value of the London Psychogeriatric Rating Scale. J Am Geriatr Soc 26: 348–354
Hoffmann GMA, Gouze JC, Mendlewicz J (1985) Speech pause time as a method for the evaluation of psychomotor retardation in depressive illness. Br J Psychiatry 146: 535–538
Hughes CP, Berg L, Danziger WL, Coben LA, Martin RL (1982) A new clinical scale for the staging of dementia. Br J Psychiatry 140: 566–572
Hüppe M (1987) Emotionsausdruck im Alter: Experimentelle Untersuchungen zur Bedeutung von Gestik und Sprechaktivität als Emotionsindikatoren bei alten Frauen. Dissertation, Julius-Maximilians-University, Würzburg
Isaacs B, Kennie AT (1973) The Set Test as an aid to the detection of dementia in old people. Br J Psychiatry 123: 467–470
Janke W (1984) Emotionalität. In: Oswald WD, Herrmann WM, Kanowski S, Lehr U, Thomae H (eds) Gerontologie. Kohlhammer, Stuttgart, pp 78–95
Janke W, Baltissen R (1979) Critical considerations on methods of assessing emotional and motivational characteristics of old persons. In: Hoffmeister F, Mueller C, Krause HP (eds) Brain function in old age. Evaluation of changes and disorders. Springer, Berlin Heidelberg New York, pp 214–227. (Bayer symposium, vol 7)
Janke W, Debus G (1978) Die Eigenschaftswörterliste. Hogrefe, Göttingen
Janke W, Hüppe M (in press) Emotionalität bei alten Personen. In: Scherer KR (ed) Enzyklopädie der Psychologie, vol. IV (3): Psychologie der Emotion. Hogrefe, Göttingen
Janke W, Debus G, Hüppe M (1984) Die Selbstbeschreibungsform der Eigenschaftswörterliste (EWL 60-S) nach Janke und Debus. Psychologisches Institut I, Würzburg
Janke W, Debus G, Hüppe M (1987) Die Eigenschaftswörterliste zur Fremdbeurteilung des Befindens (EWL 60-F). Psychologisches Institut I, Würzburg
Katzman R, Brown T, Fuld P, Peck A, Schechter R, Schimmel H (1983) Validation of a short orientation-memory-concentration test of cognitive impairment. Am J Psychiatry 140: 734–739
Kazniak A (1986) The neuropsychology of dementia. In: Grant I, Adams K (eds) Neuropsychological assessment of neuropsychiatric disorders. Oxford University Press, New York, pp 172–220
Klos T, Ellgring H (1985) Sprechgeschwindigkeit und Sprechpausen von Depressiven. In: Hautzinger M, Staunz R (eds) Psychologische Aspekte depressiver Störungen. Roderer, Regensburg, pp 4–26
Kochansky GE (1979) Psychiatric rating scales for assessing psychopathology in the elderly: a critical review. In: Raskin A, Jarvik LF (eds) Psychiatric symptoms and cognitive loss in the elderly. Wiley, New York, pp 125–156
Kramer NA, Jarvik LF (1979) Assessment of intellectual changes in the elderly. In: Raskin A, Jarvik LF (eds) Psychiatric symptoms and cognitive loss in the elderly. Wiley, New York, pp 221–271
La Rue, D'Elia, Clark E, Spar J, Jarvik L (1986) Clinical tests of memory in dementia, depression and healthy aging. Psychology and Aging. 1: 69–77
Laux L, Glanzmann P, Schaffner P, Spielberger CD (1981) Das State-Trait-Angstinventar. Theoretische Grundlagen und Handanweisung. Beltz, Weinheim
Lawson JS, Rodenburg M, Dykes JA (1977) A dementia rating scale for use with psychogeriatric patients. J Gerontol 32: 153–159
Lehmann E (1984) Klinische und psychologische Skalen zur Erfassung „gewünschter und unerwünschter Arzneimittelwirkungen bei Hirnleistungsstörungen". Beltz, Weinheim
Lezak MD (1983) Neuropsychological assessment, 2nd edn. Oxford University Press, New York
Maurer K, Dierks T (1987) Brain mapping – Topographiedarstellung des EEG und der evozierten Potentiale in Psychiatrie und Neurologie. Z. EEG-EMG 18: 4–12
McNair DM, Lorr M, Droppleman LF (1971) Eits manual for the profile of mood states. Educational and Industrial Testing Service, San Diego

Miller E (1980) Cognitive assessments in older adult. In: Birren JE, Sloane RE (eds) Handbook of mental health and aging. Prentice-Hall, Englewood Cliffs: pp 520–536

Neugarten BL, Havighurst RJ, Tobin SS (1961) The measurement of life satisfaction. J Gerontol 16: 134–143

Orsini DL, van Gorp WG, Borne KB (1988) The neuropsyogy casebook. Springer, Berlin Heidelberg New York

Oswald WD (1979) Psychometrische Verfahren und Fragebogen für gerontopsychologische Untersuchungen. Z Gerontol 12: 341–350

Oswald WD, Fleischmann UM (1985) Psychometrics in aging and dementia. Advances in gerontopsychological assessments. Arch Gerontol Geriatr 4: 299–309

Oswald WD, Fleischmann UM (1986) Nürnberger-Alters-Inventar. NAI. Psychologisches Institut, Erlangen–Nürnberg

Overall JE, Gorham DR (1962) The Brief Psychiatric Rating Scale (BPRS). Psychol Rep 10: 799–812

Plutchik R, Conte H, Lieberman M, Bakur M, Grossman J, Lehmann N (1970) Reliability and validity of a scale for assessing the functioning of geriatric patients. J Am Geria Soc 18: 419–500

Pope B, Blass T, Siegman AW, Raher J (1970) Anxiety and depression in speech. J Consult Clin Psychol 35: 128–133

Porish AD, Sbordone RJ (1986) The Luria-Nebraska Neuropsychological Battery. In: Goldstein G, Tarter RT (eds) Advances in clinical neuropsychology, vol 3. Plenum, New York, pp 291–316

Radloff LS (1977) The CES-D scale: a self-report depression scale for research in the general population. J Appl Psychol Meas 1: 385–401

Reisberg B, Ferris SH, DeLeon MJ, Crook T (1982) The Global Deterioration Scale for assessment of primary degenerative dementia. Am J Psychiatry 139: 1136–1139

Reisberg B, Ferris SH, DeLeon MJ (1985) Senile dementia of the Alzheimer type: diagnostic and differential diagnostic features with special reference to functional assessment staging. In: Traber J, Gispen WH, Willem H (eds) Senile dementia of the Alzheimer type. Springer, Berlin Heidelberg New York, pp 18–37 (Advances in applied neurological sciences, vol 2)

Rosen WG, Mohs RC, Davis KL (1984) A new rating scale for Alzheimer's disease. Am J Psychiatry 141: 1356–1360

Salzman C, Kochansky GE, Shader RI (1972) Rating scales for geriatric psychopharmacology: a review. Psychopharmacol Bull 8: 3–50

Shader RJ, Harmatz JS, Salzman C (1974) A new scale for clinical assessment in geriatric populations: Sandoz Clinical Assessment Geriatric (SCAG). J Am Geriatr Soc 22: 107–113

Spielberger CD, Gorsuch RL, Lushene RE (1970) STAI. Manual for the State-Trait-Anxiety Inventory. Consulting Psychologists, Palo Alto CA

Tobacyk J, Dixon JC, Dixon JS (1983) Two brief measures for assessing mental competence in the elderly. J Pers Assess 47: 648–655

Ulrich G (1981) Videoanalyse depressiver Verhaltensaspekte. Enke, Stuttgart

von Zerssen D (1976a) Die Befindlichkeits-Skala (Bf-S). Beltz, Weinheim

von Zerssen D (1976b) Depressivitäts-Skala (D-S). Beltz, Weinheim

Wiendieck G (1970) Entwicklung einer Skala zur Messung der Lebenszufriedenheit im höheren Lebensalter. Z Gerontol 3: 215–224

Wittling WW (1983) Neuropsychologische Diagnostik. In: Groffmann KJ, Michel L (eds) Enzyklopädie der Psychologie, vol II (4): Verhaltensdiagnostik. Hogrefe, Göttingen, pp 193–335

Zuckerman M, Lubin B (1965) Manual for the Multiple Affect Adjective Checklist. Educational and Industrial Testing Service, San Diego

Zung WWK (1965) A self-rating depression scale. Arch Gen Psychiatry 12: 63–70

Zung WWK (1976) SAS. Self-rating Anxiety Scale. In: Guy W (ed) ECDEU Assessment manual for psychopharmacology. Rockville, Maryland, pp 337–340

The SKT – A Short Cognitive Performance Test as an Instrument for the Assessment of Clinical Efficacy of Cognition Enhancers

H. Erzigkeit

One of the main issues in clinical psychology deals with the documentation and control of therapeutic effects. Especially if we try to measure of the effects of drugs expected to influence cognitive performance, we sometimes find conditions that restrict the application of psychometric tests as they exist in general psychology.

When in the early 1970s we started to work on problems concerning the measurement of the severity of cerebral disturbances caused by organic brain diseases, many psychological tests were already available. So we applied some of them in our daily routine and empirical studies. The patients we tested at the Neurological and Psychiatric Hospital of the University of Erlangen suffered from mildest to severest grades of almost all possible organic mental disorders.

Some theoretical and practical problems were bound to emerge because most of the tests available were not constructed and evaluated for patients with moderate or severe disturbances in cognitive performance. Many tests, for example, paper-and-pencil tests, were too difficult to handle; tremor, disturbed motor abilities or simply forgetting a pair of spectacles sometimes made it impossible to test a patient.

To imagine the situation, one should keep in mind that the more a "subject" turns into a "patient", certain variables – which are not of practical relevance in general psychology – become more and more important. For example, it is quite obvious that patients suffering from organic brain syndromes or dementia in general are less motivated to pass psychological tests or to do their very best to attain good results. Without additional assumptions the differences between patients with mild and severe degrees of dementia cannot be compared in the sense of a psychological test.

In my opinion diagnoses of patients suffering from severe forms of dementia can be classified by neurological variables. Rating scales are adequate instruments to estimate the severity of the dementia or its course. Psychological tests are usually not applicable. Personality factors are not variables which sufficiently describe the severity of the diagnoses because – concerning the clinical relevance – in disturbances of this degree, neurological symptoms are predominant and the extreme cognitive deficits seem to exist almost independently of interpersonal differences.

We find quite a different situation when testing patients suffering only from mild to moderate degrees of cognitive disturbances. Interindividual differences in, for example, intelligence, education or other variables still determine the whole personality more than the disease, so interpersonal differences obviously should be controlled in order to avoid artificial results when estimating the severity of the disturbance. A young, intelligent, and well-educated patient with only mild to moderate cognitive

Bergener, Reisberg (Eds.)
Diagnosis and Treatment
of Senile Dementia
© Springer-Verlag Berlin Heidelberg 1989

disturbances, for instance, will still be able to perform memory tasks as well as or even better than an elderly healthy person with less education and lower intelligence (Erzigkeit 1977, 1986b).

And it is also a well-known fact that the clinical manifestations of a patient – let us say a university graduate or a top manager who is well educated and has enjoyed professional success – might reveal how difficult differential diagnoses and estimation of cognitive disturbances can be and how easily young assistants and psychologists can be fooled. These patients know how to behave, how to care for themselves and play their role, and they often have learned to converse using the very best "small talk" in order to appear friendly, polite and well. In other words they have learned to hide symptoms like deficits in memory and attention or their inability to learn new things. Rather often we diagnosed these mildly to moderately disturbed patients as suffering from a dementia following or combined with a history of alcohol abuse.

As these are common problems with which every psychiatrist or psychologist is familiar, it does not seem to be necessary to discuss further theoretical consequences for the construction of a test that is to be applicable and reliable. When deciding which variables ought to be selected as indicators for severity we assume that clinical experience, with reference to diagnostic criteria of organic mental disorders as described in the *Diagnostic and Statistical Manual of Mental Disorders* (DSM-III R), *International Classification of Diseases* (ICD 9) or standard literature in psychiatry, points to deficits in memory and attention as the general key symptoms or indicators of the described diseases. Attention here especially means aspects of quality and speed of information processing. Other variables of personality and cognitive performance obviously also determine the clinical picture.

Although it is self-evident, it should be mentioned in this context that for medical diagnoses in most cases it is not necessary to use psychometric tests and to measure the degrees of the disturbances. Only if there is an interest in documenting the course of the disease – for example, to assess the effects of a specific treatment – will it be necessary to use tests that measure variables which are indicators of the severity of the impairment. Thus far the clinical aspects which were the basic assumptions leading to the construction of the SKT have been considered.

In consequence we had to develop a test system on the basis of evaluated subtests selected from various sources of tests used in general psychology or psychiatry and adapt them for clinical application. That meant loosening the rather strict requirements that formalize psychological test procedures and adapting the test materials to the abilities of patients suffering from different forms of dementia and to the special test situation we are often confronted with when testing patients in terms of clinical psychology, neurology, or psychiatry, and in the general practioner's routine. Applicability, that is, easy handling for both the patient and the physician, psychologist, or nurse who administers the test is especially to be taken into consideration.

This also implicates adapting the instructions as well as the efforts of the psychologist or physician to motivate the patient to do his very best to solve the test problems. Here we definitely deviate from the general standards of psychology testing: as a rule test instructions, for example, have to be given in a standardized from (Michel 1964, APA 1985).

In order to avoid measuring artefacts caused, for instance, by impaired motor or visual abilities the test materials simply must be adapted to the patients' abilities.

It should be explained why we chose test materials for the SKT that remind us of children toys. In pretests we discovered that patients refused tests less often when the "attractiveness" of the material was high. The more the test material and the reinforcing instructions created a challenging game-type situation that required cognitive efforts, without acquiring the neutral or aloof character of a typical psychological performance or intelligence test situation, the more it was accepted by our patients, and as could be proved, the reliability and validity of the test scores was higher (Lehrl and Erzigkeit 1977; Kirkilonis 1978, Fuchs 1979).

The results of clinical studies and data of reliability and validity can be found in the latest *Manual of the SKT* published in 1986. More than 8000 examinations were analyzed, mainly obtained in clinical efficacy studies with nootropic drugs or cognition enhancers (Erzigkeit 1986 a + b). Several factor analyses, for example, by Arnold (Arnold 1983, Erzigkeit 1986) have shown that the SKT mainly measures two factors which can be termed memory and attention in the sense of information processing speed.

Clinical studies have proven the SKT to be sufficiently sensitive to assess the treatment effects of so-called nootropic drugs. The ability to measure or represent treatment effects also implicates aspects of the validity and reliability of the SKT. Of course we have also computed validity coefficients, for example, correlations with other psychometric tests which were first published by Fuchs and Arnold (Fuchs 1979; Arnold 1983), but as mentioned already, these correlations with elaborated psychometric tests could only be obtained in studies with patients suffering from

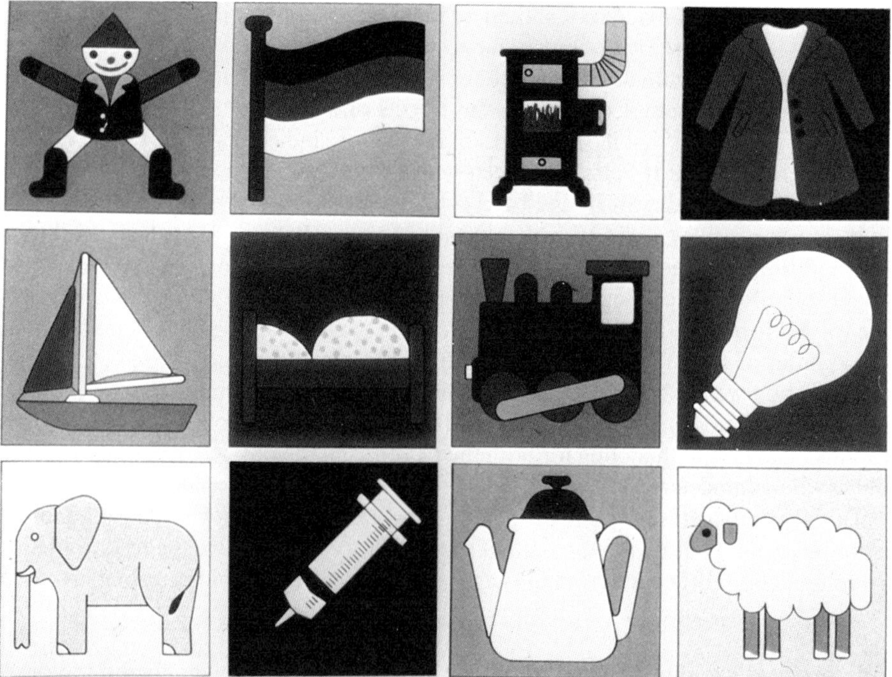

Fig. 1. Tableau used in the SKT to measure memory functions

milder disturbances of cognitive performance due to organic brain syndromes or dementia. The latest data are published by Schmage et al. in this volume.

All the computed values indicating satisfactory reliability and validity of the SKT are only valid for German-speaking patients. The practicability of the SKT should be ascertained when testing patients whose native language is not German. In this context it should be mentioned that at present the SKT is being implemented into different drug trials in the United States in order to evaluate its applicability and also to ascertain its reliability and validity. In German studies Cronbach alphas for the estimation of reliability mostly exceed values of 0.86 (Erzigkeit 1986b).

In the following the SKT test procedure is described; the figures should give an impression of the materials used.

Figure 1 shows the first subtest. The patient is asked to name 12 objects as fast as possible and to try to keep them in mind. The time needed to perform this task in seconds is the raw score of subtest I. The tableau is turned over immediately after the last object has been named.

The patient is then asked to recall the named objects. The number of objects correctly recalled within 60 s gives the raw score of subtest II as a measure of

---

Zur Erfassung von Aufmerksamkeits- und Gedächtnisstörungen

Name: _____________________ Geburtsdatum: __________ Datum: __________

Beruf: _____________________ Alter: __________ Uhrzeit: __________

Diagnose: _____________________ IQ-Gruppe: __________

Bemerkungen: _____________________

Versuchsleiter: _____________________

SUBTESTS (Höchstzeit 60 Sekunden)				Rohpunkte	Wer.-punkte*	Konfabu-lationen
I Gegenstände benennen				Sekunden		
II Gegenstände unmittelbar reproduzieren				Fehlende		

Genannte Gegenstände bitte ankreuzen:

Rübe	Fahne	Ofen	Kuh
Schiff	Bett	Lok	Kreuz
Kanne	Spritze	Engel	Schaf

Gegenstände bitte nochmals 5 Sekunden zeigen

		Rohpunkte	Wer.-punkte*	Konfabu-lationen
III Zahlen lesen		Sekunden		
IV Zahlen ordnen		Sekunden		
V Zahlen zurücklegen		Sekunden		
VI Symbole zählen　✳ ★ ☐ °44		Sekunden		
VII Interferenz　ABAB　Richtige Folge: BABBABAABBABABABAAB BBABABAAABABBABAB		Sekunden		
VIII Gegenstände mittelbar reproduzieren		Fehlende		

Genannte Gegenstände bitte ankreuzen:

Rübe	Fahne	Ofen	Kuh
Schiff	Bett	Lok	Kreuz
Kanne	Spritze	Engel	Schaf

IX Gegenstände wiedererkennen

Genannte Gegenstände bitte ankreuzen:

Rübe	Fahne	Ofen	Kuh
Schiff	Bett	Lok	Kreuz
Kanne	Spritze	Engel	Schaf

Fehlende

Gesamtpunkte

*siehe Normentabelle im Manual

© 1977 Copyright by -Vless- Verlagsgesellschaft m.b.H., Vaterstetten - München

Fig. 2. Test schedule of the SKT, Form A. The patient's personal data is noted, the tests described, and test scores recorded (German version)

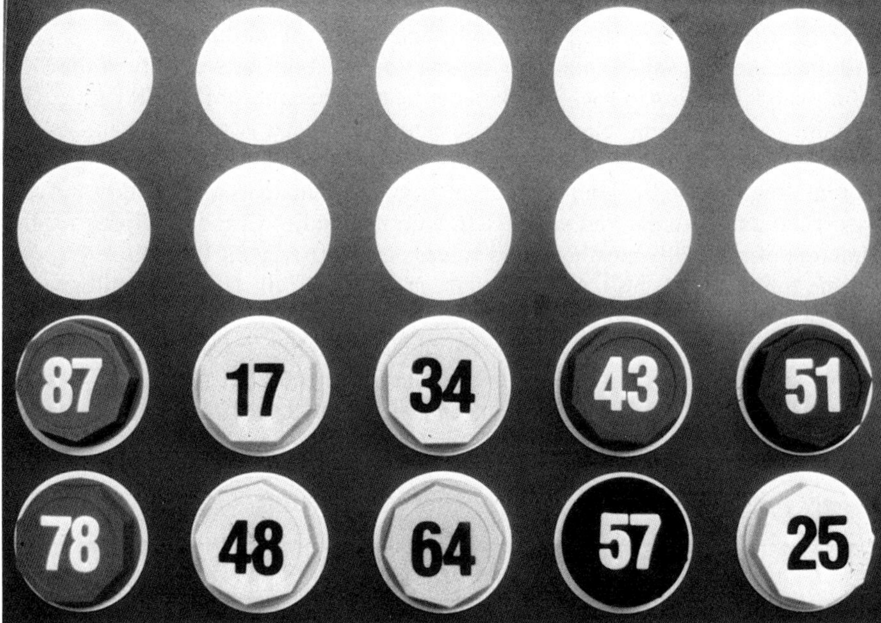

Fig. 3. Tableau for subtests III – V of the SKT

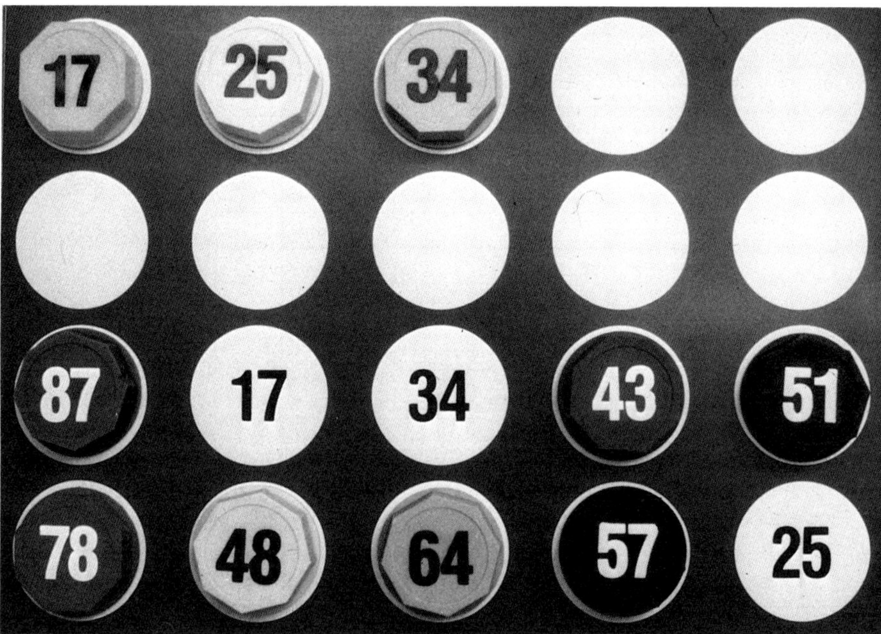

Fig. 4. Subtest IV of the SKT. Arranging numbers into a rank order

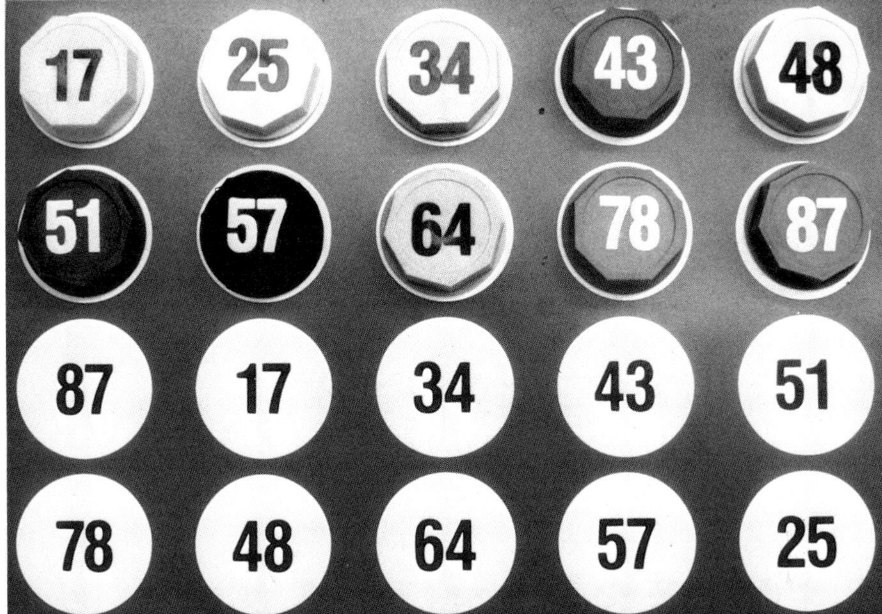

Fig. 5. The starting position of subtest V of the SKT. Replacing numbers to their original position (subtest V).

immediate recall. Figure 2 shows the schedule for the registration of the test results. After that the tableau which was shown in the beginning (Fig. 1) is presented to the patient again for a short learning-phase which gives him/her another chance to commit the 12 objects to memory.

Next, the patient has to read numbers (Fig. 3) as quickly as possible. The registered time in seconds is the raw score of subtest III. After that the patient is to try to arrange these numbers into a rank order (Fig. 4) and then put them back into their original order (Fig. 5).

For the next subtest the patient has to count symbols; Fig. 6 shows Form A of the SKT in which the patient is asked to count the squares. In subtest VII the patient is asked to read letters. Figure 7 again shows the tableau from Form A of the SKT with the capital letters A and B. This subtest is part of a group of well-known cognitive interference tests which were described by R. B. Cattell in 1946 and 1949 to measure cognitive rigidity. The patient is asked to name the letter A when he reads a B and to call it B when actually there is an A to be read. This serves to assess cognitive flexibility and aspects of concentration which are very sensitive even to mild disturbances due to organic brain diseases like dementia.

The patient is then asked again to recall the objects. The number of correct items named within 60 s is the base for subtest VIII which measures an aspect of memory performance that can be understood as delayed recall after distractions.

Finally, 48 objects are presented to the patient (Fig. 8). The last subtest serves to assess recognition, a rather stable, perhaps the most steady memory function.

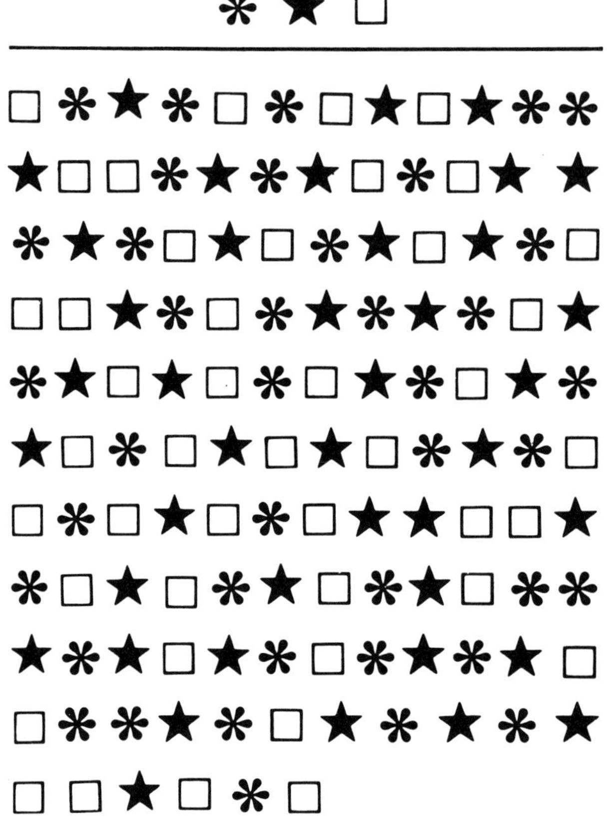

Fig. 6. Tableau for subtest VI of the SKT. Counting symbols

ABBABA

ABAABABBAABABABBA
AABABABBBABAABABA

Fig. 7. Tableau for subtest VII of the SKT. Interference test to measure cognitive rigidity

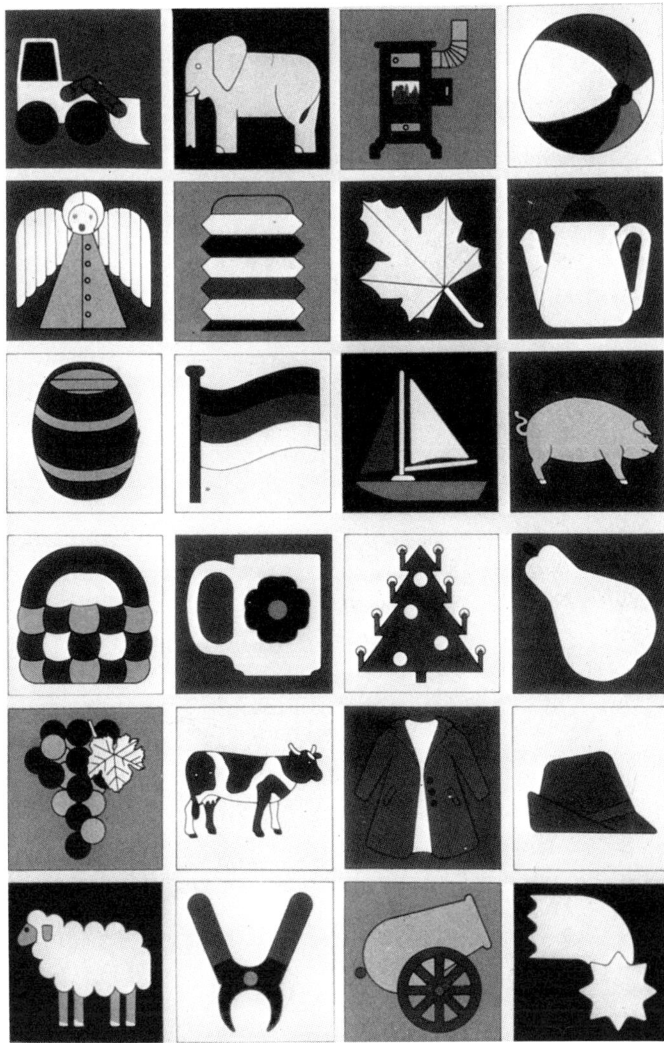

Fig. 8. Tableau for subtest IX of the SKT. Measurement of recognition

In general, the patients have exactly 60 s to pass the memory tests; for each of the other tests 60 s are the maximum: that means, if a patient needs only 10–15 s to pass a subtest he will immediately proceed to the next one. Generally, the SKT takes 10–15 min including instructions and transforming the raw scores into norm values. To do the latter, the physician or psychologist simply has to refer to the norm value tables which are available for three different intelligence and four different age groups.

The summarized score of the nine subtests serves to estimate the severity of a disturbance in terms of clinically orientated descriptions of the magnitude of organic

Fig. 9. Sample SKT data documentation of a clinical course. The patient's personal data are recorded, as are the scores of tests taken on various days (German version)

brain diseases. A total score ranging from 9 to 13 points, for example, indicates a mild organic brain syndrome and one between 14 to 18 is symptomatic of – in clinical terms – moderate disturbances due to organic brain syndromes or dementia.

Using the parallel forms of the SKT – five parallel forms called Forms A–E are available – the course of the disease can be registered in a follow-up diagram. This is only a comfortable way of presenting the test results; Figure 9, for example, shows a follow-up diagram of a patient after a severe contusio cerebri and documents the clinical course using data obtained with the SKT.

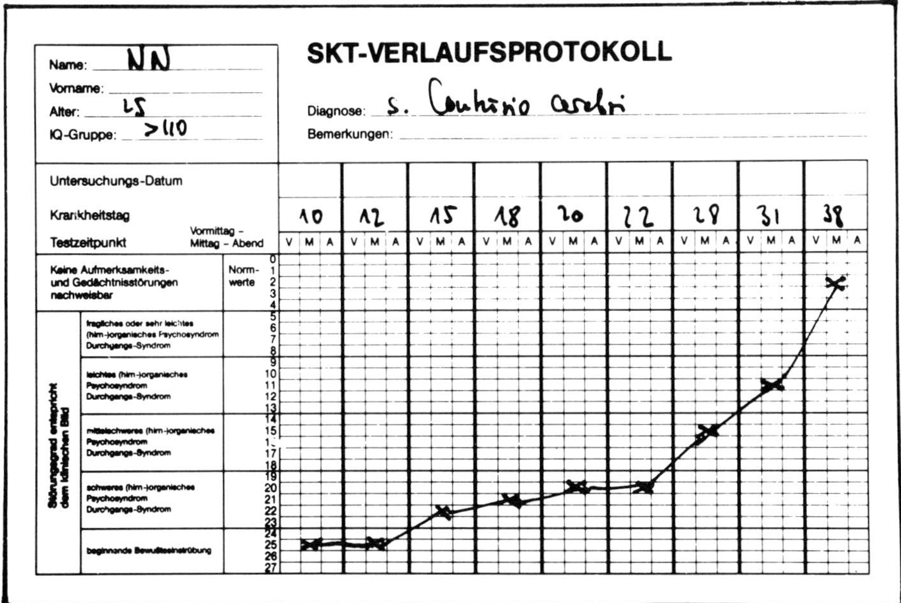

Fig. 10

Parallel test forms are useful if it is necessary to avoid learning effects. Controlling learning or avoiding ceiling effects in clinical trials will certainly be more important if the tested patients only suffer from milder disturbances. In moderate and especially in severe states of dementia learning effects will not be expected to the extent that parallel tests would be required.

The SKT was not originally intended to be used as a diagnostic instrument. However, it may contribute to the total clinical evaluation of patients suffering from dementia.

References

APA (1985) Standards for educational and psychological testing. American Psychological Association, Inc. Washington DC

Arnold KR (1983) Untersuchungen zu Aspekten der Normierung, Reliabilität und Validität eines Testsystems zur Erfassung von Aufmerksamkeits- und Gedächtnisstörungen. Dissertation, Friedrich Alexander University, Erlangen–Nürnberg

Cattell RB, Tiner L (1946) The varieties of structural rigidity. J Pers 17, p 321–341

Cattell RB (1946) The riddle of perseveration I and II. J Pers 14, p 229–267

Erzigkeit H, Lehrl S, Blaha L, Heerklotz B (1979) Messung und Meßverfahren in der Psychopathologie. Vless, Vaterstetten–München

Erzigkeit H (1977) Manual zum SKT. Formen A–E – vorläufiges Manual –. Vless, Vaterstetten – München

Erzigkeit H (1986a) Der SKT zur Beurteilung therapeutischer Effekte nootroper Substanzen. Proceedings of the 3rd symposium on nootropics 3.–5. March 1986, Dresden

Erzigkeit H (1986b) Manual zum SKT 2. neu bearbeitete Auflage. Vless, Ebersberg
Fuchs HH (1979) Validierungsuntersuchungen zum SKT. Dissertation, Friedrich Alexander University, Erlangen–Nürnberg
Kirkilonis T (1978) Empirische Untersuchung über die Anwendbarkeit psychopathometrischer Verfahren in der ärztlichen Allgemeinpraxis. Dissertation, School of Medicine, Friedrich Alexander University, Erlangen–Nürnberg
Lehrl S, Erzigkeit H (1977) Psychopathometrische Verfahren bei der Prüfung von Psychopharmaka. Zur Frage der Rentabilitätserhöhung. Pharmacopsychiatry 12: 25–37
Michel L (1969) Allgemeine Grundlagen psychometrischer Tests. In: Heiss R (ed) Handbuch der Psychologie, vol 6. Hogrefe, Göttingen

Basic Clinical and Diagnostic Characteristics of Senile Dementia

Early Diagnosis of Dementias

A. Guterman, and C. Eisdorfer

Dementia, from the Latin demens, meaning "out of one's mind" is not a single disease entity, but rather a syndrome that may be seen in over 60 different disease states (Haase 1977; Smith and Kiloh 1981). As a syndrome, it currently affects 15% of the elderly in the United States, with an estimated three million cases in 1980 alone. With the "graying" of the population, the importance of the syndrome increases. By the year 2000, it is estimated that there will be nearly 4 million persons with dementia in the United States. Of the nearly 1.5 million persons in American nursing homes, 58% suffer from one or another form of dementia, at a cost of $ 12 billion a year (Maxmen 1986). Added to the economic and social implications of such a syndrome is the immeasurable suffering, both physical and emotional, that families and caregivers as well as the demented patients themselves experience from such a disorder.

This presentation will outline the approach that we at the University of Miami take in the early diagnosis of dementia. We will also review certain salient points in the differential diagnosis of the dementias in general and dementia of the Alzheimer type (DAT, primary neuronal degeneration) in particular.

The first step in the early diagnosis of dementia is one of definition. While the effect that a misdiagnosis might have on a patient and his family can easily be appreciated, the catastrophic impact of being inappropriately diagnosed as demented is often overlooked.

Dementia is typically progressive with broad-based intellectual decline in a number of cognitive domains. The process of a dementia is diffuse in nature and the intellectual decline the result of disease in the cerebral hemispheres, in particular in the cerebral cortex and hippocampus. The amount of cerebral hemisphere involved is related to the degree of dementia.

The American Psychiatric Association's *Diagnostic and Statistical Manual of Mental Disorders,* 3rd edition revised (DSM-III-R) (APA 1987) shows the broad range of areas of impairment necessary before a diagnosis of dementia can be made (Table 1). The loss of cognitive functions must compromise or impair the patient's ability to adapt to the environment, resulting in interference with social and/or occupational functioning. Cognition is not a solitary process. It refers to an array of skills and competencies which define the range of abilities or inabilities to adapt to one's environment (Cohen and Eisdorfer 1979).

Impairment in memory is a prerequisite (Table 1). The initial memory loss is for recent events, while events and details of the past are not only retained, but frequently

Bergener, Reisberg (Eds.)
Diagnosis and Treatment
of Senile Dementia
© Springer-Verlag Berlin Heidelberg 1989

Table 1. Criteria for the diagnosis and severity of dementia

Diagnostic criteria
A. Demonstrable evidence of impairment in short- and long-term memory. Impairment in short-term memory (inability to learn new information) may be indicated by inability to remember three objects after 5 min. Long-term memory impairment (inability to remember information that was known in the past) may be indicated by inability to remember past personal information (e.g., what happened yesterday, birthplace, occupation) or facts of common knowledge (e.g., past presidents, well-known dates)
B. At least one of the following:
   1. Impairment in abstract thinking, as indicated by inability to find similarities and differences between related words, difficulty in defining words and concepts, and other similar tasks
   2. Impaired judgement, as indicated by inability to make reasonable plans to deal with interpersonal, family, and job-related problems and issues
   3. Other disturbances of higher cortical function, such as aphasia (disorder of language), apraxia (inability to carry out motor activities despite intact comprehension and motor function), agnosia (failure to recognize objects despite intact sensory function), and "constructional difficulty" (e.g., inability to copy three-dimensional figures, assemble blocks, or arrange sticks in specific designs)
   4. Personality change, i.e., alteration or accentuation or premorbid traits
C. The disturbance in and B significantly interferes with work or usual social activities or relationships with others
D. Not occurring exclusively during the course of delirium
E. Either (1) or (2):
   1. There is evidence from history, physical examination, or laboratory tests of a specific organic factor (or factors) judged to be etiologically related to the disturbance
   2. In the absence of such evidence, an etiologic organic factor can be presumed if the disturbance cannot be accounted for by any nonorganic mental disorder, e.g., major depression accounting for cognitive impairment

Severity criteria
Mild: Although work or social activities are significantly impaired, the capacity for independent living remains, with adequat personal hygiene and relatively intact judgment
Moderate: Independent living is hazardous and some degree of supervision is necessary.
Severe: Activities of daily living are so impaired that continual supervision is required, e.g., unable to maintain minimal personal hygiene, largely incoherent, or mute

dwelled upon. In the early stages the memory impairment is commonly dismissed as part of the normal aging process. Frequently the recent memory loss is preceded by a decrease in attention span, increased distractibility, and irritability. In the early stages, diurnal changes in memory are usually absent. We find that starting with a short biography of the patient permits testing of remote memory first, including address, date of birth (can be used with orientation to year to test patient's calculations, e.g., "If you were born in 1903 and this is 1988, how old are you?", school, service record (dates of entering/leaving service, presidents during these times appear to be affectively laden memories). As the dementia progresses learning for both visual and verbal material is impaired. Finally, the patient develops the inability to use cues to develop compensatory strategies.

Impairment in abstraction of thought can be seen (Table 1). This is traditionally tested using similarities/differences and abstraction of proverbs. The use of proverbs can be at times restricted by the patient's cultural, ethnic, and educational background. For this reason tests of absurdities are frequently useful (e. g., the patient is asked what, if anything, is absurd/incorrect with a statement such as "every morning we get six eggs from my father's rooster.").

When judgement is tested, one needs to proceed beyond the frequently used questions "what should you do if you find a letter with a stamp on the sidewalk." Evidence of poor impulse control, inappropriate jocularity (witzelsucht) – a sign of frontal lobe dysfunction – should be looked for. As impairment in judgement about appropriateness of behavior progresses, speech may become crude/obscene (consider however educational, socioeconomic status), genitals/breasts may be exposed in public). Paul Hoch (1972) suggests that in addition to the impairment of judgement, many patients with dementia may manifest hypersuggestibility and hence can unfortunately be manipulated by others in their environment. In very advanced and extreme cases, the judgement of the demented patient may be below that of a child (Hoch 1972).

Higher cortical function impairments in dementia generally are seen in the areas of aphasia, agnosia, and apraxia. Aphasia in the demented patient is frequently of a mixed receptive/expressive type. Speech tends to become stereotyped, slow, vague, and replete with details that are irrelevant. When this is coupled with problems in attention/concentration, the result is the inability to follow conversations or the inability to distinguish the trivial from the important. Words are frequently missed and chosen more by sound than by meaning. Appell et al. (1982) note that the inability to generate ideas in a given category is seen first, followed by word-finding difficulties, and lastly increased impairment of comprehension. The ability to read aloud and to repeat remain intact in most patients.

Agnosia is not infrequently seen in dementia. Finger agnosia, frequently as part of Gerstmann's syndrome (finger agnosia, right-left confusion, acalculia, and agraphia), can be seen with dominant parietal lobe involvement. Nondominant parietal lobe dysfunction can present with anosognosia (ignorance of the presence of disease), paragnosia (difficulty in distinguishing paired body parts), and prosopagnosia (difficulty in recognition of familiar faces). The latter is a frequent chief complaint of patients in the early stages of DAT and is generally ascribed to a "poor memory" by the patient, his family, and sometimes his doctor(s).

A variety of apraxias/dyspraxias can be seen in dementia. Dominant hemisphere involvement results in ideomotor apraxia (motor apraxia), in which the patient is unable to carry out on verbal command a motor activity that can otherwise be performed spontaneously. This form of apraxia is frequently seen in conjunction with aphasia (Benson 1979). Nondominant parietal lobe dysfunction may present with constructional apraxia and dressing apraxia. The latter is not infrequently the "first sign" to some families that something is wrong, although it is usually seen in the later stages of a dementia.

While not specifically listed in DSM-III, anomia or dysnomia should be tested in all patients as abnormalities in this higher cortical function can be detected very early in many patients with dementia. Patients should not only be asked to name an object (watch, sleeve, phone, etc.), but should be questioned about parts (e. g. sleeve, button, button hole) and function (e. g., what do you do with the watch?). The inability to name parts and/or function is usually impaired before the anomia/dysnomia for the object (as a whole) and can be seen early in a dementia. The combination of any of these higher cortical function disturbances can result in significant anxiety, irritability, and in some patients dysthymia.

· As regards changes in personality, Hoch (1972) notes that generally one sees an intensification of the patient's undesirable traits with the majority showing exaggeration or accentuation of traits that were never well received before the development of the dementia. Some patients show traits that are the opposite of premorbid personality traits. Hypochondriasis increases in some, with the risk that significant medical problems may be passed off by family and physicians. Catastrophic reactions may be seen in which the patient may respond to stimuli with excessive laughter, weeping or hostility or, by becoming dazed and immobile (Maxmen 1986). Misoneism, the dislike of or difficulty in accepting new ideas is common, as is a marked sense of possessiveness (Hoch 1972).

While not included in the diagnostic criteria, illusions, hallucinations, and delusions are common in dementia. It is important to differentiate between an illusion, the misinterpretation of a sensory stimulus, and a hallucination, which occurs without sensory input. The woman who misinterprets the sound of the fan for voices has an illusion, whereas the man who hears voices talking to him in a room devoid of sound is hallucinating. The difference is very real. Illusions are not infrequently due to disease within the sensory system involved (e. g., cataracts, hearing loss, excessive cerumen compressing the tympanic membrane) and do not respond to neuroleptic drug treatment. Hallucinations, on the other hand, are considered among the positive symptoms of psychosis and hence may respond to neuroleptic drug treatment. Note, however, that the presence of hallucinations alone is *not* sufficient to make a diagnosis of psychosis. In dementia, delusions are poorly elaborated in both their form and content and, as with hallucinations, are usually organized around misinterpretation or misidentification of everyday events. The misinterpretation/misidentification is in large part a consequence of memory deficits and impaired orientative function. In many cases the hallucinations and delusions may be fleeting. An example follows: a man, due to his memory deficit and lack of insight/judgement, finding his wife "gone" (in reality she is in the other bedroom) fails to look for her so that when a friend calls asking for her, he responds she is not home. Because of his uneasiness with this environment he believes she must be out with another man, hence, a delusion of infidelity is established.

In addition to impairment of at least one of the above areas: abstract thought, judgement, higher cortical function, or personality, (Table 1), sensorium must be clear in contrast to a delirium. Finally the etiology must either be suggested from the history and physical/laboratory examinations or other significant psychiatric disorders (e. g., schizophrenia, paranoia, depression) must be excluded.

It is important to note the following. First, that memory loss alone is not the basis for a diagnosis of dementia. In fact, while memory is an important cognitive process, empirical support for the types and extent of memory loss in dementia remain inadequate (Eisdorfer and Cohen 1982). This is a frequent problem when the patient is inadequately/incompletely evaluated for "memory loss". Dementia is *not* a normal consequence of age. The normal elderly do not have a significant generalized impairment of memory. The memory deficits of normal aging, "benign senescent forgetfulness" are not progressive and do not interfere with the individual's ability to function in everyday life (Kral 1978).

Secondly, the requirement for a clear sensorium is the primary sign that distinguishes dementia from delirium in which some level of disordered wakefulness and sensorium is sine qua non (Massy and Coffey 1983). Remembering this avoids the all too often case of a patient with a drug- or infection-induced altered level of consciousness being diagnosed, usually irreversibly, as "Alzheimer's disease".

If the first step in the diagnosing of dementia is to identify the existence and type of cognitive impairment, the second step in the early diagnosis of dementia is the determination of whether the dementia is a reversible (often called secondary) or nonreversible (primary) dementia. As many as 10%–20% of all dementia are potentially reversible (Barry and Moskowitz 1988; Table 2). The majority of these fall within four major classes, structural CNS disease, metabolic disturbances (in particular thyroid disease), medications (in particular those with anticholinergic activity), and psychiatric illness (primarily affective illness).

The nonreversible (primary) dementias listed below include DAT (Primary Neuronal Degeneration) which accounts for 50% of all cases of dementia; multi-

Table 2. Potentially reversible causes for cognitive dysfunction

I. Structural causes
   A. Subdural hematoma (secondary to head trauma)
   B. Tumors
   C. Normal pressure hydrocephalus
   D. Sensory disturbances
II. Infectious disorders
   A. Acute and subacute systemic (febrile) infections of any etiology, e.g., pneumonia
   B. Chronic infectious illness, e.g., abscess
III. Metabolic disorders
   A. Electrolyte disturbance, hyponatremia and hypernatremia, e.g., secondary to diuretic therapy, dehydration
   B. Thyroid disorders, hypothyroidism, and hyperthyroidism
   C. Diabetes mellitus, hypoglycemia, and hyperglycemia
   D. Hypocalcemia and hypercalcemia
   E. Azotemia
   F. Toxins
IV. Nutritional disorders
V. Circulatory diseases
VI. Pulmonary diseases
VII. Medications
   A. Improper use of over-the-counter medications
   B. Alcohol
   C. Illicit drugs
   D. Misuse of prescribed medications
      1. Self-medication or failure to use as prescribed
      2. Use of multiple drugs from multiple physicians without adequate communications between physicians
      3. Drug-drug interactions
VIII. Psychiatric disorders
   A. Depression
   B. Mania
   C. Anxiety
   D. Paranoia
   E. Situational disturbances

Table 3. Nonreversible primary dementias

Dementia of the Alzheimer type (primary neuronal degeneration)
Multi-infarct dementia
Mixed dementia (with features of both neuronal and vascular involvement)
Pick's disease
Parkinson's disease
Multiple sclerosis
Jakob-Creudtzfeld disease
Huntington's disease
Progressive supranuclear palsy

infarct dementia (MID, 15% all dementias; mixed (with features of both MID and DAT, another 15% of dementias), and miscellaneous forms such as Parkinson's disease, multiple sclerosis, Jakob-Creutzfeld disease, Huntington's disease, and various degenerative diseases such as progressive supranuclear palsy (PSP), and olivoponto-cerebellar degeneration. These will be discussed later.

The key to making an accurate diagnosis and hence both the reversibility of a dementia and the degree of impairment is an integrated multidisciplinary clinical approach to the evaluation of the "demented" patient. Our procedure at the University of Miami and its affiliated Wein Center at Mount Sinai Medical Center has the following component parts.

At intake a psychosocial interview is done by a social worker or psychiatric nurse. This enable us not only to obtain information about the chief complaint and history of present illness, but permits us to learn about family history in depth. It is also valuable to evaluate the impact of the patient's illness on those around him, particularly those who play a direct role in the patient's care. Information is obtained concerning family dynamics, support systems available (or not available) within the family. In addition the patient's level of functioning, including activities of daily living, are established. Patients are also evaluated using the Hamilton Depression Scale, the Blessed dementia scale, and the Folstein Mini-Mental State Examination (MMSE). Caregivers are given the CESD (Center for Epidemiological Studies of depression), Depression Scale, a self-rating scale to assess depression. Economic factors as they may relate to placement and continued treatment are evaluated at this point.

A comprehensive medical history and physical examination administered by a geriatrician/internist follows. This includes learning about current medications and their potential to precipitate either dementia or delirium. This examination is followed by a neurologic history and examination including a mental status examination and rating, and both a parkinsonism scale for extrapyramidal system disease as well as the Hachinski ischemic score (Hachinski et al. 1974). The determination of extrapyramidal features is important in a number of disorders associated with dementia, including Parkinson's disease in which up to 40% of patients may have dementia, Huntington's disease, PSP, some patients with MID, as well as up to one third of patients with DAT. The ischemic score of Hachinski is used to help separate out DAT ($\leq$ 4 points) from MID ($\geq$ 7 points).

The third portion of the evaluation to be performed by a physician is psychiatric assessment, including a mental status examination. We feel *all* patients being evaluated for a dementia require this assessment and disagree sharply with National

Institutes of Health (NIH) Consensus Conference on Dementia (NIH 1987), which suggests psychiatric evaluation in those instances "when depression is suspected." The behavioral manifestations of dementia are not limited to affective illness. Paranoia, psychosis, impaired reality testing, and delusions are all too frequent in dementia, in particular in the primary forms. Many situations arise in which the patient may be a danger to self or others. Further, the incidence of clinically significant depression in caregivers is high, Cohen and Eisdorfer (1988) having reported 55%, a finding similar to that at our center (41%); these people frequently need immediate psychiatric intervention. Even if the sole indication for psychiatric assessment was affective illness, the presentation of affective illnesses in the geriatric age group, being different from that in the young-middle aged adult, requires substantially different skills/techniques than in the younger patient (Olsen et al. 1988).

Cognitive assessment is paramount. Table 4 shows the tests we do if the patient is not severely demented. The aim of cognitive testing is to determine the patient's impairment in the following areas: memory, language, perception, praxis, problem solving, attention, and functional status. This information is useful in planning treat-

Table 4. Cognitive domains and measures used to evaluate them

A. Memory
1. Fuld object memory evaluation
2. Wechsler memory scale – passages and designs (Immediate and 30-min delay)
3. Digit span
4. Delayed condition of the Benton visual retention test or Rey-Osterreith complex and figure test
5. Memory for groceries test
B. Language
1. Vocabulary – WAIS-R
2. Boston naming test
3. FAS controlled word association test
4. Boston diagnostic aphasia examination
C. Visuospatial and visuoconstructive/perceptual
1. Copy condition of Benton visual retention test
2. Benton judgement of line orientation
3. Block design – WAIS-R
4. Object assembly – WAIS-R
D. Higher order thinking and related subskills
1. Similarities (abstract reasoning – WAIS-R)
2. Comprehension – WAIS-R
3. Trailmaking test (parts A and B)
E. Motor/psychomotor
1. Tapping
2. Double alternating hand movements
3. Computerized reaction line tests
F. Attention
1. Letter cancellation test
2. Divided attention test
3. Reaction time test with variable stimulus interval
G. Functional
1. DAFS functional scale

DAFS, direct assessment of functional status

ment and management programs for the patient as well as in determining the rate of deterioration in patients followed over a period of time and the effect of any treatment.

Routine laboratory studies should include: complete blood cell count (CBC), SMAC 23 (including glucose, electrolytes, liver function tests, blood urea nitrogen [BUN], creatinine), Thyroid function tests, serology for syphilis and if indicated by history for human immunodeficiency virus (HIV), vitamin B_{12}/folate levels, ECG, EEG, chest x-ray, and either computerized axial tomography (CAT) scan or magnetic resonance imaging (MRI) of the brain. We prefer the latter if possible because of its resolution.

Reversible (Secondary) Dementia

Table 2 lists the more common reversible causes of dementia. In a recent study, Popkin and Mackenzie (1984) reported 15% of their dementia cases as "potentially reversible." Seven specific medical disorders accounted for 90% of the reversible dementias. They and the more common psychiatric causes of a reversible dementia are discussed below.

Normal Pressure Hydrocephalus

Normal pressure hydrocephalus (NPH) or Hakim's syndrome consists of a triad of dementia, gait apraxia, and urinary incontinence. Popkin and Mackenzie reported this as the most frequent of the potentially reversible dementias, being seen in 31% of cases. The etiology is either an increase in CSF production and/or a defect in CSF reabsorption. All of the symptoms of the triad appear to result from impairment of frontal lobe function. While considered a reversible dementia, many patients, although not progressing in their impairment, do not necessarily show return to normal cognition after a shunting procedure is performed.

Mass Lesions

In the Popkin and Mackenzie studie 30% of the reversible cases of dementia were due to mass lesions. Some 21% were due to tumor and cysts of the CNS. Of the tumors responsible for dementia, the most frequent are frontal lobe, generally meningioma, and astrocytomas. Because the frontal lobes are frequently "neurologically silent" the first presentation of a mass lesion in this area may be dementia and/or seizures. These patients frequently lack other focality on the neurological exam.

The remaining 9% of the reversible dementias due to mass lesions were secondary to subdural hematomas. The possibility of subdural bleeding should be considered in all patients with dementia, in particular in those with a history of head trauma and/or alcohol abuse, as well as those receiving any form of anticoagulation.

Drug Toxicity

Popkin and Mackenzie found medication as the cause in 12% of their reversible dementias. In our experience we find this a more frequent cause, with the most common offenders being agents that have anticholinergic potential. We find that the tricyclic antidepressant amitriptyline (Elavil), the antipsychotic thioridazine (Mellaril), and the antihistamine diphenhydramine (Benadryl). These agents should also be avoided in patients with any type of dementia as we have observed a frequent worsening in the demented patient's cognition.

Thyroid Dysfunction

While both hyper- and hypothyroidism can cause dementia, dementia secondary to hypothyroidism is more frequent. Patients with impaired cognition from hypothyroidism will frequently report their initial symptom as one of "mental slowing" with some dysthymic features. Treatment in our experience has to be continued for at least 3 months before maximal improvement in cognition is seen.

Popkin and Mackenzie's study found alcohol as a cause in 5% and general paresis in 4% of patients. We have not found general paresis to be a reversible dementia. In our experience, by the time a dementia secondary to syphilis is diagnosed, treatment does not reverse the cognitive impairment.

Psychiatric Illness

Of the psychiatric disorders considered to cause a secondary dementia, the most common is depression, the so-called pseudodementia of depression (Wells 1979). While it is true that some patients with depression can be so depressed and anergic that they may appear cognitively impaired, on closer examination these patients reveal a number of differences from the truly demented patient. Depressed patients tend to correct word intrusions, typically answer "I don't know" to questions and to questions of orientation respond "don't know." Additionally, recent and remote memory loss are similar in depressed patients. In patients with dementia, however, word intrusions are frequently made and *not* corrected; answers are frequently "near misses" and orientation difficulties are seen. In testing of memory, greater loss of recent memory is seen than in remote memory. The patient with pseudodementia of depression is typically reported to have a remission of cognitive impairment with treatment of their depression.

The issue of depression as a cause of dementia, however, remains unclear. Nearly onethird of all patients meeting DSM-III criteria for primary neuronal degeneration will also meet DSM-III criteria for major depression. It is likely that the dementia-depression complex represents a subset of the primary dementia.

Nonreversible (Primary) Dementia

Alzheimer's Disease (Primary Neuronal Degeneration)

Alzheimer's disease is the most common of all dementias, accounting for at least half of all cases of dementia. The onset is classically said to be insidious, although some rare cases appear to have an abrupt onset (Loewenstein et al. 1988b). The course is slowly progressive. Both familial and nonfamilial forms appear to exist. The dementia's clinical presentation is one of impairment of recent memory. Neuropathology shows generalized cortical atrophy with ex vacuo hydrocephalus. The histopathologic hallmark of the Alzheimer's disease is the neurofibrillary tangle. A correlation appears to exist between the severity of the dementia and the density of the tangles in the hippocampus and neocortex (Ball 1976). While the tangles are most numerous in the large pyramidal cells of the hippocampus, they are frequently dispersed widely throughout the brain. The neurofibrillary tangle is composed of double-stranded twisted structures called paired helical filaments. These filaments are 10 mm in diameter and seen twisted about one another at 80 mm intervals. A second neuropathologic hallmark is the senile neuritic plaque. This structure is most common in the frontal/parietal lobes. The density of the plaques appears to correlate with the severity of the dementia (Blessed et al. 1967).

Multi-Infarct Dementia

The second most frequent form of the primary dementias is MID. It accounts for approximately 15% of all dementias. These are at least four (4) types of MID (Alexander and Geschwind 1984). The most common form results from multiple bilateral hemispheric infarcts. The infarcts are usually lacunar in nature, resulting from hypertensive disease. Among the other types of MID we find low cerebral perfusion secondary to atherosclerosis occlusion of extracranial arteries producing "water shed infarcts", progressive infarction of subcortical white matter, Binswanger's disease (subcortical arteriosclerotic leukoencephalopathy), and finally multiple infarcts due to the inflammatory arteritides. In all forms, the onset is usually more abrupt than Alzheimer's dementia, with a stepwise progression of the dementia. Hachinski's criteria include, additionally, somatic complaints, a history of stroke, focal neurologic signs/symptoms, and a history of hypertension. While the ischemic score (Hachinski et al. 1974) is useful, frequently final diagnosis rests on the presence of infarcts on the MRI/CT Scan.

The differentiation from DAT is significant for a number of reasons. MID has no hereditary basis so that accurate diagnosis of MID especially removes the fear that "my children will have Alzheimer's." Additionally, a recent study (Meyer et al. 1986) reported that in MID patients with hypertension, improvements in cognition and in the clinical course occurred if the systolic blood pressure was maintained at 135–150 mmHg. In MID patients without hypertension, improved cognition was associated with the cessation of smoking. These findings would of course not apply to DAT.

Other Primary Dementias

Mixed MID-DAT

Approximately 15% of all patients with dementia show clinical and neuropathological characteristics of a combined disease process. Since stroke is an age-related disorder and occurs most frequently in the same age group as DAT, coexistence of the two syndromes is not surprising.

Parkinson's Disease

Up to 40% of patients with Parkinson's disease may develop a dementia. While some patients may have a dementia as an "overlap" of Parkinson's disease with DAT (as with stroke, both disorders occur in the same age group), many feel that a subset of patients may exist in which both disorders exist.

Pick's Disease

Clinically Pick's disease is indistinguishable from primary neuronal degeneration. It differs pathologically in that atrophy is primarily restricted to the frontal and temporal lobes. The incidence of Pick's is 1%–2% of all dementias. Clinically most cases cannot be distinguished from dementias of the Alzheimer's type.

Huntington's Disease

Huntington's disease is hereditary, autosomal dominant with full penetrance (such that there is a one in two chance of a child being afflicted). The initial psychiatric presentation is frequently one of a schizophreniform psychosis. Dementia with extrapyramidal features generally develops in middle age and is progressive in nature. A family history usually supports the diagnosis.

Progressive Supranuclear Palsy

PSP characteristically presents with vertical gaze paralysis initially for downward gaze (the patient will frequently complain of difficulty in walking down stairs). This then involves gaze upward and late, complete ophthalmoplegia may result. Memory loss is seen with some extrapyramidal features. Because this is a "subcortical dementia" aphasia and apraxia are usually absent. The incidence is the same as that of Pick's disease.

Creutzfeldt-Jakob Disease

The progressive dementia Creutzfeldt-Jakob disease is felt to result from a viruslike agent, a small, proteinaceous particle, a prion (Prusiner 1982). The disorder usually presents with extensive focal neurologic findings, "startle myoclonus" being prominent. Death usually occurs within one year. A characteristic pattern may be seen on EEG.

New Directions in the Early Diagnosis of Senile Dementia

Having reviewed the traditional approach to the diagnosis of dementia, we wish now to present some ideas on the use of an integrated neuropsychological/neuropsychiatric program to diagnose dementia in its earliest stages.

Neuropsychological Measures

Using the DSM-III criteria it becomes apparent that the one area of impairment that traditional neuropsychological measures have difficulty in assessing is that of "occupational/social functioning." Family members frequently are not reliable informants as to the functional status of the patient with a presumed dementia. To properly evaluate day-to-day functioning, tasks must be used that can translate into information on the ability or inability to carry out activities of everyday life. Dr. David Loewenstein of our group has developed a reliable and validated scale for the assessment of functional status in patients with dementia (Loewenstein et al. 1988). Patients are evaluated on tasks of time orientation, communication abilities (using a phone, mailing a letter, taking a message), transportation (including driving skills), financial skills (identify and count currency, make change, write a check, balance a check book), shopping skills (shop from a list), eating skills, and dressing/grooming skills.

Patients with DAT have shown significant deficits in functional capacities when compared to age-equivalent normal controls and elderly patients with major depression (Loewenstein et al. 1988a). The direct assessment of functional status (DAFS) scale is likely to significantly increase our ability to objectively assess impairment of functions of everyday life, at the very earliest stages of the dementia.

Soon we will be able to compare a direct measure of functional capacity with the more sensitive neuropsychologic and information processing data. We anticipate that this will provide us with a more useful way to assess capacity to adapt at home or to any change in environment.

In the assessment of dementia cognition word intrusions have long been considered an indication of significant impairment. Recently members of our center have shown that the pattern of intrusions seen can, in the early stages, differentiate between DAT and MID (Loewenstein et al. 1988b). It remains to be seen whether a combination of word intrusion errors and the DAFS can be used to assess the course of the disorder in functional terms and can differentiate subtypes of DAT, as well as severity of the dementia.

Electrophysiological Measures

Routine EEG is generally of little value in the early diagnosis of dementia, showing at best in some cases slowing of the dominant waking background into the theta range. As a result, we are no longer relying on routine EEG. Recent studies using cognitive event-related evoked potentials (ERP), in particular the P_{300} (a positive wave occurring 250–350 msec after stimulation), suggest that the latency and/or amplitude may be changed in patients with DAT as well as mixed DAT-MID type of dementia (Brown et al. 1982; Goodin et al. 1978). Using topographic representation of the ERP as well as the routine EEG, Duffy et al. (1984) were in the earliest stages of presenile dementia (PSD) and senile dementia of the Alzheimer type (SDAT) able to differentiate these dementias from age-matched controls. Further, the topographic dissimilarities between PSD and SDAT suggested important differences between the two dementias. While both showed synchronization (increased slowing), in PSD the parietal-temporal lobes were most involved, whereas in SDAT, the synchronization occurred primarily in the frontal lobes. Additionally, increased slowing and decreased fast activity were associated with poorer performance on neuropsychological testing. Data from our group (Guterman et al. 1988) using topographic presentation of the P_{300} as well as power spectral analysis of the waking EEG activity in a group of HIV-positive homosexual males with lymphadenopathy found abnormalities in nearly 60% of these patients. The electrophysiological abnormalities were seen before the development of changes in traditional neuropsychological measures. In the more sophisticated tests involving information processing techniques, these subjects did show slowing in some cognitive processes, particularly mental rotations and complex reaction time protocol, but no other evidence for dementia (Wilkie et al. 1988). As mental status changes developed, the number and severity of abnormal electrophysiological measures increased. These findings have prompted us to use information processing techniques in our clinics and all of our patients are now being evaluated with this computer assisted battery.

In addition to changes in topographic mapping of brain activity, it appears that the sleep EEG may also be of use in enhancing our ability to diagnose dementia in its early stages. Prinz et al. (1982) found that when compared to normal elderly, patients with DAT showed less stage 3 sleep, no stage 4 sleep and little rapid eye movement (REM) sleep. Additionally the demented patients showed fragmentation of the diurnal sleep/wake pattern with frequent daytime napping and periods of nighttime wakefulness. While this study used patients with a rather advanced stage of dementia, it would be interesting to study the sleep/waking EEGs of patients with various dementias in varying stages of the illness.

Use of more elaborate electrophysiological techniques, including topographic mapping of EEG and ERP as well as that of sleep stages, may indeed give us a new perspective on physiological measures of brain function that might prove useful in the diagnosis of dementia at its earliest stages.

As we indicated earlier neuroimaging, MRI, is routinely employed at our centers. Again, here we disagree with the censuses of NIH, which suggests using CT without contrast. MRI is used routinely because
a) its resolution is better,
b) newer data being collected is done with MRI, and

c) periventricular white matter lesions are ot seen on CT and this may have predictive value. We use CT only to compare with previous studies.

Biologic Markers

Beyond the neuropsychological and electrophysiological measures discussed above, a third area of potential usefulness is that of "biologic markers." The assumption is that there exists a specific marker or, more likely, group of markers that can identify and distinguish between the various dementias. Ideally at least some of these markers should be related to the severity of the disease process and might change/progress with the dementia's progression.

The first is that of histocompatibility antigens (HLA). Henschke et al. (1978) reported DAT as one of the diseases in which an association might exist between DAT as specific HLA types. Cohen et al. (1981) studied the cognitive skills in Alzheimer patients both with and without the HLA-B7 antigen. While neither group was found to have significant differences in either memory capacity or retrieval from short-term and long-term memory, the patients with HLA-B7 antigens had selective attentional scores that were significantly lower than those without the HLA-B7 antigen.

A second biologic marker is that of imunologic factors, in particular IgG and brain reactive antibodies (BRA). In a study of patients meeting the DSM-III criteria for primary neuronal degeneration of the Alzheimer's type, Cohen et al. (1980) found that serum IgG levels were inversely correlated with the duration of illness and the levels of psychiatric symptomatology (including scores on the Folstein MMSE and the brief psychiatric rating scale, BPRS). Performance on the MMSE was positively associated with IgG serum concentrations. The authors suggested that serum IgG levels decrease with the progression of the dementia. They also raise the question as to some alteration in immune response suggestive of a more accelerated somatic change in the patient earlier in the disorder.

A recently published study by Kumar et al. (1988) studying serum IgG BRAs found them in 57% of their DAT patients, 20% age-matched controls, and 81% of older Down's syndrome patients. This finding that the BRA in DAT and Down's syndrome reacted to very different size antigens is consistent with the theory that DAT is a heterogeneous disorder and not a single biochemical entity.

Another potential biologic marker is that of platelet membrane fluidity. Increased fluidity of the membrane in DAT has been reported by Zubenko et al. (1987). This fluidity is not found in the platelets of patients with depression (Zubenko et al. 1987) or in MID (Hicks et al. 1987). Patients with increased fluidity of the platelet membranes appear to have an earlier onset of symptoms and a more rapidly progressive course (Zubenko et al. 1987). From the above, we see that there now exists a number of new techniques, neuropsychological, biochemical, and electrophysiological that have relevance to the dementias. Further studies are needed, and indeed are under way, to determine the usefulness of these in permitting us an earlier and more accurate diagnosis of senile dementia.

Studies to examine the value of specific protein markers are also underway. We feel that the newly emerging research intent in DAT will enable us not only to make more accurate positive diagnosis, but to assess the posibility that there are subtypes of the illness with different courses and potentially different modes of intervention.

References

Alexander MP, Geschwind N (1984) Dementia in the elderly. In: Alpert M (ed) Clinical neurology of aging. Oxford University Press, New York, pp 254–276

American Psychiatric Association (1987) Diagnostic and statistical Manual of mental disorders, 3rd edn., revised. APA Press, Washington

Appell J, Kertesz A, Fisman M (1982) A study of language functioning in Alzheimer patients. Brain Lang 17: 73–91

Ball MJ (1976) Neurofibrillary tangles and the pathogenesis of dementia: a quantitative study. Neuropathol Appl Neurobiol 2: 395–410

Barry PP, Moskowitz MA (1988) The diagnosis of reversible dementia in the elderly. Arch Intern Med 148: 1914–1918

Benson DF (1979) Aphasia, alexia and agraphia. Churchill-Livingstone, New York

Blessed G, Tomlinson BE, Roth M (1967) The association between quantitative measures of dementia and of senile plaque in the gray matter of elderly subjects. Br J Psychiatry 114: 797–811

Brown WS, Marsh JT, LaRue A (1982) Event-related potentials in psychiatry: differentiating depression and dementia in the elderly. Bull Los Angeles Neurol Soc 47: 91–107

Cohen D, Eisdorfer C (1979) Cognitive theory and the assessment of change in the elderly. In: Raskin A, Jarvik LF (eds) Psychiatric symptoms and cognitive loss in the elderly. Hemisphere, New York, pp 273–282

Cohen D, Eisdorfer C, Prinz P et al. (1980) Immunoglobulins, cognitive status and duration of illness in Alzheimer's disease. Neurobiol Aging 1: 165–168

Cohen D, Eisdorfer C, Walford RL (1981) Histocompatibility antigens (HLA) and patterns of cognitive loss in dementia of the Alzheimer type. Neurobiol Aging 2: 277–280

Cohen D, Eisdorfer C (1988) Depression in family members caring for a relative with Alzheimer's Disease. JAGS 36: 885–889

Duffy FH, Albert MS, McAnulty G (1984) Brain electrical activity in patients with presenile and senile dementia of the Alzheimer type. Ann Neurol 16: 439–448

Eisdorfer C, Cohen D (1982) Diagnostic criteria for primary neuronal degeneration of the Alzheimer type. J Family Prac 11: 553–557

Goodin DS, Squires KC, Starr A (1978) Long latency event-related components of the auditory evoked potential in dementia. Brain 101: 635–648

Guterman A, Ramsay RE, Resillez M et al. (1988) Multichannel cognitive evoked responses in neurologically normal HIV-positive males. Neurology 38 [Suppl 1]: 98

Haase GR (1977) Diseases presenting as dementia. In: Wells CE (ed). Dementia Ed. 2 FA Davis, Philadelphia, pp 27–67

Hachinski VC, Lassen NA, Marshall J (1974) Multi-infarct dementia; a cause of mental deterioration in the elderly. Lancet II: 207–210

Henschke PJ, Bell DA, Cape R et al. (1978) HLA antigens in Alzheimer's Disease. Tissue Antigens 12: 132–134

Hicks N, Brammer MJ, Hymas N et al. (1987) Platelet membrane properties in Alzheimer's and multi-infarct dementias. Alzheimer Dis Assoc Disorders 1: 90–97

Hoch PH (1972) Senile and Presenile Psychoses. In: Strahl MO, Lewis NCD (eds) Differential diagnosis in clinical psychiatry. Jason Aronson, New York, 361–390

Kral VA (1978) Benign senescent forgetfulness. In: Katzman R, Terry RD, Bickl CL (eds) Alzheimer's disease: senile dementia and related disorders. Raven, New York

Kumar M, Cohen D, Eisdorfer C (1988) Serum IgG brain reactive antibodies in Alzheimer disease and Down syndrome. Alzheimer Dis Assoc Disorders 2: 50–55

Loewenstein DA, Amigo E, Duara R et al. (1988a) A new scale for the assessment of functional status in Alzheimer's disease and related disorders. J Gerontology (in press)

Loewenstein D, Guterman A, Duara R et al. (1988b) Word intrusions as a means or early diagnosis of primary neuronal degeneration

Massey EW, Coffey CE (1983) Delirium: diagnosis and treatment. South Med J 76: 1147–1150
Maxmen JS (1986) Essential psychopathology. Norton, New York
Meyer JS, Judd BW, Tawaklna T et al. (1986) Improved cognition after control of risk factors for multi-infarct dementia. JAMA 256: 2203–2209
National Institutes of Health (NIH (1987) Differential diagnosis of dementing diseases. JAMA 258: 3411–3416
Olsen EJ, Guterman A, Loewenstein D et al. (1988) Depression in the older patient: common but complex. Older Patient 2: 12–18
Popkin MK, Mackenzie TB (1984) The provisional diagnosis of dementia: three phases of evaluation. In: Hall RCW, Beresford TP (eds) The handbook of psychiatric diagnostic procedures. Spectrum, New York
Prinz PN, Reskind ER, Vitaliano PP et al. (1982) Changes in the sleep and waking EEG's of nondemented and demented elderly subjects. J Am Geriatr Soc 30: 86–93
Prusiner SB (1982) Novel proteinaceous infectious particles cause scrapie. Science 216: 136–144
Smith JS, Kiloh LG (1981) The investigation of dementia: Results in 200 consecutive admissions. Lancet 1: 824–827
Wells CE (1979) Pseudodementia. Am J Psychiatry 136: 895–900
Wilkie F, Millon C, Morgan R et al. (1988) Cognitive changes in an HIV-positive population. Presented at the annual meeting of the American Psychological Association, Atlanta, August 1988
Zubenko GS, Cohen BM, Reynolds CF et al. (1987) Platelet membrane fluidity in Alzheimer's disease and major depression. Am J Psychiatry 144: 860–868

Symptomatic Changes in CNS Aging and Dementia of the Alzheimer Type: Cross-sectional, Temporal, and Remediable Concomitants*

B. Reisberg, S. H. Ferris, A. Kluger, E. Franssen, M. J. de Leon, M. Mittelman, J. Borenstein, K. Rameshwar, and R. Alba

At the beginning of this decade, there was relatively little information available regarding the clinical symptomatology of Alzheimer's disease (AD), the borders between "normal CNS aging" and AD, and the course of AD.

Considerable information has accrued in the past few years regarding the symptomatology and course of CNS aging and AD. This new information has immediate relevance not only in terms of improved diagnosis and counseling but also in terms of the improved identification of remediable concomitants. These aspects are summarized in this review.

Global Symptomatology

Efforts to describe the borders of normal and pathologic CNS aging, the course of progressive AD, management concomitants, and the separation of remediable symptomatology from presently untreatable symptoms, required first the improved description of the general or "global" symptomatology of normal CNS aging and the progressive dementia of AD. On the basis of systematic phenomenologic observations we initially described seven, major clinically distinguishable stages from normality to most severe dementia of the Alzheimer's type. Descriptions of these seven global deterioration stages (GDS stages) were initially published, together with validating information in 1982 (Reisberg et al. 1982). These stages are described in Table 1.

---

* This work was supported in part by USDHHS grant number AG03051 from the National Institute of Aging of the United States National Institutes of Health.

Table 1. Global Deterioration Scale (from Reisberg et al. 1982)[a]

1 No cognitive decline	No subjective complaints of memory deficit. No memory deficit evident on clinical interview.
2 Very mild cognitive decline	Subjective complaints of memory deficit, most frequently in following areas: (a) forgetting where one has placed familiar objects: (b) forgetting names one formerly knew well. No objective evidence of memory deficit on clinical interview. No objective deficits in employment or social situations. Appropriate concern with respect to symptomatology.

194   B. Reisberg et al.

Table 1. continued

3 Mild cognitive decline	Earliest clear-cut deficits. Manifestations in more than one of the following areas: (a) patient may have gotten lost when traveling to an unfamiliar location: (b) co-workers become aware of patient's relatively poor performance: (c) word and name finding deficit become evident to intimates: (d) patient may read a passage or a book and retain relatively little material: (e) patient may demonstrate decreased facility in remembering names upon introduction to new people: (f) patient may have lost or misplaced an object of value: (g) concentration deficit may be evident on clinical testing. Objective evidence of memory deficit obtained only with an intensive interview. Decreased performance in demanding employment and social settings. Denial begins to become manifest in patient. Mild to moderate anxiety accompanies symptoms.
4 Moderate cognitive decline	Clear-cut deficit on careful clinical interview. Deficit manifest in following areas: (a) decreased knowledge of current and recent events: (b) may exhibit some deficit in memory of one's personal history: (c) concentration deficit elicited on serial subtractions: (d) decreased ability to travel, handle finances, etc. Frequently no deficit in following areas: (a) orientation to time and person: (b) recognition of familiar persons and faces: (c) ability to travel to familiar locations. Inability to perform complex tasks. Denial is dominant defense mechanism. Flattening of affect and withdrawal from challenging situations occur.
5 Moderately severe cognitive decline	Patient can no longer survive without some assistance. Patient is unable during interview to recall a major relevant aspect of their current lives: e. g. an address or telephone number of many years, the names of close family members (such as grandchildren), the name of the high school or college from which they graduated. Frequently some disorientation to time (date, day of week, season, etc.) or to place. An educated person may have difficulty counting back from 40 by 4s or from 20 by 2s. Persons at this stage retain knowledge of many major facts regarding themselves and others. They invariably know their own names and generally know their spouse's and children's names. They require no assistance with toileting and eating, but may have some difficulty choosing the proper clothing to wear.
6 Severe cognitive decline	May occasionally forget the name of the spouse upon whom they are entirely dependent for survival. Will be largely unaware of all recent events and experiences in their lives. Retain some knowledge of their past lives but this is very sketchy. Generally unaware of their surroundings, the year, the season, etc. May have difficulty counting from 10, both backward and sometimes forward. Will require some assistance with activities of daily living, e.g., may become incontinent, will require travel assistance but occasionally will display ability to travel to familiar locations. Diurnal rhythm frequently disturbed. Almost always recall their own name. Frequently continue to be able to distinguish familiar from unfamiliar persons in their environment. Personality and emotional changes occur. These are quite variable and include: (a) delusional behavior, e. g., patients may accuse their spouse of being an impostor, may talk to imaginary figures in the environment, or to their own reflection in the mirror, (b) obsessive symptoms, e. g., person may continually repeat simple cleaning activities: (c) anxiety symptoms, agitation, and even previously nonexistent violent behavior may occur, (d) cognitive abulia i. e., loss of willpower, because an individual cannot carry a thought long enough to determine a purposeful course of action.
7 Very severe cognitive decline	All verbal abilites are lost over the course of this stage. Early in this stage words and phrases are verbalized, but speech is very circumscribed. Later in this stage there is no speech at all – only grunting. Incontinence of urine; requires assistance toileting and feeding. Basic are lost with the progression of this stage psychomotor skills, e. g., ability to walk. The brain appears to no longer be able to tell the body what to do. Generalized and cortical neurologic signs and symptoms are frequently present.

[a] Reisberg B, Ferris SH, de Leon MJ, Crook T (1982) The global deterioration scale for assessment of primary degenerative dementia. Am J Psychiatry 139: 1136–1139

Current data on the validity and reliability of this staging procedure has recently been summarized (Reisberg et al. 1988e; Foster et al. 1988; Gottlieb et al. 1988, Reisberg et al. 1988d). Table 2 shows the correlation between these global assessments of progressive cognitive impairment and independently developed mental status assessments (Folstein et al. 1975; Kahn et al. 1960), rating scale assessments (Blessed et al. 1968), memory tests (Gilbert et al. 1968; Wechsler 1958), a composite psychometric variable (Reisberg et al. 1988d), a vocabulary measure (Wechsler 1958), a measure of perceptual motor skills (Wechsler 1958), pure motor skills, and computerized tomographic assessments of the magnitude of brain change (de Leon et al. 1980).

As can be seen from Table 2, strong significant relationships can be demonstrated between the GDS global assessments of progressive cognitive impairment and all behavioral assessments examined. It should be noted that the strongest relationships can be observed between the GDS measures and the most comprehensive behavioral assessment measures. Specifically, the strongest correlation (.89) was observed between GDS assessments and Mini-Mental State Examination (MMSE) scores (Folstein et al. 1975). The latter incorporates measures of initial and delayed recall, orientation, concentration and calculation, language and vocabulary, comprehension, and praxis. Consequently, it is not surprising that this excellent and widely utilized tool relates strongly to global assessments of progressive deficit in aging and Alzheimer's disease.

Similarly, a robust relationship was observed between the global GDS assessments and the combination psychometric variable, i.e., the Psychometric Deterioration Score (PDS). The PDS represents a combined score derived from equal weighting of six tests. Tests 1–3 are taken from the Guild Memory Test (Gilbert et al. 1968) and tests 4–6 are taken from the Wechsler Adult Intelligence Scale (WAIS) (Wechsler 1958). The PDS is calculated by taking the sum of the percent correct performances for:

Table 2. Relationship between Global Deterioration Scale (GDS) score assignments and other behavioral and in vivo assessments of brain change in community-residing subjects presenting to an outpatient research program with normal aging and Alzheimer's disease[a]

Assessment measure	N	Pearson correlation coefficient with GDS assignment
Mental status assessments		
Mini-Mental State Examination (Folstein et al. 1975)	170	0.89[b]
Mental Status Questionnaire (Kahn et al. 1960)	273	0.83[b]
Rating scale assessments (Blessed et al. 1968)		
Dementia scale	122	0.67[b]
Information test	121	0.75[b]
Memory test	121	0.79[b]
Concentration test	120	0.68[b]

Table 2. continued

Assessment measure	N	Pearson correlation Coefficient with GDS Assignment
Cognitive tests		
A. Memory		
Memory for paragraphs (Gilbert et al. 1968)		
Initial recall	260	0.79[b]
Delayed recall	260	0.78[b]
Paired-associate word recall (Gilbert et al. 1968)		
Initial recall	260	0.65[b]
Delayed recall	260	0.63[b]
Designs recall (Gilbert et al. 1968)	258	0.75[b]
Digit recall (Wechsler 1958)		
Forward	261	0.66[b]
Backward	261	0.71[b]
Buschke Selective Reminding Test		
Recall (mean score, trials 1–5)	202	0.79[b]
B. Composite psychometric variable		
Psychometric deterioration score (PDS)[a]	251	0.86[b]
C. Language Function		
WAIS vocabulary score (Wechsler 1958)	261	0.67[b]
D. Perceptual motor skills		
Digit symbol substitution test (Wechsler 1958)	256	0.78[b]
E. Motor skills		
Finger tapping (average score, right and left hands)	213	0.49[b]
Computerized tomographic assessments of brain change		
Cortical sulcal widening (de Leon et al. 1980)	213	0.33[b]
Cerebral ventricular dilatation (de Leon et al. 1980)	213	0.31[b]

[a] Adapted from Reisberg et al. Drug Dev Res (1988)
[b] $p < 0.001$.

1. immediate recall and delayed recall of paragraphs;
2. immediate recall and delayed recall of paired associates;
3. recall of designs;
4. WAIS vocabulary;
5. the digit symbol substitution test, and
6. digits forward and backward; the obtained sum is then divided by the total number of tests.

This score is then converted into a continuous scale, with low absolute scores representing relatively little deterioration and high scores denoting very deteriorated psychometric test performance. The combined psychometric measure correlates with the GDS very robustly ($r = 0.86$, $N = 251$).

Not surprisingly, less comprehensive assessments of mental status such as the ten-item Mental Status Questionnaire of Kahn et al. (1960), and tests of specific memory and cognition modalities relate strongly ($r_s = 0.6$ to 0.8), but somewhat less robustly to the GDS global assessments of deterioration in aging and Alzheimer's disease. Interestingly, vocabulary decline seems to relate quite robustly to the progressive dementia of Alzheimer's disease ($r = 0.67$, $N = 261$, for WAIS vocabulary scores). Similarly, even a relatively "pure" motor task, i. e., finger tapping, shows a significant and moderately strong relationship to progressive global deterioration in aging and dementia ($r = 0.49$, $N = 213$).

It is also not surprising that significant, though weaker relationships can be seen between structural measures of brain change and global deterioration in aging and dementia ($r_s = 0.33$ and 0.31, respectively, for computerized tomographic assessments of progressive sulcal widening and progressive ventricular dilatation; $N = 213$). That changes in these structural measures relate significantly to global changes in aging and Alzheimer's disease is noteworthy, and has been reported previously (Brinkman et al. 1986; de Leon et al. 1979; de Leon et al. 1980; de Leon et al. 1983; Fox et al. 1975).

Since the GDS assessments relate particularly strongly to the widely used MMSE measure, a more detailed examination of this relationships may be instructive and can be seen for a larger subject sample in Table 3. The MMSE scores show very subtle differences and do not reliably distinguish between subjects with and without subjective complaints of cognitive impairment (i. e., GDS categories 1 and 2). Similarly, some subjects with cognitive impairment sufficient to interfere with complex occupational or social functioning (i. e., at the third GDS level) continue to achieve perfect or near-perfect MMSE scores and the mean score of these subjects remains within the so-called "normal range." Hence, the MMSE alone does not effectively distinguish a subject with cognitive deterioration of this general magnitude from a subject with, for example, a poor educational background (Folstein 1983). In the range from GDS levels 3 to 6, the MMSE is an excellent tool for discriminating various levels of cognitive impairment in subjects with AD. However, unlike the GDS, which describes the progression of this particular dementing disorder (AD) in detail, the MMSE, provides no information about the source of cognitive disability.

The MMSE differs from the GDS in other fundamental ways. As a "test measure," rather than a clinical assessment, a useful MMSE score may not be obtainable on patients who are uncooperative or who exhibit behavioral disturbances. Such patients may nevertheless be clinically staged globally and accurate GDS level assignments

198   B. Reisberg et al.

Table 3. Relationship Between Global Deterioration Score (GDS) assignments and Mini-Mental State Examination (MMSE) scores in subjects with normal aging and Alzheimer's disease ($n = 298$, $r = 0.9$[a])

GDS level	n	MMSE (mean ± SD)
1	18	29.6 ± 0.7
2	49	28.9 ± 1.3
3	42	24.6 ± 3.5
4	75	20.0 ± 3.8
5	67	14.3 ± 3.4
6[b]	40	8.3 ± 4.8
7[b]	7	0.0 ± 0.0

[a] $p < 0.001$

[b] It should be noted that by the 6th GDS stage, many subjects are institutionalized and others are considered by their caregivers too difficult to manage or too behaviorally disturbed to be brought to an outpatient research center. In the 7th stage, most subjects are institutionalized and many others are considered too impaired to travel to an outpatient setting. Consequently, MMSE scores for the GDS = 6 and GDS = 7 subjects tend to be obtained on the least impaired subjects in their respective categories and the mean scores for the GDS = 6 subjects most of whom were seen in outpatient settings, are probably considerably higher than the true means for all subjects at this stage. The true means can be obtained by outreach efforts in which subjects are followed into their residential or nursing home residences, and taxi and/or ambulette services are arranged for patient transport to the research center. Using these latter measures, the true mean for MMSE scores in the 6th stage is observed to be approximately 5.

obtained. The GDS incorporates aspects of the patient's functional condition (e. g., ability to travel independently, dress, feed themselves, toilet independently, ambulate, etc.), as well as cognitive status. The MMSE and other mental status and psychometric assessments do not assess functional deterioration. The MMSE also bottoms out at a relatively early point in the evolution of AD (late sixth stage to early seventh stage).

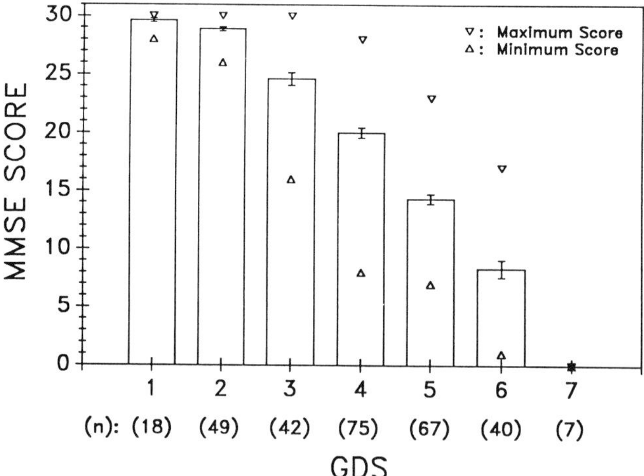

Fig. 1. Mini-Mental State Examination (MMSE) score (mean ± SEM) as a function of Global Deterioration Scale (GDS) score. $r = -0.90$, $p < 0.001$, $n = 298$

Detailed, stage-specific relationships between each GDS level and individual mental status, behavioral and in vivo brain change measures have recently been examined in great detail in community-residing subjects presenting to an outpatient research center with normal aging, AAMI, and AD (N_s = 120 to 260) (Reisberg et al. 1988d). These relationships are illustrated in Figures 1 to 8. As can be seen from these figures, most behavioral measures demonstrate significant deterioration in performance

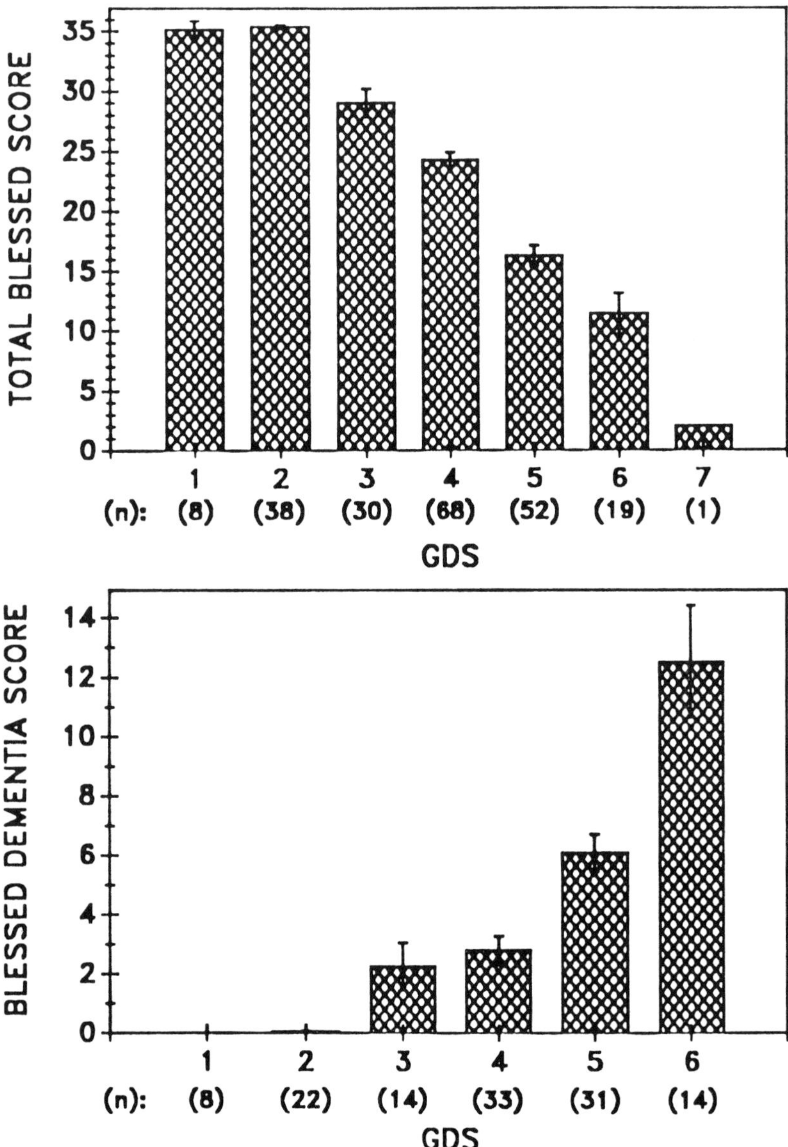

Fig. 2. Total Blessed (I + M + C) test score (*top*) and Blessed dementia scale score (*bottom*) (mean ± SEM) as functions of GDS score. Total score, $r = -0.81$, $p < 0.001$, $n = 216$; dementia score, $r = 0.67$, $p < 0.001$, $n = 122$. (Adapted from Reisberg et al. 1988d)

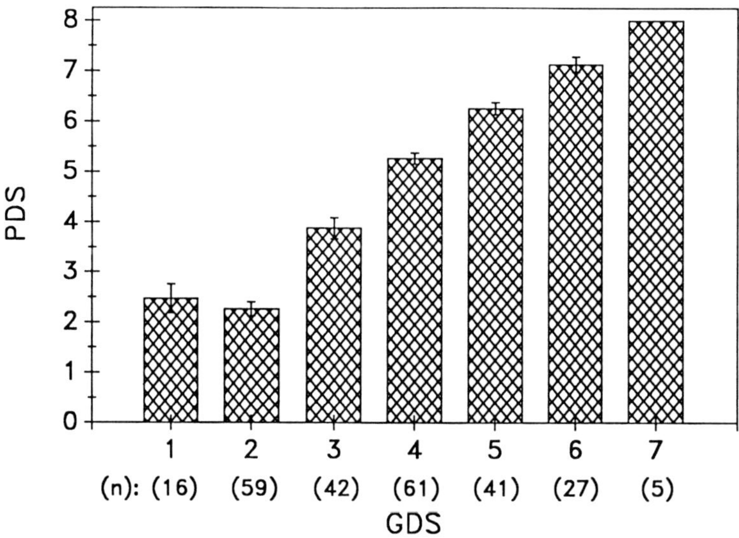

Fig. 3. Psychometric Deterioration Score (PDS; mean ± SEM) as a function of GDS score. $r = 0.86$, $p < 0.001$, $n = 251$. (Adapted from Reisberg et al. 1988d)

between consecutive stages of the GDS from levels 2 to 6. By the sixth GDS stage, most behavioral measures show bottoming effects and these bottoming effects are virtually complete by the 7th GDS stage. At the other end of the GDS spectrum, the behavioral and neuroimaging measures studied did not differentiate between normal aged controls (GDS = 1 subjects) and aged subjects with subjective complaints of cognitive impairment (GDS = 2 subjects).

The component elements incorporated in the GDS have also been investigated for validity of ordinal change and concurrence across stages. Present research supports the optimal validity of the stage-specific elements embodied in the GDS including progressive changes in concentration, recent and remote memory, orientation, functioning, language, mood, and motor capacity in subjects with AAMI and PDD (Reisberg et al. 1986b). Some of this research on ordinal change and concurrence across stages is summarized below.

Ordinal and Concordant Clinical Symptomatology

At least two independent hierarchic dementia assessment instruments have been developed. The first of these is the Dementia Rating Scale of Cole and Dastoor (Cole and Dastoor 1980; Cole et al. 1983; Cole and Dastoor 1987). This scale was developed on the basis of observations of French-speaking clinicians that deterioration in dementia appears to be a reversal in many ways of Piaget's descriptions of cognitive and intellectual development in infancy and childhood (de Ajuriaguerra et al. 1964; Constantinidis et al. 1978; de Ajuriaguerra and Tissot 1975). These observations are remarkably similar to those of Leeds (1960) mentioned above, but appear to have

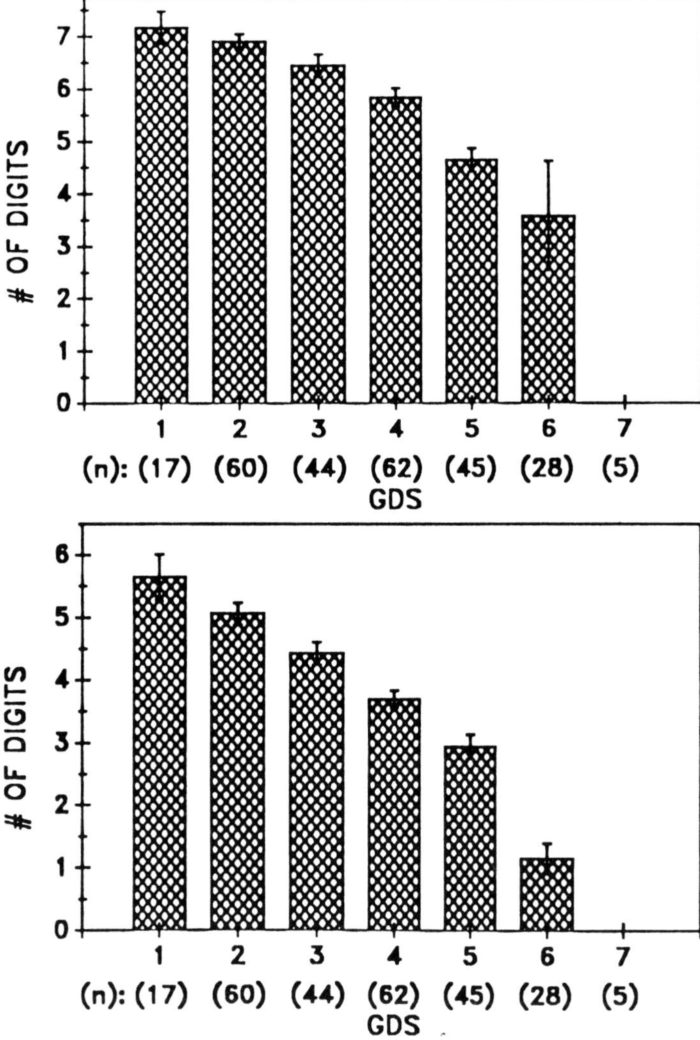

Fig. 4. Recall of digits (mean ± SEM) as a function of GDS score. *Top*, forward, $r = -0.66$, $p < 0.001$, $n = 261$; bottom, backward, $r = -0.71$, $p < 0.001$, $n = 261$. (Adapted from Reisberg et al. 1988d)

been entirely independently derived. As finally constituted (Cole and Dastoor 1987), the Hierarchic Dementia Scale contains twenty categories each with its own hierarchic scale, assessing cognitive abilities, praxis, recent and remote memory, orientation, reading and writing abilities, calculation skills, ability to follow instructions, and prefrontal neurologic reflexes. An initial goal in the construction of the Hierarchic Dementia Scale was the development of hierarchic scale categories which would be optimally concordant, and thereby diagnostic, for dementia of the Alzheimer's type, and perhaps for other dementing disorders as well. Although items are enumerated

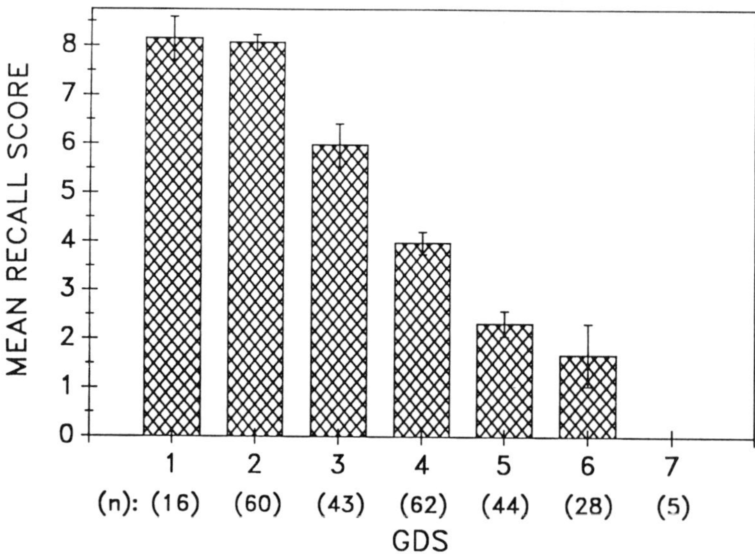

Fig. 5. Recall on selective reminding task (mean ± SEM) as a function of GDS score. $r = -0.79$, $p < 0.001$, $n = 202$. (Adapted from Reisberg et al. 1988d)

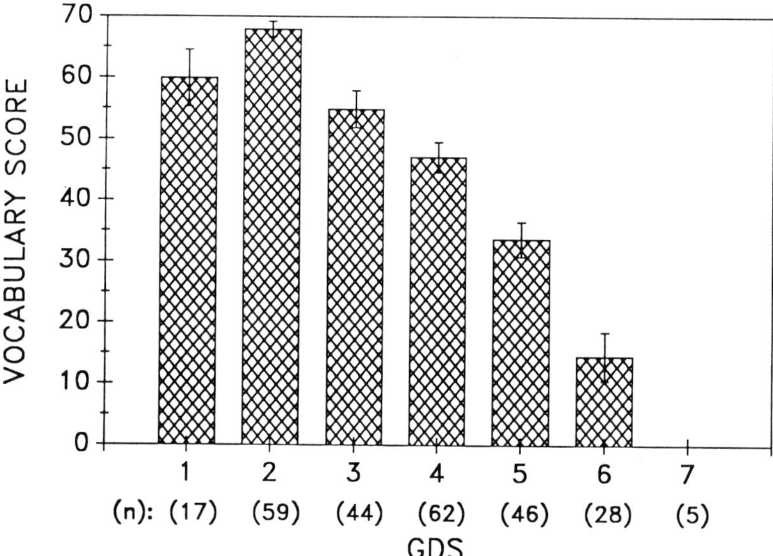

Fig. 6. WAIS vocabulary score (mean ± SEM) as a function of GDS score. $r = -0.67$, $p < 0.001$; $n = 261$. (Adapted from Reisberg et al. 1988d)

along Piagetian lines, roughly in order of difficulty in terms of the timecourse of developmental acquisition, it appears that the goals of optimal concordance across categories with continuing deterioration in AD and precise concordant data in AD have not yet been achieved. However, the authors state that "inasmuch as different functions deteriorate at different rates in different dementias, the scale may be useful

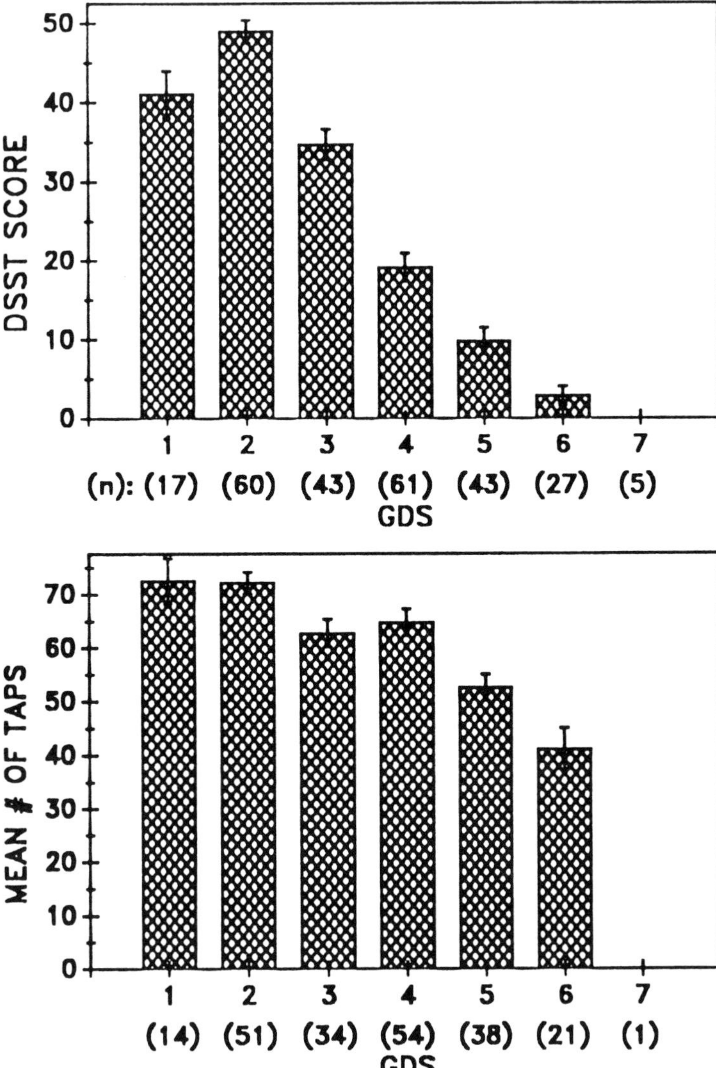

Fig. 7. Digit symbol substitution test (DSST; *top*) and finger tapping speed (*bottom*) (means ± SEM) as functions of GDS score. DSST, $r = -0.78$, $p < 0.001$, $n = 256$; finger tapping, $r = 0.49$, $p < 0.001$, $n = 213$. (Adapted from Reisberg et al. 1988d)

in differentiating various types of dementias" (Cole and Dastoor 1987). These goals may ultimately be achievable. In the interim the developers of the Hierarchic Dementia Scale have been investigating the longitudinal course of Alzheimer's disease using these measures (Cole and Dastoor 1987; Dastoor and Cole 1986).

Meanwhile, in the United States, the previously developed Global Deterioration Scale (GDS) (Reisberg et al. 1982), was divided into several seven-stage ordinal assessments representing dimensions or axes of progressive change in normal CNS aging and progressive AD. Initial constituent measures or "axes" on this Brief

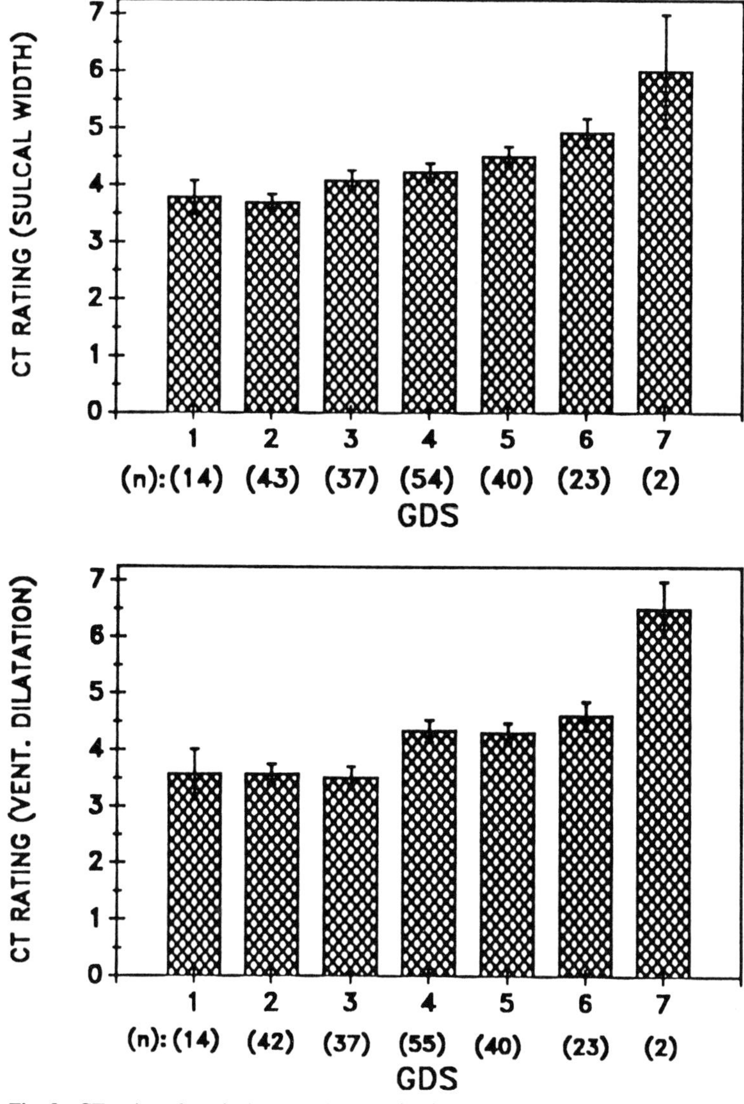

Fig. 8. CT rating of cortical sulcal widening (*top*) and cerebral ventricular dilatation (*bottom*) (means ± SEM) as functions of GDS score. Sulcal widening, $r = 0.33$, $p < 0.001$, $n = 213$; ventricular dilatation, $r = 0.31$, $p < 0.001$, $n = 213$. (Adapted from Reisberg et al. 1988d)

Cognitive Rating Scale (BCRS) included assessments of progressive changes in concentration, recent memory, past memory, orientation, and functioning and self-care (see Table 4) (Reisberg et al. 1983a). These five assessment modalities or axes on the BCRS are sometimes referred to as the "major axes" and the five ordinal scales as the "BCRS: Part I". The subscales were empirically devised and designed to be optimally concordant across levels of ability and progressive disability in normal aged and AD patients. Consequently, in an AD patient with a score of "4" on, for example,

Table 4. Concomitant ordinal changes in normal aging and progressive Alzheimer's disease

Level	Concentration	Recent memory	Past memory	Orientation	Functioning and self-care
1	No objective or subjective evidence of deficit.	No objective or subjective evidence of deficit.	No subjective or objective impairment.	No deficit in memory for time, place, identity of self or others.	No difficulty, either subjectively or objectively.
2	Subjective decrement.	Subjective impairment only (e. g., forgetting names more than formerly).	Subjective impairment only. Can recall two or more primary schoolteachers.	Subjective impairment only. Knows time to nearest hour, location.	Complains of forgetting location of objects. Subjective work difficulties.
3	Minor objective signs of poor concentration (e. g., on serial 7s from 100).	Deficit in recall of specific events evident upon detailed questioning. No deficit in the recall of major recent events.	Some gaps in past memory upon detailed questioning. Able to recall at least one childhood teacher and/or childhood friend.	Any mistake in time by 2h or more; day of the week by 1 day or more; date by 3 days or more.	Decreased job functioning evident to co-workers. Difficulty in traveling to new locations.
4	Definite concentration deficit for persons of their background (e. g., marked deficit on serial 7s; frequent deficit in serial 4s from 40).	Cannot recall some major events of previous weekend or week. Scanty knowledge of current events, favorite TV shows, etc.	Clear-cut deficit. Spouse recalls more of patient's past than the patient; can't recall childhood friends/ teachers but knows the names of schools attended.	Mistakes day of month by 10 days or more, and/or confuses month of the year by 1 month or more.	Decreased ability to perform complex tasks (e. g., planning dinner for guests, handling finances, shopping).
5	Marked concentration deficit (e. g., giving months backwards or serial 2s from 20).	Unsure of weather, may not know current president or current address.	Major past events sometimes not recalled (e. g., names of some of the schools attended).	Unsure of month and/or year and/or season; unsure of locale.	Requires assistance in choosing clothing.
6	Forgets the concentration task. Frequently begins to count forward when asked to count backwards from 10 by ls.	Occasional knowledge of some recent events. Little or no idea of current address, weather, etc.	Some residual memory of past (e. g., may recall country of birth, former occupation, mother's and/or father's name).	No idea of date. Identifies spouse but may not recall name. Knows own name.	Requires assistance in feeding, and/or toileting, and/or bathing.
7	Marked difficulty counting forward to 10 by ls.	No knowledge of any recent events.	No memory of past.	Cannot identify spouse. May be unsure of personal identity.	Requires constant assistance in all activities of daily life.

Adapted from Reisberg et al. (1983a)

the functional axis, the most probable score on the recent memory, past memory, orientation, or functioning and self-care axes would also be a "4", and the most probable corresponding global deterioration scale score would be "4". Ratings on each axis were indeed found to be highly correlated with ratings on each of the others in subjects with normal aging or AD (r_s = 0.88 to 0.93) (Reisberg et al. 1983a).

Current data regarding the validity of these BCRS concordant ordinal measures has recently been reviewed (Reisberg and Ferris 1988a). An example of the magnitude of consistency of these measures across the axes can be seen in Figure 9 which represents the scores on the first four BCRS axes for subjects who were at level 4 on BCRS Axis V assessing functioning and self-care. As can be seen from Figure 9, these axes do appear to be optimally weighted for the magnitude of pathology across measures. Figure 9 also permits an estimate of the consistency of deterioration across various assessment modalities. As can be seen by reference to Figure 9, more than a third of AD patients who functionally are at a level where they have difficulty handling their personal finances but still have the capacity to choose the proper clothing for the season and the occasion (i. e., Level 4 on Axis V), have a deficit in concentration and calculation (Axis I), whereby they cannot accurately subtract serial 4s from 40, but can still subtract serial 2s from 20 (Level 4 on Axis I). Similarly, nearly half of all AD patients scoring at Level 4 on Axis V manifest a recent memory deficit at this same level on the BCRS. Specifically, they have difficulty recalling major events of the past

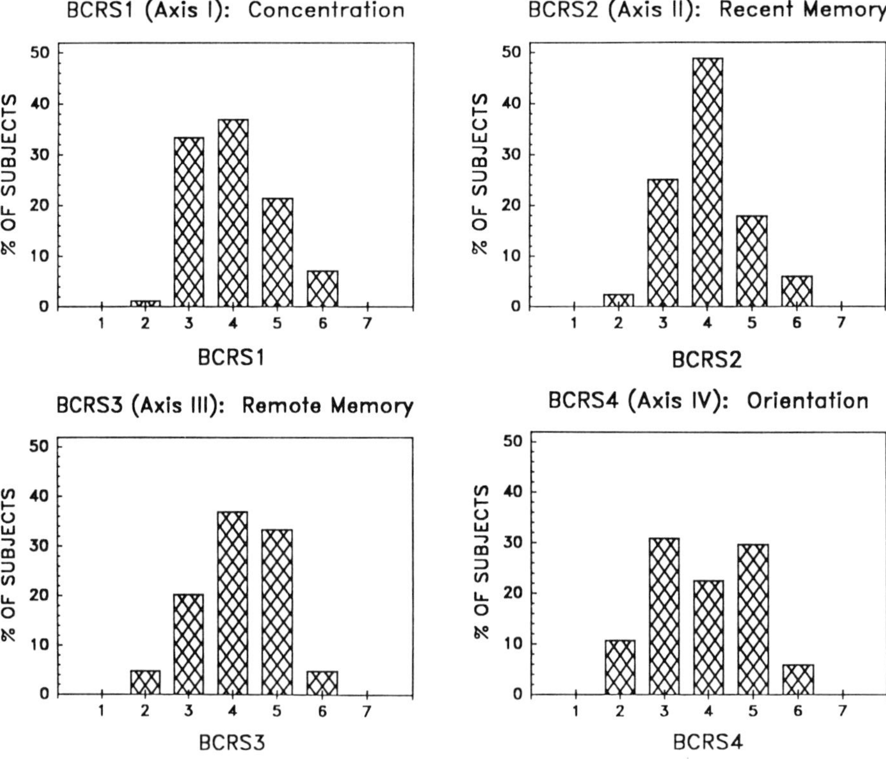

Fig. 9. Percentage of subjects scoring at various severity levels on BCRS axes I–IV in 84 patients with Alzheimer's disease at BCRS axis V (functioning and self-care) level 4

week, but can still accurately state the present weather conditions, the name of the current national leader, and their current address. More than a third of all AD patients scoring at level 4 on Axis V manifest a past memory deficit at this same level. Specifically, the spouse's memory of the patient's past appears better than the patient's own memory of their personal history. However, the patient can still recall such major past events as the names of the schools which they attended. On Axis IV of the BCRS, measuring orientation, it will be noted that there is a greater scatter of scores for AD subjects scoring at Level 4 on Axis V. Nevertheless, the median orientation score for Axis V, Level 4 AD patients is also 4.

In summary, as Figure 9 demonstrates quite dramatically, the progressive deficits in AD can be described using the BCRS as proceeding in a relatively consistent pattern across various clinical modalities. This consistency of deterioration across dimensions is not seen in most other clinical disorders.

It was initially hoped that these strong interrelationships would prove of diagnostic utility in the differential diagnosis of dementing disorders, since other dementias apart from AD would not necessarily follow this relatively homogeneous pattern. This hypothesis in many ways was identical to that posited for the hierarchic dementia scale (Cole and Dastoor, 1980). However, despite the apparently robust magnitude of the intercorrelations between deterioration scores on various parameters and global impairment in AD, the differential diagnostic utility of these interrelationships when examined cross-sectionally must still be further clarified.

Ordinal Asessments of Progressive Functional Change in Degenerative Dementia of the Alzheimer Type

As noted above, one of the axes of the BCRS (Reisberg et al. 1983a), evaluated seven-stage ordinal functional changes in normal aging and AD. Later, the functional descriptions of progressive changes were elaborated upon and ultimately evolved into a sixteen-stage ordinal scale of progressive functional change in dementia of the Alzheimer type known as Functional Assessment Staging or "FAST" staging of AD (Reisberg et al. 1984; Reisberg et al. 1985a; Reisberg et al. 1985b; Reisberg 1986e).

These functional stages were enumerated to correspond optimally to the respective global stages of aging and AD on the GDS. In addition, FAST stages 6 and 7 have been subdivided into a total of 11 substages. The FAST stages are as follows:

1. No objective or subjective functional deficit.
2. Subjective functional deficit, e.g., in recalling the location of objects.
3. Deficit in demanding occupational and social tasks generally observable to intimates and co-workers.
4. Observable deficits in complex tasks such as managing personal finances or planning dinner for guests.
5. Decreased ability to choose proper clothing to wear for the season, or the occasion.
6. Decreased ability to dress, bathe, and toilet; specifically, five substages of stage 6 can be identified as follows:
    a) Decreased ability to put on clothing independently.
    b) Decreased ability to bathe independently.
    c) Decreased cleanliness in toileting.

   d) Decreased urinary continence.
   e) Decreased fecal continence.
7. Loss of speech and motor capacity. Specifically, six substages of stage 7 can be identified as follows:
   a) Speech ability limited to approximately a half-dozen intelligible words in an average day.
   b) Speech ability limited to a single intelligible word in the course of an average day.
   c) Loss of ability to ambulate without assistance.
   d) Loss of ability to sit up without assistance.
   e) Loss of ability to smile.
   f) Loss of ability to hold up one's head independently.

A recent cross-sectional study examined the extent to which this precise functional degenerative order of loss of capacity occurred in consecutive AD patients (Borenstein and Reisberg 1987). Fifty-six patients with AD were prospectively studied, all of whom had GDS scores of "4" or greater. Fifty of the fifty-six AD patients, followed the FAST functional deterioration course precisely. In six of the cases there were slight variations, limited to a single substage variation in four cases (i.e., a one-point reversal on the sixteen FAST stages), and a variation of two substages or a two-point reversal in two cases. A Guttman analysis (Nie et al. 1975) confirmed that the results observed were not due to chance and substantiated the statistical validity of the FAST scale.

These results lend support for the presence of a characteristic pattern of progressive functional deficit in AD. There appears to be only a small, statistically insignificant variability in the ordinal appearance of these deficits in AD.

Clearly, these functional disabilities can be produced by pathologic conditions other than AD. For example, arthritis, a stroke, normal pressure hydrocephalus, or trauma from a vehicular accident can all lead to loss of ambulatory ability. However, the specific order of functional loss is characteristic of AD. Differential diagnostic aspects of the FAST stages have been discussed elsewhere in detail (Reisberg et al. 1985a; Reisberg et al. 1985b; Reisberg 1986e). Briefly, the order of functional losses in AD, as enumerated in the FAST, is of considerable diagnostic utility. When combined with information on the temporal course of the FAST stages (described below), the FAST can be a very powerful diagnostic tool for the clinician.

The Temporal Course of AD

Because of the relatively precise nature of the sixteen FAST stages, it has been possible to follow subjects prospectively and empirically to determine the estimated mean duration of each of the FAST stages. Temporal estimates of the duration of these stages in AD were published in 1986 (Reisberg 1986e). The estimated mean time course of the FAST stages can be seen in Table 5.

These data can now be combined with the stage-specific cross-sectional mental status and psychometric data which have been alluded to earlier in this paper and published elsewhere in detail (Reisberg et al. 1988d), and a time-line of AD can be

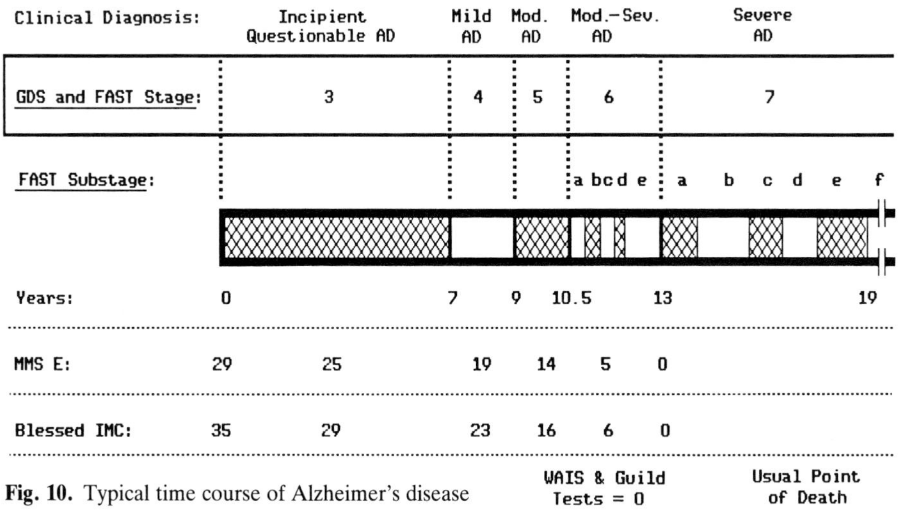

Clinical Diagnosis:	Incipient Questionable AD	Mild AD	Mod. AD	Mod.-Sev. AD	Severe AD
GDS and FAST Stage:	3	4	5	6	7
FAST Substage:				a bc d e	a b c d e f

Years: 0   7   9   10.5   13   19

MMS E: 29   25   19   14   5   0

Blessed IMC: 35   29   23   16   6   0

WAIS & Guild Tests = 0   Usual Point of Death

Fig. 10. Typical time course of Alzheimer's disease

constructed with unprecedented precision. This time-line of AD can be seen in Figure 10.

It should be noted that this time-line of AD refers to the commonly encountered, late onset form of AD. The relatively rare autosomal dominant familial form of AD which may be encountered in patients as early as the third or fourth decades of life, may proceed more rapidly (Reisberg et al. 1988b).

Some important aspects of the temporal course of AD are apparent from Figure 10. Specifically, it should be noted that approximately one-third of the total potential time course of AD (i.e., the third GDS stage) can be identified as a clear-cut harbinger of the AD pathologic process only in retrospect. Also, only 6 years of the more than twelve-year course of AD which can be prospectively charted is measurable using currently available mental status assessments including MMSE and the IMC of Blessed et al. (1968). Presently utilized psychological test measures chart an even more restricted range of the total course of the disease. Clearly, death can occur at any point in the disease process. However, empirical observations indicate that AD patients commonly succumb after ambulatory ability is lost (stages 7c or 7d).

Other tentative observations regarding the temporal course of AD include the following:
1. There is no current convincing evidence that age of onset (above age 50), or sex affect the course of the disease (Reisberg et al. 1986d). In this regard AD appears to be analogous to many forms of malignancy in that when an otherwise healthy person contracts a malignancy, the malignant process is the major determinant of five-year survival, at virtually any age. Similarly, whenever an AD patient enters the beginning of the fourth stage, the life expectancy of the patient is determined by the inexorable progression of the disease process. This progression appears to be the same in a fifty-year-old as in an eighty-five-year-old, and the same in women as in men.
2. The development of an intercurrent illness process may result in an apparently staccatic jump in the otherwise gradual progression of AD. When the seemingly

Table 5. Time course of functional loss in Alzheimer's disease (Functional Assessment Staging)[a]

FAST Stage	Characteristics	Clinical diagnosis	Estimated duration in AD[b]
1	No decrement	Normal adult	
2	Subjective deficit in word finding or recalling location of objects	Normal aged adult	
3	Deficits noted in demanding employment settings	Compatible with incipient AD	7 years
4	Requires assistance in complex tasks, e.g., handling finances, planning dinner party	Mild AD	2 years
5	Requires assistance in choosing proper attire	Moderate AD	18 months
6a	Requires assistance dressing	Moderately severe AD	5 months
b	Requires assistance bathing properly		5 months
c	Requires assistance with mechanics of toileting (such as flushing, wiping)		5 months
d	Urinary incontinence		4 months
e	Fecal incontinence		10 months
7a	Speech ability limited to about a half-dozen words	Severe AD	12 months
b	Intelligible vocabulary limited to a single word		18 months
c	Ambulatory ability lost		12 months
d	Ability to sit up lost		12 months
e	Ability to smile lost		18 months
f	Ability to hold head up lost		12 months or longer

[a] Adapted from Reisberg B (1986) Geriatrics 41: 30–46
[b] In subjects without other complicating illnesses who survive and progress to the subsequent deterioration stage.

rapid jump in progression in illness is irreversible, the AD disease process must "catch up," and then resume its gradual inexorably progressive course.
3. Decompensating processes – including stress, unfamiliar surroundings, major surgical procedures and intercurrent illness – produce potentially reversible disability which tends to proceed along the lines of the FAST progression.
For example, an AD patient who is hospitalized at FAST stage 6b or 6c, will frequently develop urinary incontinence (FAST stage 6d), which may remit when the patient is returned to their home. Similarly, patients in the late 6th FAST stage

have a marked tendency to lose ambulatory capacity in response to psychotropic extrapyramidal side-effects, arthritis, etc.

4. Progression of the disease tends to produce stage specific regression to the mean across modalities.

   As noted, stage specific data on concentration ability, recent memory capacity, past memory capacity, orientation ability, mental status test performance, and other measures, as well as functional capacity has been published (Reisberg et al. 1988d; Reisberg et al. 1983a; Reisberg et al. 1985a; Reisberg et al. 1983b). Although all of these measures correlate strongly with GDS and/or FAST scores, there is, of course, individual variability. When such variability is present, this rule states that progression of the disease produces regression to the stage-specific mean on the measure.

5. The magnitude of temporal disparity of the FAST stages is mirrored by the magnitude of temporal disparity of the acquisition of the same functions in normal development.

   In this regard, it is useful to note that a one to one inverse relationship between the 16 FAST degenerative stages of AD and reciprocal normal human developmental functions has been observed (Reisberg et al. 1986c). The developmental analogy is also useful in predicting the temporal course of AD in various ways. For example, even the absolute time course of functional loss in AD from FAST stages 3 to 6e is almost precisely the same as the absolute time course of acquisition of these same functions in normal development. In the final 7th stage of AD, functions which are acquired in normal development over a period of only approximately 1.5–2 years, are lost over a period of seven or more years in the degenerative course of AD. An approximation of the extent to which the time course of functional loss in AD is mirrored by the time course of functional acquisition in normal development can be seen in Figure 11.

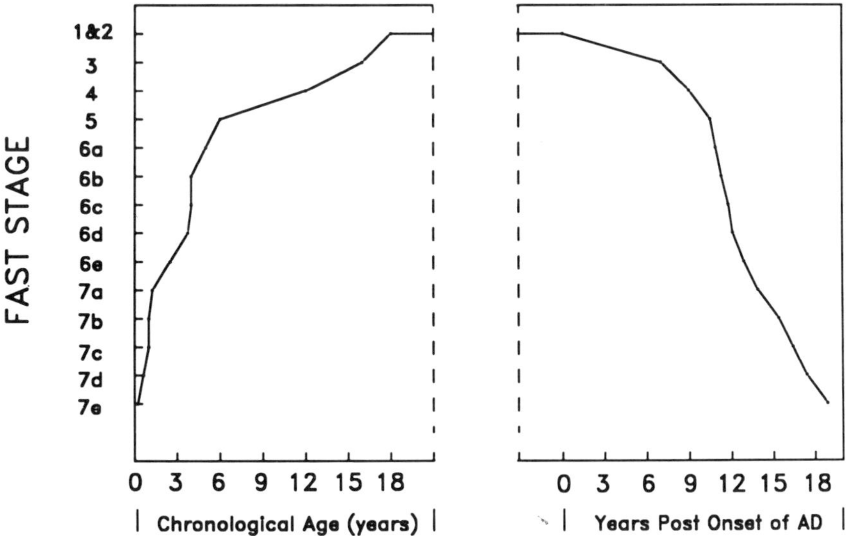

Fig. 11. Changes in functional Assessment Staging (FAST) as a function of age in normal aging and Alzheimer's disease

6. The longer the time interval, the greater the certainty with which the course of AD can be predicted.

   Just as in normal human development, predictions of time course of skill acquisition are increasingly certain the longer the observation interval, similarly, in AD, the time course of skill degeneration is increasingly certain, the longer the observation interval. For example, it is very difficult to predict when a two year old child who has achieved fecal continence will attain urinary continence. It could be in two days, or two months, or in two years or more. Predictions vary by a factor of greater than 100. However, we can predict with much greater certainty that the two year old child will be putting on clothing properly in approximately 5 years and will be able to handle money in approximately 10 years. Predictions over the much longer term vary by a factor of less than 1.

   Similarly, it is very difficult to predict when an AD patient at FAST stage 6d who is incontinent of urine, will lose fecal continence. It may occur in 2 days or in one year. Predictions vary by a factor of greater than 100. However, we can predict with much greater certainty that the AD patient who has difficulty putting on clothing properly at stage 6a will be incontinent of feces in approximately 2 years and that the AD patient in stage 4 who has difficulty handling money properly will be incontinent of feces in approximately 5 years. Predictions of course of degeneration over those intervals vary by a factor of approximately 1.

7. The data in Figure 10 and other stage specific cross-sectional data (e. g., Reisberg et al. 1988d, permit explicit predictions of the mean temporal course of AD which are amenable to empirical testing. For example, on the MMSE, the following mean time intervals of AD progression would be projected as follows:

MMSE Change	Projected mean time interval in Uncomplicated AD
19–14	1.75 years
14 to 5	2.00 years
5 to 0	1.25 years
23 to 0	6.00 years

Etiologic Implications of the Temporal Course of AD

Current observations regarding the temporal course of AD have clear etiologic import. Two important hypotheses can be formulated on this basis at the present time:

1. A unitary final common pathway is strongly suggested by the stereotypic symptomatology and course of AD.
2. The developmental analogies regarding the course of AD may have etiologic and treatment import.

Perhaps these striking analogies indicate that AD results from a fundamental disorder of developmental physiologic central nervous system processes. In this regard it is interesting to note that natural cell death has been shown to be a normal concomitant of nervous system embryogenesis (Hamburger and Levi-Montalcini 1949; Oppenheim 1981; Cowan et al. 1984; Oppenheim 1985). It is believed that neuronal survival in normal development is dependent, at least in part, upon competition for neurotrophic factors (Hamburger and Oppenheim 1982). Presently, the best characterized neurotrophic factor is nerve growth factor (NGF), a polypeptide. Exogenously administered NGF decreases cell death during development (Hendry and Campbell 1976; Hamburger et al. 1981) or after axotomy (Hendry and Campbell 1976; Yip and Johnson Jr. 1984). Antisera to NGF has also been shown to increase cell death in sympathetic and sensory neurons (Levi-Montalcini and Booker 1960). Recently, Martin et al. (1988) have provided evidence that the cell death which is decreased by NGF in sympathetic neurons is due to a trophic factor. They believe the NGF trophic factor "suppresses an active suicide response" of sympathetic neurons. As evidence for this, they demonstrated that the death of NGF-deprived neurons was entirely prevented by inhibiting protein or RNA synthesis (Martin et al. 1988).

This latter finding is particularly interesting in the light of concurrent observations regarding neurometabolic changes in AD. Ferris et al. (1980) first demonstrated a decrease in cerebral metabolism using the then newly developed positron emission tomographic (PET) scanning techniques. This work has been subsequently confirmed. Recent work indicates that these metabolic deficits may be among the earliest identifiable changes occurring in AD (Haxby et al. 1986; Hoyer et al. 1988). Other work provides evidence for a close association between the metabolic changes in AD and neuroendocrine events. Specifically, animal studies have demonstrated that elevated corticosterone is associated with decreased cerebral blood flow (Lasbennes et al. 1986) and brain glucose utilization (Landgraf et al. 1978). De Leon et al. (1988) have recently demonstrated a consistent abnormal, abrupt elevation in serum cortisol levels in AD patients in comparison with controls, in response to a glucose tolerance testing protocol. Furthermore, they found an association between the altered neuroendocrine function in AD and both the hippocampal lesions and the reductions in the brain glucose metabolism.

Consequently, it is tempting to speculate that the brain's initial physiologic homeostatic response to a decrease in NGF in AD might be to decrease cerebral metabolism through neuroendocrine mechanisms such as increased cortisol secretion.

This hypothesis would be consistent with the observation that endocrine factors prevent neuronal cell death under other circumstances (Nordeen et al. 1985). Naturally, any endocrine hemostatic changes may have various CNS consequences (Long and Holaday, 1985).

There is other evidence that NGF may be implicated in the microscopically visible pathologic changes in AD. The NGF-responsive PC12 pheochromocytoma cell line has provided a convenient model for the investigation of the process of neuronal differentiation (Greene and Tischler 1976). In the presence of NGF, PC12 cells differentiate from a chromaffin-like phenotype to a sympathetic neuron-like phenotype. Fibroblast growth factor (FGF) also promotes the neuronal differentiation of PC12 cells. Differential screening of a c DNA library from the PC12 rat pheochromocytoma cell line reveals a clone, called clone 73, whose corresponding mRNA is induced by NGF. Clone 73 encodes an intermediate filament protein, which is distinct from other known intermediate filament proteins (Leonard et al. 1987). NGF or FGF increase the mRNA recognized by clone 73 by a factor of 5. Interestingly, dexamethasone also regulates the mRNA, however in an opposite direction, causing a two- to threefold decrease in its level (Leonard et al. 1988).

NGF has also been demonstrated to effect various microtubule associated proteins (MAPs), including their expression (Brugg and Matus 1988) and phosphorylation (Aletta et al. 1988). The effects of NGF have been related to possible roles in microtubule assembly, stability, cross-linking, and nuclear signaling (Aletta et al. 1988).

In view of de Leon et al.'s observation of an abnormal cortisol response to glucose in AD (de Leon et al. 1988) and studies demonstrating decreased brain glucose utilization in response to elevated corticosterone (Landgraf et al. 1978), the observation that glucocorticoids and NGF have been demonstrated to have opposing actions in various models may have partricular significance. The opposing actions of NGF and dexamethasone, in the regulation of mRNA encoding an intermediate filament protein, have already been mentioned (Leonard et al. 1988). Additionally, NGF and glucocorticoids have been observed to have opposing actions in the differentiation decisions of neural crest-derived precursor cells, which can give rise to chromaffin cells under the influence of glucocorticoids, or to sympathetic neurons in the presence of NGF (Bjerre and Bjorklund 1973; Doupe et al. 1985b; Doupe et al. 1985a; Anderson and Axel 1986). Consequently, experiments examining the effects of NGF on the abnormal cortisol response to glucose in AD might be worthwhile, and might prove to be of etiopathogenic import.

In summary, independent recent observations regarding:
1. the sequence and time course of degeneration in AD,
2. the neurochemistry of neuronal growth and development, and
3. the metabolic and neuroendocrine factors associated with both AD and normal neuronal growth and development, may be interrelated.

An examination of these interrelationships leads to various hypotheses notably including:
1. a hypothesized role of NGF and/or FGF in the etiology and/or pathology of AD, and
2. the specific hypothesis that decreased CNS metabolism in AD produces an abnormal cortisol response, which produces a decrease in NGF, which in turn results in the observed pathologic and clinical changes in AD.

Pharmacologically Remediable Symptomatology

Another very important group of clinical symptoms which are in many ways characteristic of AD are potentially remediable behavioral symptoms. These symptoms occur in the context of the progressive neurochemical changes in AD, the progressive cognitive changes in AD, and more generalized mood changes accompanying the progression of AD.

The neurochemical and neurotransmitter changes in AD are characteristic and have been increasingly well described (Davies 1988). Deficits in choline acetyltransferase have been repeatedly observed in the brains of Alzheimer's patients and have been shown to correlate with the severity of the illness (Davies and Maloney 1976; Perry et al. 1977, Perry et al. 1978a; Bowen et al. 1979). Other deficits in the cholinergic system (Perry et al. 1978b; Marsh et al. 1985) and other central neurotransmitter systems (Francis et al. 1985; Rossor et al. 1984) have been noted to occur in Alzheimer's patients. Notable amongst these are noradrenergic deficits (Bondareff et al. 1982), and perhaps decrements in cerebral neuronal functioning. Increments in MAO-B activity have also been noted to occur centrally and peripherally in Alzheimer's patients (Adolfsson et al. 1980). Collectively, these changes are likely to produce characteristic neurochemical milieus of phenomenologic and pharmacologic relevance in the brains of AD patients.

The progressive cognitive deficits in AD have already been described in detail in this review. Mood changes are less constant features of the progression of AD than are changes in cognitive abilities and functioning. Nevertheless, such changes tend to occur in a somewhat characteristic pattern with the progression of Alzheimer's disease (Reisberg et al. 1983a). More specifically, the fourth Global Deterioration Scale stage (GDS = 4) is most frequently marked by a flattening of affect and withdrawal from previously challenging situations. In the fifth GDS stage tearful episodes are a frequent occurrence, in addition to the flattening of affect observed earlier in the illness. In the sixth GDS stage overt symptoms of agitation and psychosis are frequently noted, whereas in the final stage of Alzheimer's disease – the seventh stage – a pathologic passivity frequently replaces the agitation and psychosis which may have been observed earlier in the illness.

The behavioral symptoms of Alzheimer's disease, in particular the agitation and psychosis referred to above, are an enormous source of anguish to caregivers of victims of the disease. Our research indicates that concerns about these symptoms, and the medications which are prescribed to treat these symptoms, are the most frequently voiced by caregivers in support group settings (Shulman and Steinberg 1984). Issues with respect to these agitation symptoms are also the most frequently cited reasons provided by caregivers for placing their beloved spouses or relatives in institutional settings (Ferris et al. 1987).

Despite the importance of these symptoms, and the frequent use of psychotropic medications by physicians to treat these symptoms, very few studies have systematically examined the utility of psychotropic medications in treating these symptoms in Alzheimer's patients. Before adequate investigations can proceed, the nature of potentially remediable behavioral symptomatology in Alzheimer's patients must be described and appropriate rating instruments for measuring such symptoms must be available.

The nature of these symptoms in the Alzheimer's patient appear to be the result of two primary interacting processes:
1. the characteristic neurotransmitter changes which occur in the brains of the Alzheimer's patient, and
2. the cognitive changes occurring in the Alzheimer's patient.

For example, it has been noted that Alzheimer's patients frequently have the delusions, that "people are stealing things from them," that "the spouse is an impostor" and that their "house is not their home" (Reisberg and Ferris 1985). It appears that the delusional content in these patients is related to the presence of cognitive deficit. For example, with increasing cognitive deficit, Alzheimer's patients no longer remember where they have placed things as well as formerly. Consequently, when they become delusional, they may have a tendency to develop the delusion that people are stealing things from them. Similarly, with the evolution of cognitive deficit, Alzheimer's patients no longer recognize their spouse or their home environment with the same facility. Accordingly, when they develop delusional tendencies, these may frequently be manifested in content as the false belief that their spouse is not truly their spouse or that they are not, in actuality, in their domicile.

Another behavioral syndrome frequently noted in Alzheimer's patients is purposeless activity or cognitive abulia (literally, a loss of will power resulting from decreased cognitive abilities). Decreased cognition results in decreased ability to channel one's energy in specific, goal-oriented, behavior. Since motoric functioning is relatively well-preserved until the very last substages of the illness, Alzheimer's patients begin to exhibit purposeless behavior such as pacing.

In order to develop more information about the precise nature and incidence of potentially remediable symptoms of outpatients with specifically diagnosed Alzheimer's disease, we conducted a retrospective chart review (Reisberg et al. 1987). Fifty-seven patients with a diagnosis of Alzheimer's disease and Global Deterioration Scale (GDS) scores of 4 or greater were studied. The mean age ($\pm$ 1 SD) of the patients was 75 $\pm$ 9.1 years (range = 55–93 years) and they consisted of 24 men and 33 women.

On the basis of the phenomenologic and pharmacologic treatment data from this study, we have developed a rating scale – The Behavioral Pathology in Alzheimer's Disease Rating Scale (BEHAVE-AD). It differs from other rating measures in several important ways. Specifically:

1. All assessment measures are designed to specifically reflect and measure the characteristic behavioral symptoms which commonly occur in the Alzheimer's patient.
2. All assessment measures are largely independent of the primary, presently unremediable, cognitive symptomatology of Alzheimer's disease.
3. All assessment measures reflect behaviors which are frequently disturbing to caregivers of the Alzheimer's patient.
4. All assessment measures reflect behaviors which present clinical and research experience indicates are potentially remediable in the Alzheimer's patient, through pharmacologic and perhaps other interventions. Collectively, these advantages should enable clinical investigators to utilize this quantified assessment tool in prospectively designed studies of pharmacologically remediable symptoms in the Alzheimer's patient. Since virtually no such prospective studies have yet been conducted, this would appear to be an opportune time for the introduction of such a measure. It should be noted that this scale incorporates information and experience from a previous measure designed by us which we found to be underinclusive (Reisberg and Ferris 1985).

The BEHAVE-AD consists of 25 items which fall within 7 categories. The categories are
a) Paranoid and Delusional Ideation,
b) Hallucinations,
c) Activity Disturbances,
d) Aggressivity,
e) Diurnal Rhythm Disturbances,
f) Affective Disturbance, and
g) Anxieties and Phobias.

Each item is rated on a 4-point scale. In addition, the scale contains a global rating of the degree to which the behaviors are troubling to the caregiver. Pharmacologic intervention is based primarily upon the global assessment. A listing of the nature of the most important potentially remediable symptoms from the BEHAVE-AD can be found in Table 6. This listing is modified from a previously published description of the nature of those remediable symptoms (Reisberg et al. 1986a).

The relative incidence of specific remediable behavioral symptoms in AD patients had not been studied. Since these symptoms are likely to respond to pharmacologic intervention, the precise delineation of the nature and frequency of these symptoms is of considerable relevance. Accordingly, we examined the relative occurrence of these symptoms in 52 outpatients (20 men and 32 women) with AD (mean GDS = 5.2 ± 0.8; mean MMSE = 13.7 ± 6.8) and one or more of the behavioral symptoms (Reisberg et al. 1988c).

The results of this study are illustrated in Table 7. Eighteen specific symptoms were identified which occurred in 10% or more of all patients. The most common remediable symptom was purposeless activity, occurring in 58% of patients studied. Verbal repetitive behavior, tearfulness, and verbal outbursts occurred in 46%, 42%, and 42% of patients, respectively. The specific delusions that "people are stealing things" and that "one's house is not one's home" each occurred in 37% of patients. Collec-

Table 6. Pharmacologically remediable behavioral symptomatology in Alzheimer's disease[a, b]

A. **Paranoid and Delusional Ideation**

1. *The "people are stealing things" delusion.* Alzheimer's patients can no longer recall the precise whereabouts of household objects. This is probably the psychological explanation for what apparently is the most common delusion of AD patients, that someone is hiding or stealing objects. More severe manifestations of this delusion include the belief that persons are actually coming into the home to hide or steal objects; the patient may actually speak with or listen to the intruders.

2. *The "House is Not One's Home" delusion.* AD patients, as a result of their cognitive deficits, may no longer recognize their home. This appears to account, in part, for the common conviction of the AD patient that the place in which they are residing is not their home. Consequently, while actually at home, AD patients commonly request that their caregiver "take me home." They may also pack their bags for their return home. More disturbing to the caregiver, and of greater potential danger to the patient, are actual attempts to leave their house to go "home". Occasionally, attempts to prevent the patient's departure may result in anger or even violence toward the caregiver on the part of the patient. Such violence is extremely upsetting to the spouse or other caregiver.

3. *The "Spouse (or other caregiver) is an Impostor" delusion.* With the evolution of cognitive deficit, AD patients no longer recognize their caregivers as well as previously. Perhaps for this reason, a frequent delusion in the AD patient is that persons are impostors. In some instances anger and even violence may result from this conviction.

4. *The delusion of "Abandonment."* With the evolution of intellectual deficit in AD, a degree of insight into their condition remains relatively preserved. Although AD patients are largely aware of their cognitive deficits, denial protects them from the emotional consequenses of this awareness. Similarly, they may be aware of the burden which they have become. These insights are probably related to the common delusion of abandonment, institutionalization, or of a conspiracy or plot to institutionalize the patient.

5. *The Delusion of "Infidelity."* The insecurities described above are also related to the AD patient's occasional conviction that their spouse is unfaithful to them, sexually or otherwise. This conviction of infidelity may also apply to other caregivers.

6. *Other suspicions, paranoid ideation, or delusions.* Although the above specific delusions are the most commonly observed in AD, others may also be present.

Table 6. continued

B. **Hallucinations**

1. *Visual hallucinations.* These can be vague or clearly defined. Commonly, AD patients will see intruders or dead relatives at home or have similar hallucinatory experiences.

2. *Auditory hallucinations.* Occasionally, in the presence or absence of visual hallucinations, AD patients may hear dead relatives, intruders, or others whispering or speaking to them. Sometimes the voices are only heard when caregivers are not present.

3. *Other hallucinations.* Less commonly, other forms of hallucinations may be observed in AD patients (e. g., smelling a fire).

C. **Activity Disturbances**

AD patients' decreased cognitive capacity renders them less capable of channeling their energies in socially productive ways. Since motor abilities are not severely compromised until the final stage of the illness, the patient may develop various psychological/motoric solutions for their need to channel their energies. A few of the most common examples are the following:

1. *Wandering.* For a variety of reasons including inability to channel energies, anxieties, delusions such as those described above, and the decreased cognitive abilities per se, AD patients frequently wander away from the home or caregiver. Restraint may be necessary and this, in turn, may provoke anger or violence in the patient.

2. *Purposeless activity (cognitive abulia).* AD patients may not be able to carry a thought long enough to complete a purposeful movement. This results in a variety of purposeless, frequently repetitive activities including: opening and closing a purse or pocketbook; packing and unpacking clothing; repeatedly putting on and removing clothing; opening and closing drawers; incessant repeating of demands or questions; or simply pacing. Among the most severe manifestations of this syndrome is repetitive self-abrading.

3. *Inappropriate activities.* These occur primarily as a result of decreased cognitive capacities, increased anxieties and suspiciousness, and excess physical energies. They include storing and hiding objects in inappropriate places, such as throwing clothing in the wastebasket or putting empty plates in the oven. Attempts by the caregiver to prevent these inappropriate activities may be met by anger or even violence.

D. **Aggressivity**

1. *Verbal outbursts.* As already noted, these can occur in association with many of the behavioral symptoms already described. They can also occur as an isolated phenomenon. For example, an AD patient may begin to use unaccustomed foul or abusive language with intimates and/or with strangers.

2. *Physical outbursts.* These also can occur as part of the aforementioned syndromes or as an isolated manifestation. The AD patient may, in response to frustration or seemingly without cause, strike out at the spouse or caregiver.

E. **Diurnal Rhythm Disturbance**

Sleep problems are a frequent and significant part of the behavioral syndrome of AD. They may, in part, be the result of decreased cognition which upsets habitual and other diurnal cues, the energy and motoric changes occurring in the illness, and the neurochemical processes predisposing to agitation and psychosis.

1. *Day/night disturbance.* The most common sleep problem in AD patients is multiple awakenings in the course of the evening. These can occur in the context of an overall decrease in sleep or in association with increased daytime napping.

F. **Affective Disturbance**

The depressive syndrome of AD is primarily reactive in nature. The syndrome tends to occur somewhat earlier in the course of AD than many of the other symptoms described above and appears to be related to the pattern of insight and denial in the patient.

Table 6. continued

1. *Tearfulness.* This predominant depressive manifestation generally occurs in brief periods. If queried as to the reason for their tearfulness, the patient might respond that they are crying "because of the person whom they once were," or "because of what is happening to them," or that they "forgot the reason." This tearfulness frequently may be a precursor of more severe behavioral symptomatology.

2. *Other depressive manifestations.* A depressive syndrome may coexist with AD just as other illnesses may coexist with AD. A full discussion of this conjunction is beyond the scope of this summary. However, thoughts of death, generally not accompanied by overt affective symptoms or dysphoria, do occur as part of the depressive behavioral syndrome of AD. In some instances, these thoughts can be accompanied by suicidal threats or gestures.

G. **Anxieties and Phobias**

These may be related to the previously described behavioral manifestations of AD. They also can occur independently.

1. *Anxiety regarding upcoming events (Godot syndrome).* This common syndrome appears to result from decreased cognitive and, more specifically, memory abilities in the AD patient, and from their inability to channel their remaining thinking capacities productively. Consequently, the patient will repeatedly query with respect to an upcoming event. These queries may be so incessant and persistent as to be intolerable.

2. *Fear of being left alone.* This is the most commonly observed phobia in AD. As a phobic phenomenon it is entirely out of proportion to any real danger. For example, the anxieties may become manifest as soon as the spouse goes into another room.

[a] Reisberg B, Borenstein J, Franssen E, Shulman E, Steinberg C, Ferris SH (1986) Remediable behavioral symptomatology in Alzheimer's disease, Hosp Community Psychiatry 37: 1199–1201

[b] Adapted from "Behavioral Pathology in Alzheimer's Disease (BEHAVE-AD)" © 1986 by Barry Reisberg, M.D.

Table 7. Nature and incidence of specific behavioral symptoms in 52 AD patients who manifest one or more behavioral symptoms

Symptoms	N	%
Purposeless activity (cognitive abulia)	30	58
Verbal repetitive behavior	24	46
Tearfulness	22	42
Verbal outbursts	22	42
"People are stealing things" delusion	19	37
"One's house is not one's home" delusion	19	37
Day/night disturbance	19	37
Visual hallucinations	18	35
Depressed mood	18	35
Agitation	18	35
Delusions, unspecified type	16	31
Suspiciousness	15	29
Wandering	15	29
Physical threats/violence	12	23
Auditory hallucinations	10	19
Delusion of abandonment	10	19
"Spouse is an impostor" delusion	8	15
Delusion of infidelity	5	10
Other hallucinations	1	2

Adapted from Reisberg et al. (1988c)

tively, these results indicate that a specific symptomatologic profile of potentially remediable behavioral symptoms in AD can be described in considerable detail. This symptomatic syndrome is common and should be carefully assessed in all pharmacologic trials of the treatment of cognitive or behavioral symptoms of AD. This recommendation applies to cognitive as well as behavioral AD trials because current data are consistent with the hypothesis that all observed positive cognitive changes which have been produced by pharmacologic agents in AD patients have been the secondary resultant of improvements in mood and BEHAVE-AD symptoms.

Conclusion

Clearly, information regarding the symptomatic course of AD has been rapidly accruing. These symptoms should be conceptualized in global terms as well as in terms of the ordinal and temporal course of loss of specific cognitive, psychologic, psychometric, and functional elements. Information regarding current knowledge of these factors has been reviewed briefly in this chapter. Possible etiologic implications of the symptomatic and temporal course of AD have also been discussed.

It is particularly important for the present-day clinician and/or investigator to recognize and separate out, commonly occurring potentially remediable symptoms in the course of AD. Precise interventions for these remediable symptoms can now be systematically studied using available methodologic instruments.

References

Adolfsson R, Gottfries CG, Oreland L (1980) Increased activity of brain and platelet monoamine oxidase in dementia of the Alzheimer type. Life Sci 27: 1029–1034

Aletta JM, Lewis SA, Cowan NJ, Greene LA (1988) Nerve growth factor regulates both the phosphorylation and steady-state levels of microtubule-associated protein 1.2 (MAP1.2). J Cell Biol 106: 1573–1581

Anderson DJ, Axel R (1986) A bipotential neuroendocrine precursor whose choice of cell fate is determined by NGF and glucocorticoids. Cell 47: 1079–1090

Bjerre B, Bjorklund A (1973) The production of catecholamine-containing cells in vitro by young chick embryos: effects of nerve growth factor (NGF) and its antiserum. Neurobiol (Copenh) 3: 140–161

Blessed G, Tomlinson BE, Roth M (1968) The association between quantitative measures of dementia and senile change in the cerebral gray matter of elderly subjects. Br J Psychiatry 114: 797–811

Bondareff W, Mountjoy CQ, Roth M (1982) Loss of neurons of origin of the adrenergic projection to cerebral cortex (nucleus locus ceruleus) in senile dementia. Neurology (NY) 32: 164–168

Borenstein J, Reisberg B (1987) Functional deficits in Alheimer's disease. 1987 New Research Program & Abstracts, American Psychiatric Association, 140th Annual Meeting 56 (Abstract)

Borenstein J, Franssen E, de Leon MJ, Sinaiko E, Ferris SH, Reisberg B (1987) Predictors of course in Alzheimer's disease. The Third Congress of the International Psychogeriatric Association 34 (Abstract)

Borenstein J, Reisberg B, Sinaiko E, Ferris SH (1987) Use of functional assessment as a diagnostic technique. The Third Congress of the International Psychogeriatric Association 34–35 (Abstract)

Bowen DM, Spillane JA, Curzon G, Meier-Ruge W, White P, Goodhardt MJ, Iwangoff P, Davison AN (1979) Accelerated ageing or selective neuronal loss as an important cause of dementia. Lancet 1: 11–14

Brinkman SD, Largen JW, Cushman L, Sarwar M (1986) Anatomical validators: progressive changes in dementia. In: Poon LW (ed) Handbook for clinical memory assessment of older adults. American Psychological Assoc., Washington (DC), pp 359–366

Brugg B, Matus A (1988) PC12 cells express juvenile microtubule-associated proteins during nerve growth factor-induced neurite outgrowth. J Cell Biol 107: 643–650

Cole MG, Dastoor DP (1980) Development of a dementia rating scale: Preliminary communication. J Clin Exp Gerontol 2: 46–63

Cole MG, Dastoor DP (1987) A new hierarchic approach to the measurements of dementia. Psychosomatics 28: 298–304

Cole MG, Dastoor DP, Koszycki D (1983) The hierarchic dementia scale. J Clin Exp Gerontol 5: 219–234

Constantinidis J (1978) Is Alzheimer's disease a major form of senile dementia? Clinical, anatomical and genetic data. In: Katzman R, Terry RD, Bick KL (eds) Alzheimer's disease: senile dementia and related disorders (Aging, Vol. 7) Raven Press, New York

Constantinidis J, Richard J, de Ajuriaguerra J (1978) Dementias with senile plaques and neurofibrillary changes. In: Isaacs AD, Post F (eds) Studies in geriatric psychiatry. John Wiley, New York, pp 119–152

Cowan WM, Fawcett JW, O'Leong DDM, Stanfield BB (1984) Regressive events in neurogenesis. Science 225: 1258–1265

Dastoor DP, Cole MG (1986) The course of Alzheimer's disease: An uncontrolled longitudinal study. J Clin Exp Gerontol 7: 289–299

Davies P (1988) Neurochemical studies: update in Alzheimer's disease. J Clin Psychiatry 49 [5, Suppl.]: 23–28

Davies P, Maloney AJF (1976) Selective loss of central cholinergic neurons in Alzheimer's disease. Lancet 2: 1403

de Ajuriaguerra J, Tissot R (1975) Some aspects of language in various forms of senile dementia: comparisons with language in childhood. In: Lennenberg EH, Lennenberg E (eds) Foundations of language development, (Vol. 1) Academic Press, New York

de Ajuriaguerra J, Rey M, Bellete-Muller M (1964) A propos de quelques problèmes posées par le déficit opératoire des viellards atteints de démence dégénerative en debut d'evolution. Cortex 1: 232–256

de Leon MJ, Ferris SH, Blau I, George AE, Reisberg B, Kricheff II, Gershon S (1979) Correlations between CT changes and behavioral deficits in senile dementia. Lancet 2: 859–860

de Leon MJ, Ferris SH, George AE, Reisberg B, Kricheff II, Gershon S (1980) Computed tomography evaluations of brain-behavior relationships in senile dementia of the Alzheimer's type. Neurobiol Aging 1: 60–69

de Leon MJ, Ferris SH, George AE, Reisberg B, Christman DR, Kricheff II, Wolf AP (1983) Computed tomography and positron emission transaxial tomography evaluations of normal aging and Alzheimer's disease. J Cereb Blood Flow Metab 3: 391–394

de Leon MJ, McRae T, Tsai JR, George AE, Marcus D, Freedman M, Wolf AP, McEwen B (1988) Abnormal cortisol response in Alzheimer's disease associated with CT and PET temporal lobe changes. Lancet 2 (8607): 391–392

Doupe AJ, Landis SC, Patterson PH (1985b) Environmental influence in the development of neural crest derivatives: glucocorticoids, growth factors and chromaffin cell plasticity. J Neurosci 5: 2119–2142

Doupe AJ, Patterson PH, Landis SC (1985a) Small intensely fluorescent (SIF) cells in culture: role of glucocorticoids and growth factors in their development and phenotypic interconversions with other neural crest derivatives. J Neurosci 5: 2143–2160

Ferris SH, de Leon MJ, Wolf AP, Farkas T, Christman DR, Reisberg B, Fowler JS, MacGregor R, Goldman A, George AE, and Rampal S (1980) Positron emission tomography in the study of aging and senile dementia. Neurobiol Aging 1: 127–131

Ferris SH, Steinberg G, Shulman E, Kahn R, Reisberg B (1987) Institutionalization of Alzheimer's disease patients: reducing precipitating factors through family counseling. Home Health Care Services Quarterly 8: 23–51

Folstein MF (1983) The Mini-Mental State exam. In: Crook T, Ferris SH, Bartus R (eds) Assessment in geriatric psychopharmacology. Mark Powley Associates, New Canaan, Ct. p 47–51

Folstein MF, Folstein SE, McHugh PR (1975) Mini-mental state: a practical method for grading the cognitive state of patients for the clinician. J Psychiatr Res 12: 189–198

Foster JR, Sclan S, Welkowitz J, Boksay I, Seeland I (1988) Psychiatric assessment in medical longterm care facilities: Reliability of commonly used rating scales. Intern. J of Geriatric Psychiatry 3: 229–233

Fox JH, Topel JL, Huckman MS (1975) Use of computerized tomography in senile dementia. J Neurol Neurosurg Psychiatry 38: 948–953

Francis PT, Palmer AM, Sims NR, Bowen DM, Davison AN, Esiri MM, Neary D, Snouden JS, Wilcock GK (1985) Neurochemical studies of early-onset Alzheimer's disease: Possible influence on treatment. N Engl J Med 313: 7–11

Gilbert JG, Levee RF, Catalano FL (1968) A preliminary report on a new memory scale. Percept Mot Skills 27: 277–278

Gottlieb GL, Gur RE, Gur RC (1988) Reliability of psychiatric scales in patients with dementia of the Alzheimer type. Am J Psychiatry 45: 857–859

Greene LA, Tischler AS (1976) Establishment of a noradrenergic clonal line of rat adrenal pheochromocytoma cells which respond to nerve growth factor. Proc Natl Acad Sci USA 73: 2424–2428

Hamburger V, Levi-Montalcini R (1949) Proliferation, differentiation and degeneration in the spinal ganglia of the chick embryo under neuronal experimental conditions. J Exp Zool 111: 451–452

Hamburger V, Oppenheim RW (1982) Naturally occuring neuronal death in vertebrates. Neurosci Comment 1: 39–55

Hamburger V, Brunso-Bechtold JK, Yip JW (1981) Neuronal death in the spinal ganglia of the chick embryo and its reduction by nerve growth factor. J Neurosci 1: 60–71

Haxby JV, Grady CL, Duara R, Schlageter N, Berg G, Rappaport SI (1986) Neocortical metabolic abnormalities precede nonmemory cognitive defects in early Alzheimer's-Type dementia. Arch Neurol 43: 882–885

Hendry IA, Campbell J (1976) Morphometric analysis of rat superior cervical ganglion after axotomy and nerve growth factor treatment. J Neurocytol 5: 351–360

Hoyer S, Oesterreich K, Wagner O (1988) Glucose metabolism as the site of the primary abnormality in early-onset dementia of the Alzheimer type? J Neurol 235: 143–148

Kahn RL, Goldfarb AI, Pollack M, Peck A (1960) Brief objective measures for the determination of mental status in the aged. Am J Psychiatry 117: 326–328

Landgraf R, Mitro A, Hess J (1978) Regional net uptake of 14C-glucose by rat brain under the influence of corticosterone. Endocrinol Exp 12: 119–129

Lasbennes F, Lestage P, Bobillier P, Seylaz J (1986) Stress and local cerebral blood flow: studies on restrained and unrestrained rats. Exp Brain Res 63: 163–168

Leeds M (1960) Senile recession: A clinical entity? J Am Geriatr Soc 8: 122–131

Leonard DGB, Ziff EB, Green LA (1987) Identification and characterization of mRNA's regulated by nerve growth factor in PC12 cells. Mol Cell Biol 9: 3156–3167

Leonard DGB, Gorham JD, Cole P, Greene LA, Ziff EB (1988) A nerve growth factor-regulated messenger RNA encodes a new intermediate filament protein. J Cell Biol 106: 181–193

Levi-Montalcini R, Booker B (1960) Destruction of the sympathetic ganglia in mammals by an antiserum to the nerve-growth promoting factor. Proc Natl Acad Sci USA 42: 384–391

Long JB, Holaday JW (1985) Blood-brain barrier: endogenous modulation by adrenal-cortical function. Science 227: 1580–1583

Mash DC, Flynn DD, Potter LT (1985) Loss of M2 muscarinic receptors in the cerebral cortex in Alzheimer's disease and experimental cholinergic denervation. Science 228: 1115–1117

Martin DP, Schmidt RE, Di Stefano PS, Lowry OH, Carter JG, Johnson Jr EM (1988) Inhibitors of protein synthesis and RNA synthesis prevent neuronal death caused by nerve growth factor deprivation. J Cell Biol 106: 829–844

Nie NH, Hull CH, Jenkins JG, Steinbrenner K, Bent DH (1975) Statistical Package for the Social Sciences, McGraw-Hill, 2nd edn New York, pp 531–533

Nordeen EJ, Nordeen KW, Sengelaub DR, Arnold AP (1985) Androgens prevent normally occurring cell death in a sexually dimorphic spinal nucleus. Science 229: 671–673

Oppenheim RW (1981) Neuronal cell death and some related regressive phenomena during neurogenesis. In: Cowan WM (ed) Studies in developmental neurobiology: Essays in honor of Victor Hamburger. Oxford University Press, London, pp 74–132

Oppenheim RW (1985) Naturally occuring cell death during neural development. Trends Neurosci 17: 487–493

Perry EK, Perry RH, Blessed G, Tomlinson BE (1977) Necropsy evidence of central cholinergic deficits in senile dementia. Lancet 1: 189

Perry EK, Perry RH, Blessed G (1978b) Changes in brain cholinesterases in senile dementia of the Alzheimer type. Neuropathol Appl Neurobiol 4: 273–277

Perry EK, Tomlinson BE, Blessed G, Bergmann K, Gibson PH, Perry RH (1978a) Correlation of cholinergic abnormalities with senile plaques and mental test scores in senile dementia. Br Med J 2: 1457–1459

Reisberg B (1986e) Dementia: A systematic approach to identifying reversible causes. Geriatrics 41: 30–46

Reisberg B, Ferris SH (1985) A clinical rating scale for symptoms of psychosis in Alzheimer's disease. Psychopharmacol Bull 21: 101–104

Reisberg B, Ferris SH (1988a) The Brief Cognitive Rating Scale (BCRS). Psychopharmacol Bull 24: 629–636

Reisberg B, Ferris SH, de Leon MJ, Crook T (1982) The global deterioration scale for assessment of primary degenerative dementia. Am J Psychiatry 139: 1136–1139

Reisberg B, London E, Ferris SH, Borenstein J, Scheier L, de Leon MJ (1983b) The Brief Cognitive Rating Scale: Language, motoric, and mood concomitants in primary degenerative dementia. Psychopharmacol Bull 19: 702–708

Reisberg B, Schneck MK, Ferris SH, Schwartz GE, de Leon MJ (1983a) The brief cognitive rating scale (BCRS): Findings in primary degenerative dementia (PDD). Psychopharmacol Bull 19: 47–50

Reisberg B, Ferris SH, Anand R, de Leon MJ, Schneck MK, Buttinger C, Borenstein J (1984) Functional staging of dementia of the Alzheimer's type. Ann NY Acad Sci 435: 481–483

Reisberg B, Ferris SH, de Leon MJ (1985a) Senile dementia of the Alzheimer type: Diagnostic and differential diagnostic features with special reference to functional assessment staging. In: Traber J, and Gispen WH (eds) Senile dementia of the Alzheimer type, Vol. 2. Springer, Berlin Heidelberg New York, pp 18–37

Reisberg B, Ferris SH, Franssen E (1985b) An ordinal functional assessment tool for Alzheimer's-type dementia. Hosp Community Psychiatry 36: 593–595

Reisberg B, Borenstein J, Franssen E, Shulman E, Steinberg G, Ferris SH (1986a) Remediable behavioral symptomatology in Alzheimer's disease. Hosp Community Psychiatry 37: 1199–1201

Reisberg B, Ferris SH, Borenstein J, Sinaiko E, de Leon MJ, Buttinger C (1986b) Assessment of presenting symptoms. In: Poon LW (ed) The handbook for clinical memory assessment of older adults. American Psychological Association, Washington (DC), pp 108–128

Reisberg B, Ferris SH, Franssen E (1986c) Functional degenerative stages in dementia of the Alzheimer's type appear to reverse normal human development. In: Shagass C et al. (eds) Biological Psychiatry 1985, Vol. 7. Elsevier, Science Publishing Co, New York, pp 1319–1321

Reisberg B, Ferris SH, Shulman E, Steinberg G, Buttinger C, Sinaiko E, Borenstein J, de Leon MJ, Cohen J (1986d) Longitudinal course of normal aging and progressive dementia of the Alzheimer's type: A prospective study of 106 subjects over a 3.6 year mean interval. Prog Neuropsychopharmacol Biol Psychiatry 10: 571–578

Reisberg B, Borenstein J, Salob SP, Ferris SH, Franssen E, Georgotas A (1987) Behavioral symptoms in Alzheimer's disease: phenomenology and treatment. J Clin Psychiatry 48 (Suppl): 9–15

Reisberg B, Borenstein J, D'Andrea N, Ferris SH (1988c) Phenomenology of pharmacologically remediable neuropsychiatric symptoms in Alzheimer's disease (AD). Psychopharmacology 96 (Suppl): 224 (Abstract)

Reisberg B, Ferris SH, de Leon MJ, Crook T (1988e) The Global Deterioration Scale (GDS). Psychopharmacol Bull 24: 661–663

Reisberg B, Ferris SH, de Leon MJ, Sinaiko E, Franssen E, Kluger A, Mir P, Borenstein J, George AE, Shulman E, Steinberg G, Cohen J (1988d) Stage-specific behavioral, cognitive, and in vivo changes in age-associated memory impairment (AAMI) and primary degenerative dementia of the Alzheimer type. Drug Dev Res 15: 101–114

Reisberg B, Ferris SH, Franssen E, Jenkins EC, Wisniewski KE (1988b) Clinical features of a neuropathologically verified familial Alzheimer's cohort with onset in the fourth decade: comparison with senile onset Alzheimer's disease and etiopathogenic implications. In: Proceedings: First International Conference on Alzheimer's Disease and Related Disorders (in press)

Rossor MN, Iversen LL, Reynolds GP (1984) Neurochemical characteristics of early and late onset types of Alzheimer's disease. Br Med J 288: 961–964

Shulman E, Steinberg G (1984) Emotional reactions of Alzheimer's caregivers in support group settings. Gerontologist (special issue October): 102

Wechsler DA (1958) The Measurement and Appraisal of Adult Intelligence, Williams and Wilkins, 4th edn. Baltimore

Yip HK, Johnson Jr EM (1984) Developing dorsal root ganglion neurons require trophic support from their control processes: evidence for a role of retrogradely transported nerve growth factor from the central nervous system to the periphery. Proc Natl Acad Sci 81: 6245–6249

Diagnosis and Treatment of Senile Dementia: Early Diagnosis and Differential Diagnosis*

C. G. Gottfries

Introduction

Organic psychosyndromes can be due either to a selective disturbance of brain function or to more general degenerative disorders or a disturbed metabolism of the brain. The term dementia is a more narrow concept. It is not applied to isolated focal loss of function such as occurs in amnesia, aphasia, agnosia, or apraxia. Historically, dementia has meant an acquired, irreversible, global deterioration of mental functions. The disorder was thought to be progressive and due to organic brain damage. In this definition, different aspects of the disease are brought together in a way which, in the light of present knowledge, is difficult to accept.

Definition of Dementia

At present dementia is defined as a disorder characterized by mental impairment acquired in later life, independent of course, extent, or etiology. According to the DSM-III, the mental impairment in dementia should be of such a degree that it interferes with the social life or health of the patient. The distinction of disabling and nondisabling mental impairment is, however, difficult and perhaps unnecessary. In dementia, memory impairment should be present together with impairment of at least one other main cognitive capacity or adaptive behavior. According to the DSM-III, there should be no major alteration of consciousness. This may be difficult to differentiate, as confusion and dementia overlap.

Diagnosis of Dementia

At our institute dementia is diagnosed on the basis of symptoms according to DSM III and the diagnostic process presented in Fig. 1. In this diagnostic process the severity of

* This study was supported by grants from The Old Servant's Foundation, The Medical Research Council, Greta and Johan Kock's Foundation, Hjalmar Svensson's Research Foundation, The Söderström-König Nursing Home Foundation, The Pfannenstill Foundation, The Lundbeck Foundation, and Fredrik and Ingrid Thuring's Foundation.

Bergener, Reisberg (Eds.)
Diagnosis and Treatment
of Senile Dementia
© Springer-Verlag Berlin Heidelberg 1989

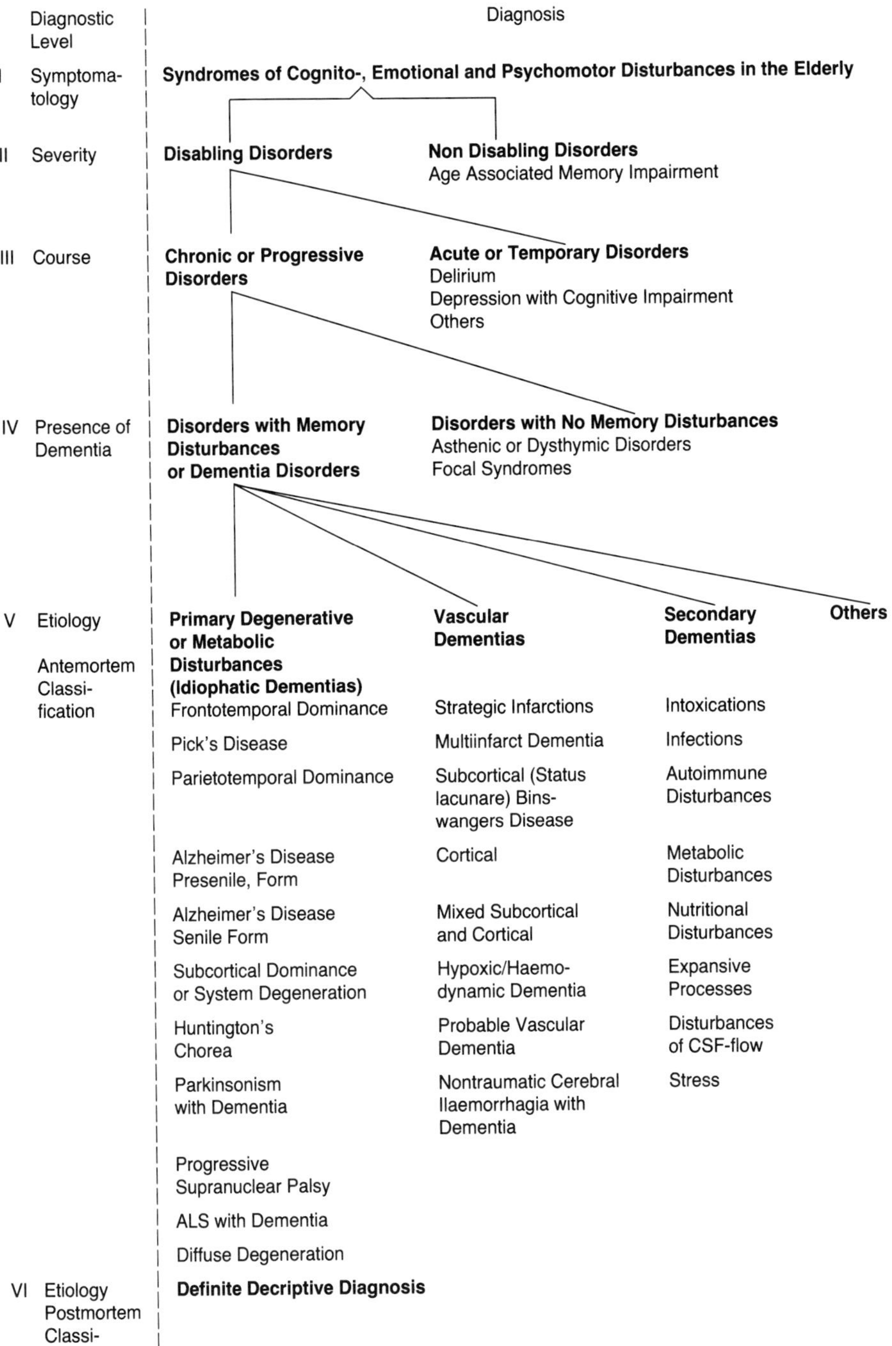

Fig. 1. The classification of dementias

the disorder, the course of the disorder, and the assumed etiology of the disorder are taken into account. As is evident in the figure, aquired mental impairment in old age can be divided into disabling and nondisabling disorders. To the group of nondisabling disorders belong age-associated memory impairment (AAMI) or benign senile forgetfulness. Whether this benign form of mental impairment in old age is due to the normal aging process, a special entity, or a dementing process which may progress to a more malignant form of dementia, is at present not known (see Crook et al. 1986).

According to the course of the illness, the disabling disorders are classified as long-standing or temporary disorders. The latter group includes those forms which in some textbooks are named pseudodementias. The most important forms of cognitive impairment in this group are those seen together with delirium or depression.

According to their etiology, the long-standing disorders can be subdivided into four groups:
a) primary dementias, in which the etiology is assumed to be a primary degeneration or dysfunction of the brain;
b) vascular dementias, in which the blood supply to the brain is assumed to be disturbed;
c) secondary dementias, in which a known somatic disorder causes the dementia; and
d) "nonspecified dementias."

Primary Dementias

The primary or idiopathic dementias are the quantitatively most important group. This group can be subdivided according to assumed etiology, in descriptive diagnoses as Pick's disease, Alzheimer's disease, senile dementia of Alzheimer type, parkinsonism with dementia, Huntington's chorea, etc. As most of these diagnoses cannot be confirmed until autopsy, it would perhaps be of interest, due to the development in brain imaging techniques, to divide the group according to the findings with these techniques. To some extent, concepts such as frontal lobe dementias, cortical dementias, and subcortical dementias are already used.

Alzheimer described already in 1906 a disorder with onset in presenile age with specific lesions in the brain, which was later named after him. Originally this concept was used only for disorders with early onset, but as neuropathologists found that the same type of brain lesions were found also in brains of patients with late-onset dementia and with the same type of symptomatology as patients with Alzheimer's disease (AD), these forms were named senile dementia of Alzheimer type (SDAT). It is obvious, however, that there are late-onset dementias, senile dementias (SD) without Alzheimer lesions, for which the term SDAT is not appropriate.

In this chapter the term SD is used for primary dementias with onset after the age of 65, including SDAT but excluding descriptive diagnoses such as Huntington's chorea, parkinsonism with dementia, etc.

Differential Diagnostic Problems

Senile Dementia – Dementia of Alzheimer Type

A few comments must be made regarding the concepts of SD, SDAT and AD. The differentiation between AD and SDAT is based on the age at onset (before or after 65). In several investigations the two forms are collapsed into one group called dementia of Alzheimer type (DAT). There is, however, still no justification for grouping these two forms together. In studies of familial aggregation, Heston and Mastri (1977) found that relatives of AD patients had a markedly increased risk for AD. Sjögren et al. (1952) and Sourander and Sjögren (1970) found that there is a fourfold increased risk for SD in siblings of SD patients. No instance of AD was found in the family members investigated. These family studies thus indicate that the two disorders are separate from each other. Investigations of neurotransmitters, their metabolites, and enzyme activities involved in the metabolism of neurotransmitters indicate that the changes recorded are more severe in the cases with early onset than in those with late onset (Gottfries et al. 1983; Rossor et al. 1984). In an investigation by Mayeux et al. (1985) the frequency distribution of age at onset of symptoms was recorded for patients with AD and SD. In this investigation a bimodal distribution was found, again indicating that there are two disorders with different age at onset.

Brun and Gustafson (1978) reported white matter changes in brains from patients with dementia. They found these changes mostly in SD patients but to a lesser extent in patients with AD. Blennow et al. (1988a) reported a study with computed tomography imaging of the brain. In the AD patients there was cortical atrophy and almost complete absence of periventricular white matter attenuation and central atrophy, whereas patients with SDAT, SD or vascular dementia showed moderate to severe changes. These findings also indicate that AD is a distinct clinical entity.

From these studies it can be concluded that SD, SDAT and AD should not be collapsed into one group. AD is a small, perhaps rather homogenous group, but SD is a very large group delimited by the age at onset and the absence of evident explanation for the mental impairment. The diagnosis of SDAT cannot be made until after death; therefore it can be asked whether the concept of SD not is to be prefered. SD thus should include SDAT and other forms of primary dementias with onset after the age of 65. Those forms that can be diagnosed according to special symptoms, e. g., Huntington's chorea, should of course not be included.

Senile Dementia – Age-Associated Memory Impairment

Epidemiological data indicate that there is a high correlation between age and dementia disorders (Gottfries 1986). The strong relationship may indicate that dementia is inevitable. At present it is difficult to distinguish mental impairment due to normal aging from that due to pathological processes in the brain, by psychological tests or rating scales. Nor do morphological changes clearly delimit normal aging from SD. Atrophy of the brain, neuron loss, and the Alzheimer lesions do not always differentiate SD from normal aging although there often are quantitative differences. Postmortem human brain studies have been performed for studying neurotransmitter metabolism. These investigations have shown that several of the neurotransmitters are reduced with age, at least at ages above 60 (Carlsson and Winblad 1976). As these findings are obtained in brains from normally aged individuals, an involution phase with onset in the 60s can be assumed to take place. It is well known that the brain has a very large reserve capacity. The behavioral consequences of the aging process therefore do not become evident until the reserves run out at the age of approximately 80–90. One important feature, however, of the involution process is that the thresholds for insufficiency reactions are lowered. This is clinically reflected by the increased rates of delirium states, affective disorders/suicides, and memory disturbances. It has also been shown that environmental factors have an importance for the development of disabling dementia (Karlsson et al. 1988). The normal aging process together with negative environmental factors may give rise to memory disturbances. Whether these behavioral disturbances can be separated from a special entity, the so-called age-associated memory impairment (AAMI), and the pathological process SD, is at present not possible to say. According to the author, it can be assumed that there is a continuity between the normal aging process, AAMI, and SD.

Senile Dementia – Temporary Disorders

Delirium states are usually rather easy to diagnose, and the differential diagnosis between SD and delirium states is not difficult. However, ratings with the GBS scale (Andersson and Gottfries 1988) have shown that in many demented patients, although they have no delirium, a mild to moderate confusion often is present. At our institute we assume that disturbed clearness of mind may be an important factor in the pathophysiology of SD.

It is well known that the differential diagnosis between depression and SD may offer problems. A careful psychiatric status of the patient, psychological investigations, and electroencephalogram may, however, distinguish between the two disorders.

Senile Dementia – Vascular Dementias

The most well-known form of vascular dementia is multi-infarction dementia (MID). In this disorder there is an abrupt onset and a stepwise course, which clearly differentiates this form from SD. Wallin et al. (1988) found in autopsy studies, however, that there are forms of vascular dementia with no abrupt onset and with a slow progression. Later in the course of the illness there may be vascular insults. Neuropathological and neurochemical investigations of the brains of these patients have shown that there are rather general disturbances, e. g., reduced concentrations of choline acetyltransferase activity and reduced concentrations of 5-hydroxytryptamine and 5-hydroxyindolacetic acid (5-HIAA), in cortical as well as subcortical areas. In these vascular dementias there are no Alzheimer lesions. Vasculitis or hemodynamic disturbances in the form of blood pressure falls or heart rhythm disturbances are assumed to be of importance for the dementia.

Senile Dementia – Secondary Dementias

Vitamin B_{12} deficiency is known to be associated with dementia and confusion even in the absence of hematologic change. Regland et al. (1988) investigated 155 patients with dementia for the concentration of vitamin B_{12} in serum. Values of S-B_{12} below 130 pmol/l were considered pathologic. Such low levels were found in 50% (5/10) in the group of confusional states and in 23% (13/56) in the SD group. In the AD group 6% (2/35), in the vascular group 9% (5/54), and in a control group 0% (0/16) had S-B_{12} concentrations lower than 130 pmol/l. It was concluded that in the group described as SD there was a significant increase of pathologically reduced concentrations of vitamin B_{12}. A significant negative correlation was found between the S-B_{12} levels and the activity of monoamine oxidase in platelets. This finding was interpreted as indicating that in the patients with low vitamin B_{12} levels there were immature platelets. A pathophysiological role of vitamin B_{12} for the dementia process cannot be excluded.

Immunological aberrations have been suggested as critical factors in the pathogenesis of neurodegenerative diseases. Results reported by McRae-Degueurce et al. (1988) show that patients with AD and SDAT in their CSF contain antibodies which recognize acetylcholine-like epitopes in cholinergic neurons in the rodent central nervous system. These findings indicate that in AD and SDAT there may be autoimmune processes which perhaps can be diagnosed by investigation of the CSF. If such a subgroup exists, it should be counted to the group of secondary dementias.

Early Diagnosis

Monoamine Metabolites in CSF

As biopsies are not usually carried out in the diagnosis of dementia disorders, biological markers for dementia must be sought in the body fluids. Over the past decade there has been increasing interest in the transmitter changes in dementia disorders. In studies by Parnetti et al. (1987) and Bråne et al. (1988), the monoamines and their metabolites were investigated in CSF. It was shown that only the main metabolites homovanillic acid (HVA), 3-methoxy-4-hydroxyphenylglycol (MHPG) and 5-HIAA gave valid information when controls were compared with patients with dementia disorders. A consistent finding is that HVA is significantly reduced in patients with AD when compared to those with SD and to controls. Also 5-HIAA was significantly reduced, however this reduction was less evident between the AD and the SD patients. MHPG was significantly increased in the SD patients when compared to controls. These findings are in accordance with other studies (Gottfries et al. 1969; Soininen et al. 1981). The HVA and 5-HIAA concentrations in CSF were, according to Bråne et al. (1988), significantly correlated with rated impairment.

Neuropeptides in CSF

CSF studies may also give information about disturbances of neuropeptides in the brain. In AD and SD patients somatostatin and corticotropin releasing factor are shown to be reduced in brain tissue as well as in CSF (Widerlöv et al. 1988). Delta sleep inducing peptide is reduced in serum as well as in CSF (Ernst et al. 1987). It may be of value to further study the concentrations of neuropeptides in CSF in the search for markers for dementia disorders. Such studies are in progress.

γ-Globulins in CSF

According to Blennow et al. (1988b) there is an intrathecal synthesis of immuno-globulin in patients with AD and SD. The intrathecal synthesis of IgM is somewhat more frequent and pronounced than IgG synthesis. The intrathecal immunoglobulin synthesis is not related to sex, age, or severity of disease; neither is it correlated to blood-brain barrier damage. The changes are not associated with other markers of infection of CNS and cannot be explained by common infectious agents. It is inter-preted either as an indication of a dysfunction of the immune system (autoimmune process), an indication of infectious agent, or as secondary to cerebral degeneration. IgG was found in 11% and IgM in 16% of patients with AD or SD. The further study of immunoglobulins in CSF may be of diagnostic value.

Neuroendocrinological Studies in Dementia

The dexamethasone suppression test (DST) is a laboratory test in patients with melancholia. However, it has also been shown that 50%–70% of patients with dementia disorders have a pathological response to DST (Balldin et al. 1983). These data indicate that demented patients have a disturbed activity in the hypothalamus-pituitary-adrenal (HPA) axis.

Other neuroendocrinological parameters can be used for the diagnosis and the elucidation of the pathophysiological substrate of dementia disorders. One method for assessing the postsynaptic noradrenaline (NA) sensitivity in patients is to give the NA agonist clonidine, known to stimulate the secretion of growth hormone (GH) in animals as well as in humans. The maximum GH response can be considered a marker for the postsynaptic NA sensitivity. In melancholia there is a blunted GH response to clonidine. According to Balldin et al. (1988), clonidine did not stimulate GH, yet depressed blood pressure levels were recorded in the investigated patients. Thus, there seems to be a change in the α_2-receptor sensitivity involved in GH secretion in patients with dementia disorders, while receptors which regulate blood pressure are unchanged.

Another neuroendocrin test is a challenge with thyrotropine-releasing hormone (TRH). In normals this test produces a TSH response. In melancholia 25% of patients have a blunted TRH response. In a study performed at our institute (J. Balldin, unpublished data) it was found that in 12 demented patients four had a blunted response to TRH loading as marked by a low TSH increase.

It is evident that the neuroendocrinologic studies provide information about the pathophysiology of dementia disorders and may also be of diagnostic value. Of interest are the considerable similarities between neuroendocrine disturbances in melancholia and dementia disorders. These tests can therefore not be used in the differential diagnosis between dementia and depression with dementia.

Serum Investigations

It is obvious from the data presented above that the concentration of vitamin $S-B_{12}$ shoud be investigated in patients with SD. As vitamin B_{12} is actively transported over membranes, it may perhaps also be of value to investigate the vitamin B_{12} concentration in CSF. As the vitamin B_{12} deficiency may be a marker for reduced transport over membranes, perhaps other essential nutrients that are actively transported must also be checked in old-age dementias, e. g., folic acid, vitamin B_6, amino acids such as tryptophane and tyrosine, and metals such as zinc.

Summary

The concept of SD refers to a group of primary dementias with onset over the age of 65. This is a large group of dementias, and from an etiologic point of view it can be assumed to be a heterogeneous group. There may be a continuity between the physiological aging process, AAMI, and SD. The differential diagnosis between SD and temporary disorders is difficult. Patients with no dementia symptoms in their history and with an acute onset of a delirium attack are easily diagnosed. Ratings have, however, shown that mild to moderate degrees of confusion are very often present in the SD syndrome. The differential diagnosis between SD and vascular dementias is, in typical cases, not difficult. However, there are vascular dementias with an insidious onset and a slow progression which may offer difficulties when separating them from SD.

At present there are no good markers for the diagnosis of SD. CSF studies of monoamine metabolites have shown altered concentrations when comparing AD and SD patients with age-matched controls. The neuropeptides somatostatin, corticotropin-releasing factor, and δ-sleep-inducing peptides are reduced in CSF. In patients with AD and SD, 25% also have altered concentrations of γ-globulins in CSF. CSF investigations must therefore be recommended in the early diagnosis of SD.

Neuroendocrinologic studies have shown disturbed functions in AD and SD which are very similar to those found in melancholia. These investigations can be considered in the early diagnosis of SD but cannot be used for the differential diagnosis between SD and affective disorders. Serum investigations in SD should focus on vitamin B_{12} deficiency and possibly also on deficiency of other essential nutrients.

References

Alzheimer A (1907) Über eine eigenartige Erkrankung der Hirnrinde Cbl. Nervenheilk Psychiat 18: 177–179. In: Wells C (ed) Dementia. FA Davies Co, Philadelphia, 1970

Andersson M, Gottfries CG (1988) Levels of motor and intellectual function in patients in nursing homes and being nursed at home (in Swedish). Lakartidningen (to be published)

Balldin J, Gottfries CG, Karlsson I, Lindstedt G, Långström G, Wålinder J (1983) Dexamethasone suppression test and serum prolactin in dementia disorders. Br J Psychiatry 143: 277–281

Balldin J, Gottfries CG, Lindstedt G, Långström G, Svennerholm L (1988) The clonidine test in patients with dementia disorders: relation to clinical status and cerebrospinal fluid metabolite levels. Int J Geriatr Psychiatry 3: 115–123

Blennow K, Gottfries CG, Uhlemann C, Wallin A (1988a) Periventricular white matter low attenuation on CT in dementia of the Alzheimer type and vascular dementia. Abstracts first international conference on Alzheimer Disease and related disorders, Las Vegas, Nevada, Sept 6–9, 1988. Alzh Dis Ass Disord 2: 162

Blennow K, Fredman P, Gottfries CG, Svennerholm L, Wallin A (1988b) Intrathecal synthesis of immunoglobulin M and G in patients with Alzheimer's disease (to be published)

Bråne G, Gottfries CG, Karlsson I, Lekman A, Parnetti L, Svennerholm L (1988) Monoamine metabolites in CSF correlated to psychological variables in patients with dementia of Alzheimer type. Alzh Disease Ass Disorders (to be published)

Brun A, Gustafson L (1978) Limbic lobe involvement in presenile dementia. Arch Psychiatr Nervenkr 226: 76–93

Carlsson A, Winblad B (1976) Influence of age and time interval between death and autopsy on dopamine and 3-methoxytyramine levels in human basal ganglia. J Neural Transm 38: 271–276

Crook T, Bartus RT, Ferris SH, Whitehouse P, Cohen GD, Gershon S (1986) Age-associated memory impairment: proposed diagnostic criteria and measures of clinical change – report of a National Institute of Mental Health work group. Dev Neuropsychol 2(4): 261–276

Ernst A, Cramer H, Strubel D, Kuntzmann F, Schoenenberger GA (1987) Comparison of DSIP (Delta Sleep-Inducing Peptide) and P-DSIP-like (Phosphorylated) immunoreactivity in cerebrospinal fluid of patients with senile dementia of Alzheimer type, multi-infarct syndrome, communicating hydrocephalus and Parkinson's disease. J Neurol 235: 16–21

Gottfries CG (1986) Nosological aspects of differential typology of dementia of Alzheimer type. In: Bergener M (ed) Dimensions in aging. Academic, London, pp 207–219

Gottfries CG, Gottfries I, Roos B (1969) Homovanillic acid and 5-hydroxyindolacetic acid in the cerebrospinal fluid of patients with senile dementia, presenile dementia and parkinsonism. J Neurochem 16: 1341–1345

Gottfries CG, Adolfsson R, Aquilonius SM, Carlsson A, Eckernäs SÅ, Nordberg A, Oreland L, Svennerholm L, Wiberg Å, Winblad B (1983) Biochemical changes in dementia disorders of Alzheimer type (AD/SDAT). Neurobiol Aging 4: 261–271

Heston LL, Mastri AR (1977) The genetics of Alzheimer's disease: associations with hematologic malignancy and Down's syndrome. Arch Gen Psychiatry 34: 976–981

Karlsson I, Bråne G, Melin E, Nyth AL, Rybo E (1988) Effects of environmental stimulation on biochemical and psychological variables in dementia. Acta Psychiatr Scand 77: 207–213

Mayeux R, Stern Y, Spanton S (1985) Heterogeneity in dementia of the Alzheimer type. Evidence of subgroups. Neurology 35: 453–461

McRae-Degueurce A, Bööj S, Rosengren L, Haglid K, Gottfries CG, Wallin A, Blennow K, Dahlström A (1988) Antibodies in the CSF of a subgroup of patients with Alzheimer's disease recognize cholinergic neurons in the rat forebrain. In: Neurochemistry international, vol 13 (Suppl 1). Abstracts of 7th general meeting of the European Society for Neurochemistry, Gothenburg, Sweden, 12–17 June 1988, Pergamon, Oxford, p 52

Parnetti L, Gottfries J, Karlsson I, Långström G, Gottfries CG, Svennerholm L (1987) Monoamines and their metabolites in cerebrospinal fluid of patients with senile dementia of Alzheimer type using high performance liquid chromatography and gas chromatography-mass spectrometry. Acta Psychiatr Scand 75: 542–548

Regland R, Gottfries CG, Oreland L, Svennerholm L (1988) Low B12 levels related to high activity of platelet MAO in patients with dementia disorders. Acta Psychiatr Scand 78: 451–457

Rosser MN, Iversen LL, Reynolds GP, Mountjoy CQ, Roth M (1984) Neurochemical characteristics of early and late onset types of Alzheimer's disease. Br Med J 288: 961–964

Sjögren T, Sjögren H, Lindgren AGH (1952) Morbus Alzheimer and morbus Pick. A genetic, clinical and patho-anatomical study. Acta Psychiatr Neurol Scand [Suppl] 82

Soininen H, MacDonald E, Rekonen M, Riekkinen PJ (1981) Hamovanillic acid and 5-hydroxy-indoleacetic acid levels in cerebrospinal fluid of patients with senile dementia of Alzheimer type. Acta Neurol Scand 64: 101–107

Sourander P, Sjögren H (1970) The concept of Alzheimer's disease and its clinical implications. In: Wolstenholme GEW, O'Connor M (eds) Alzheimer's disease and related conditions. Churchill Livingstone, London, pp 11–36

Wallin A, Alafuzoff I, Carlsson A, Eckernäs SÅ, Gottfries CG, Karlsson I, Svennerholm L, Winblad B (1988) Neurotransmitter deficits in a non-multiinfarct category of vascular dementia. Acta Neurol Scand (to be published)

Widerlöv E, Gottfries CG, Lindström L, Ekman R (1988) Brain and CSF neuropeptide alterations in schizophrenia. In: Neurochemistry international, vol 13 (Suppl 1). Abstracts of 7th general meeting of the European Society for Neurochemistry, Gothenburg, Sweden, 12–17 June 1988, Pergamon, Oxford, p 66

Strategies for Treating Alzheimer's Disease and Age-Associated Memory Impairment

T. H. Crook

Introduction

Alzheimer's disease (AD) and age-associated memory impairment (AAMI) are well-defined clinical entities in which the cardinal symptom is impairment of memory for recent events (McKhann et al. 1984; Crook et al. 1986a). The neurochemical bases of the two conditions appear to be similar or identical, although the magnitude of the neurochemical deficits, as well as the behavioral deficits seen in AD is greatly exaggerated over those seen in AAMI (Gottfries 1985).

In view of their common neurochemical underpinnings it may be that the same compounds will be found effective in treating both AD and AAMI. On the other hand, it may be that compounds found effective in AAMI will not prove efficacious in AD because of structural neuronal changes in the latter condition. The greatly restricted behavioral repertoire of AD patients may also complicate detection of modest drug effects in that population (Crook and Larrabee 1988). An important distinction between AD and AAMI relevant to drug development is that behavioral symptomatology is considerably more severe in the former condition and, thus, drug side effects that may be acceptable in treating AD may be wholly unacceptable in treating AAMI (Leber 1986).

A number of diverse and creative strategies have been developed to guide the development of effective treatments for AD and AAMI (e.g., Crook et al. 1986b). The following paragraphs focus largely on classes of compounds in which data from clinical trials have been published or in which clinical studies in AD or AAMI are now underway.

Cholinergic Compounds

The cholinergic hypothesis has passed into its second decade, and aside from findings by Summers and coleagues (1986) in a methodologically faulty study (Pirozzolo et al. 1987), attempts at treatment baed on the hypothesis have been largely disappointing. Following reports in 1976 by Davies and Maloney and by Bowen and colleagues of a depletion of choline acetyltransferase (an enzyme-marking acetylcholine) in the brains of AD patients, literally dozens of trials with cholinergic agents were conducted. Trials with the acetylcholine precursors choline and phsophatidylcholine (lecithin) were conducted initially, and with very few exceptions, these studies were clearly negative (Bartus et al. 1982).

Bergener, Reisberg (Eds.)
Diagnosis and Treatment
of Senile Dementia
© Springer-Verlag Berlin Heidelberg 1989

A second approach to cholinergic augmentation is administration of cholinesterase inhibitors such as THA, physostigmine, or oxotremorine. Findings with these compounds have been of greater interest from an academic perspective, but, with the exception of the methodologically flawed Summers et al. (1986) study, clinically disappointing. Certainly the most widely studied of the cholinesterase inhibitors have been physostigmine, administered intravenously in early studies (e.g., Davies et al. 1978) and orally in more recent ones (e.g., Mohs et al. 1985). In general, physostigmine may affect attentional processes other than memory (Beller et al. 1985), and any effects appear to be of very modest magnitude and duration in a small subgroup of AD patients (Stern et al. 1987). Thus, the compound does not appear to be of clinical utility, particularly in view of concerns about safety (Cain 1986; Dysken and Janowsky 1985).

A third approach to cholinergic treatment is administration of compounds that directly stimulate postsynaptic acetylcholine receptors. An early, preliminary report by Christie and colleagues (1981) of improvement in some AD patients with parenteral administration of the muscarinic agonist arecoline was somewhat encouraging, but subsequent carefully controlled trials with another agonist, RS-86, were negative (Bruno et al. 1986). Two other muscarinic agonists, oxotremorine and pilocarpine, have also been studied (Caine 1980; Davis et al. 1987) and found ineffective. In general, side effects with these compounds have been highly problematic.

Exceptional, pioneering studies with the muscarinic agonist bethanecol have been conducted during the past several years by Harbaugh and colleagues (1984). In these studies the drug was delivered directly to the brain through a continuous infusion device implanted in the abdomen. The studies were successful in demonstrating the feasibility of intrathecal drug delivery, but recent findings suggest that bethanecol administration does not significantly improve memory in AD (Harbaugh 1986).

Taken together, clinical trials conducted with cholinergic compounds in AD indicate that some cognitive processes are minimally modifiable in some patients through cholinergic intervention. It is possible that more potent and specific cholinesterase inhibitors or agonists would prove more effective than the compounds now available.

With regard to AAMI, it should be noted that
a) cholinergic deficits occur as a function of normal aging (Bartus et al. 1986),
b) selected cholinergic compounds produce significant effects on memory in healthy aged animals (Bartus et al. 1982),
c) trials with appropriate cholinergic agents have not been reported.

Such trials may not be advisable with currently available cholinesterase inhibitors or muscarinic agonists because of side effects, but safer, more selective compounds may merit attention in AAMI. The acetylcholine precursor phosphatidylcholine (lecithin) does not appear to present safety problems, but precursor treatment alone may be less appealing from a theoretical perspective.

Compounds Affecting Other Neurotransmitter Systems

In addition to changes in cholinergic function, both noradrenergic and serotonergic changes occur in normal aging and in AD, and both neurotransmitter systems may be implicated in memory impairment (Zornetzer 1986; Altman and Normile 1986). Loss of nonadrenergic cells in the locus coeruleus has been reported in some AD patients (Bondareff et al. 1982; Cross et al. 1981), as has loss of serotonergic cells in the raphe nuclei (Bowen et al. 1983; Mann and Yates 1983).

The most reasonable compounds for noradrenergic intervention may be alpha$_2$ agonists such as clonidine or guanfacine (Zornetzer 1986). Animal studies with these compounds have been encouraging (Arnsten et al. 1989), but clinical data are limited largely to studies in Korsakoff's disease (McEntee and Nair 1980) where clonidine has been shown to improve memory in some patients. Problems with sedation are frequently noted with clonidine and, thus, guanfacine has become the primary alpha$_2$ agonist of interest. Clinical trials with guanfacine are now underway in both AD and AAMI.

There is reasonable evidence that correcting a serotonergic (5-HT) deficit in AD and AAMI may improve memory (Altman and Normile 1986). Clinical trials with the 5-HT reuptake inhibitors alaproclate and zimelidine have produced equivocal, generally negative, results in AD (Cutler et al. 1985; Dehlin et al. 1985), but the compounds have not been studied in AAMI. Future trials with reuptake inhibitors or 5-HT antagonists, particularly 5-HT3 antagonists such as zacopride (AHR 11190B), may be of interest in both AD and AAMI. It may also be of interest to examine such compounds in combination with drugs affecting other relevant neurotransmitter systems (Carlsson 1981).

Other neurotransmitter systems implicated in AD include both dopamine (Yates et al. 1979) and gammaaminobutyric acid (GABA; Rossor et al. 1982). Clinical trials based on augmenting these neurotransmitter systems have been quite limited in comparison to the many studies untertaken with cholinergic agents, but the results have been generally disappointing. GABA-agonist therapy in AD was evaluated in a recent, well-controlled trial that produced negative results (Mohr et al. 1986). Multiple trials with dopaminergic compounds have also resulted in largely negative findings (e.g. Fleischhacker et al. 1986). Thus, direct intervention through either of these neurotransmitter systems alone does not appear promising at the present time.

Alteration of monoaminergic (MAO) neurotransmission may also hold some promise in treating AD and AAMI. Increased MAO-B activity has been reported in critical brain regions in normal aging as well as in AD, and clinical evaluation of MAO-B inhibitors such as deprenyl has been proposed (Carlsson 1983). Empirical evidence for some effects in AD is provided by a study of Tariot and his colleagues (1987) demonstrating cognitive and behavioral improvement in AD patients with deprenyl at a low dosage level (at which only MAO-B is thought to be inhibited) and not at a higher level (at which MAO-A is also thought to be inhibited). This line of clinical inquiry may merit further exploration in AAMI as well as AD.

Neuropeptides

Numerous studies demonstrate a decline with age in the brain levels of peptides that affect learning and memory (for a review, see Banks and Kastin 1986). There has also long been a body of evidence demonstrating that administration of various neuropeptides or their analogs can facilitate learning and memory in animals under various experimental conditions (De Wied and Gispen 1977). Less is known about peptide levels in AD, but decreased levels of at least one peptide, somatostatin, have repeatedly been found in the brains of AD patients at postmortem (Davies et al. 1980; Rossor et al. 1980) and also in cerebrospinal fluid taken from AD patients (Wood et al. 1982).

Many effects of specific neuropeptides are relevant to the treatment of AD. For example, within the brain, adrenocorticotropic hormone (ACTH), thyrotropin-releasing hormone (TRH), and arginine vasopressin (AVP) are critical in maintaining acetylcholine and catecholamine activity (Banks and Kastin 1986). Thus, several neuropeptides have been thought to merit consideration as possible treatments for cognitive deficits in both AD and AAMI.

Relatively few clinical trials have been conducted with appropriate neuropeptides in AAMI or comparable populations, and trials conducted in AD have been generally disappointing. Among the compounds tested most extensively in AD is a synthetic ACTH 4–9 analog, Organon 2766, found to possibly affect mood, but not cognition (Berger and Tinklenberg 1981; Soininen et al. 1985). Similar results were reported in early studies with ACTH 4–10 (Ferris et al. 1976). Studies have also focused on vasopressin (VP) and various VP analogs, including 1-desamino-8-D-arginine vaso-pressin (DDAVP) and desglycinamide-9-arginine-8-vasopressin (DGAVP) in the treatment of AD. As in the case of ACTH, small changes in behavioral performance have been repeatedly observed, but these changes have generally been ascribed to changes in attention or mood rather than learning or memory (Peabody et al. 1985).

Trials in AD with TRH or TRH analogs (such as MK-771) have been suggested, based in part on the unique facilitative effects of the peptide on cholinergic neurons (Davies 1981; Yarbrough and Pomara 1985). Clinical evidence is extremely limited, but a small preliminary study of TRH has been reported, with negative results (Peabody et al. 1986).

As noted previously, somatostatin has consistently been found to be reduced in postmortem brain tissue from AD patients. Somatostatin is widely distributed throughout the brain and has been described as both a peptide and a neurotransmitter (Luft et al. 1978), however, its significance in learning and memory is not well understood. One clinical trial has been reported with a potent somatostatin analog, L363, 586, infused intravenously in ten AD subjects (Cutler et al. 1985). No significant improvement in cognitive performance was noted, although the authors argued that studies of higher dosage levels may be warranted.

Two compounds that received widespread attention several years ago are the opiate receptor antagonist naloxone and its oral analog naltrexone. Opiate antagonists have been shown to influence attention, learning, and memory in different animal and human paradigms (e. g., Arnsten et al. 1983; Gallagher 1982), and it was hypothesized that they may be effective compounds for treating AD (Roberts 1986). On these bases, a preliminary study was undertaken by Reisberg and colleagues (1983), and improved cognitive performance was reported in some AD patients. However, subsequent, carefully controlled trials examining a wide range of doses have failed to support this early finding (Pomara et al. 1985; Tariot et al. 1986).

In general, then, clinical trials conducted to date with neuropeptides in AD have not been encouraging. It may be that insufficient quantities of the investigational compounds enter the brain, and thus simultaneous manipulation of the blood-brain barrier or carrier-mediated transport systems may be necessary in clinical trials to determine if available neuropeptides influence memory in AD (Banks and Kastin 1986). Of course, another alternative is direct delivery of compounds to the brain through an implanted infusion device, as was done by Harbaugh and colleagues (1984) with bethanecol. In addition to AD, trials of selected peptides in AAMI would appear to be of interest, in view of their effects in reversing age-related cognitive deficits in animals.

Nootropics

The term "nootropics" was coined by Giurgea (1976) to describe compounds that directly affect higher brain function and metabolism and have virtually no physiologic effects at other body sites. Piracetam, the prototypical nootropic, is a GABA analog that has diverse effects on brain chemistry and facilitates performance on various learning and memory paradigms in both humans and animals (Giurgea 1976). A number of trials have been conducted with piracetam in AD and, in general, results have been equivocal or negative (Ferris et al. 1982). However, carefully controlled trials with the compound have not been reported in AAMI. This would seem a reasonable undertaking in view of the diverse, potentially facilitative, neurochemical effects of piracetam and its demonstrated effects in reversing age-related behavioral deficits in animals (Bartus et al. 1981).

Various analogs of piracetam have been developed, including pramiracetam, aniracetam, oxiracetam, and others. Compounds such as CI-911 and CI-933, vincamine and its analogs, and other compounds may also be referred to as nootropics although they are not related to piracetam and may affect sites outside the brain. Numerous clinical trials have been conducted with such compounds in diverse patient populations, including AD and related disorders. It appears unlikely from this body of evidence that these compounds are of greater utility than piracetam in AD and that, like piracetam, clinical trials in AAMI may be more appropriate than trials in AD.

A compound sometimes classified as a nootropic, although it is not free of effects outside the brain, is dihydroergotoxine, a combination of three ergot alkaloids in their dihydrogenated forms. The compound affects cerebral metabolism and noradrenergic, serotonergic, and dopaminergic neurotransmission. More than 60 studies have been reported with the compound, and in general, it appears to have modest, but consistent effects on mood and activation, but not direct effects on learning and memory (Goodnick and Gershon 1984). Similar effects are also reported when dihydroergotoxine is combined with lecithin (Jenike et al. 1986).

In general, the concept of a nootropic agent is extremely appealing, but efficacy has not been demonstrated with existing compounds in AD. New compounds such as L059 may be more promising, and careful clinical trials in AAMI would be of interest.

Other Treatment Strategies

Among other approaches to treatment that may be considered in AD and AAMI are the following:

1. Compounds that alter membrane phospholipids may hold promise in the treatment of AAMI (Rotrosen 1986). A formulation of phosphatidylserine from bovine cortex (BC-PS) has been shown to exert clinical effects in AD (Delwaide et al. 1986; SMID group 1988) and is now being carefully evaluated in AAMI and AD.
2. Alteration of the brain angiotensin-renin system with compounds such as captopril may exert effects on memory (Sudilovsky et al. 1988). Studies with captopril and other angiotensin converting enzyme (ACE) inhibitors such as SQ29852 are now underway in AAMI and AD.
3. Compounds such as milacemide (Saletu and Grunberger 1984) that affect N-methyl-d-aspartate (NMDA) receptors may be of interest in both AD and AAMI.
4. A number of novel compounds are being evaluated in AAMI or in related populations. Among these drugs is sabeluzole, a benzothiazol derivative, shown to improve memory in a small study of "healthy elderly volunteers" (Clincke et al. 1988).
5. Compounds that affect calcium hemostasis have been developed and may merit evaluation in both AAMI and AD (Gibson and Peterson 1986). A preliminary study of 4-aminopyridine in AD was encouraging (Wesseling et al. 1984). 3-4-Diaminopyridine is said to be one thousand times more potent than 4-aminopyridine and less toxic (Gibson and Peterson 1986). Thus, this compound may merit clinical evaluation. Aside from the aminopyridines, the calcium channel blocker nimodipine is being studied in AAMI and AD. As discussed by Dr. Landfield and others in this volume, the compound has diverse metabolic effects that are of considerable interest in AAMI and of interest in AD. Clinical data presented herein also suggest that the compound is a candidate of major interest for the treatment of late-life cognitive disorders.

Summary

Diverse and creative neurochemical strategies have been proposed to guide the development of effective treatments for AD and AAMI. The task of the clinical investigator is to evaluate compounds that derive from these strategies in a systematic and judicious manner. Clinical investigators must also remain alert to the possibility that serendipitous clinical observation, rather than neurochemical theory, will once again provide the route through which neuropharmacology advances. Clear diagnostic criteria have been specified, sensitive new psychometric instruments are available (Crook and Larrabee 1988), and the opportunity is at hand to undertake clinical trials that may lead to therapeutic advances of major significance in man's long struggle to minimize the effects of aging and diseases of old age.

References

Altman HJ, Normile HJ (1986) Serotonin, learning, and memory: implications for the treatment of dementia. In: Crook T, Bartus R, Ferris S, Gershon S (eds) Treatment development strategies for Alzheimer's disease. Powley, Madison, pp 361–383

Arnsten AFT, Segal DS, Neville HJ (1983) Naloxone augments electrophysiological signs of selective attention in man. Nature 304: 725–727

Arnsten AFT, Xia CAI, Goldman-Rakic PS (1989) The alpha-2 adrenergic agonist guanfacine improves memory in aged monkeys without sedative or hypotensive side effects: evidence for alpha-2 receptor subtypes. J Neuroscience (in press)

Banks WA, Kastin AJ (1986) Aging, peptides, and the blood-brain barrier: implications and speculation. In: Crook T, Bartus R, Ferris S, Gershon S (eds) Treatment development strategies for Alzheimer's disease. Powley, Madison, pp 245–265

Bartus RT, Dean RL, Sherman KA, Friedman E, Beer B (1981) Profound effects of combining choline and piracetam on memory. Neurobiol Aging 2: 105–111

Bartus RT, Dean RL, Beer B, Lippa AS (1982) The cholinergic hypothesis of geriatric memory dysfunction. Science 217: 408

Bartus RT, Dean R, Fisher SK (1986) Cholinergic treatment for age-related memory disturbances: dead or barely coming of age? In: Crook T, Bartus R, Ferris S, Gershon S (eds) Treatment development strategies for Alzheimer's disease. Powley, Madison, pp 421–450

Beller SA, Overall JE, Swann AC (1985) Efficacy of oral physostigmine in primary degenerative dementia. Psychopharmacology 87: 147–151

Berger P, Tinklenberg JR (1981) Neuropeptides and senile dementia. In: Crook T, Gershon S (eds) Strategies for the development of an effective treatment for senile dementia. Powley, New Canaan, pp 155–171

Bondareff W, Mountjoy CQ, Roth M (1982) Loss of neurons of origin of the adrenergic projection to cerebral cortex (nucleus locus coeruleus) in senile dementia. Neurology 32: 164

Bowen DM, Allen SJ, Benton JS, Goodhart MJ, Haan EA, Palmer AM, Sims NR, Smith CCT, Spillane JA, Esiri MM, Neary D, Snowdon JS, Wilcock GK, Davison AN (1983) Biochemical assessment of serotonergic and cholinergic dysfunction and cerebral atrophy in Alzheimer's disease. J Neurochem 41: 266–271

Bruno G, Mohr E, Gillespie M, Fedio P, Chase TN (1986) Muscarinic agonist therapy of Alzheimer's disease. Arch Neurol 43: 659–661

Cain JW (1986) Hypertension associated with oral administration of physostigmine in a patient with Alzheimer's disease. Am J Psychiatry 143 (7): 910–912

Caine ED (1980) Cholinomimetic treatment fails to improve memory disorders. N Engl J Med 303: 585

Carlsson A (1981) Aging and brain neurotransmitters. In: Crook T, Gerson S (eds) Strategies for the development of an effective treatment for senile dementia. Powley, New Canaan, pp 93–104

Carlsson A (1983) Changes in neurotransmitter systems in the aging brain and in Alzheimer's disease. In: Reisberg B (ed) Alzheimer's disease: the standard reference. Free Press, New York, pp 100–107

Christie JE, Shering A, Ferguson J, AIM (1981) Physostigmine and arecoline: effects of intravenous infusions in Alzheimer presenile dementia. Br J Psychiatry 138: 46–50

Clincke GHC, Tritsmans L, Idzikowski C, Amery WK, Janssen PAJ (1988) The effect of R 58 735 (sabeluzole) on memory functions in healthy elderly volunteers. Psychopharmacoloty 94: 52–57

Crook T (1988) Pharmacotherapy of cognitive deficits in Alzheimer's disease and age-associated memory impairment. Psychopharmacol Bull 24 (1): 31–38

Crook TH, Larrabee GJ (1988) Interrelationships among everyday memory tests: stability of factor structure with age. Neuropsychology 2: 1–12

Crook T, Bartus RT, Ferris SH, Whitehouse P, Cohen GD, Gershon S (1986) Age-associated memory impairment. Proposed diagnostic criteria and measures of clinical change – report of a National Institute of Mental Health work group. Dev Neuropsychol 2 (4): 261–276

Crook T, Bartus R, Ferris S, Gershon S (eds) (1986b) Treatment development strategies for Alzheimer's disease. Powley, Madison

Crook T (1988) Pharmacotherapy of cognitive deficits in Alzheimer's disease and age-associated memory impairment. Psychopharmacology Bulletin, 24: 31–38

Cross AJ, Crow TJ, Perry EK, Perry RH, Blessed G, Tomlinson BE (1981) Reduced dopamine betahydroxylase activity in Alzheimer's disease. British Medical Journal, 282: 93–94

Cutler NR, Haxby J, Kay AD, Narang PK, Leska LJ, Costa JL, Nimos M, Linnoila M, Potter WZ, Renfrew JW (1985) Evaluation of zimelidine in Alzheimer's disease. Arch Neurol 42 (8): 744–748

Davies P (1981) Theoretical treatment possibilities for dementia of the Alzheimer type: the cholinergic hypothesis. In: Crook T, Gershon S (eds) Strategies for the development of an effective treatment for senile dementia. Powley, New Canaan, pp 19–32

Davies P, Katzman R, Terry HD (1980) Reduced somatostatin-like immunoreactivity in cerebral cortex from cases of Alzheimer's disease and Alzheimer senile dementia. Nature 288: 279

Davis KL, Mohs RC, Tinklenberg JH, Pfefferbaum A, Hollister LE, Kopell BS (1978) Physostigmine: enhancement of long-term memory processes in normal subjects. Science 201: 272

Dehlin O, Hedenrud B, Jansson P, Norgard J (1985) A double-blind comparison of alaproclate and placebo in the treatment of patients with senile dementia. Acta Psychiatr Scand 71: 190–196

Delwaide PL, Gyselynck-Mambourg AM, Hurlet A, Ylieff M (1986) Double-blind randomized controlled study of phosphatidylserine in senile demented patients. Acta Neurol Scand 73: 136–140

De Wied D, Gispen WH (1977) Behavioral effects of peptides. In: Gainer H (ed) Peptides in neurobiology. Plenum, New York, pp 397–422

Dysken MW, Janowsky DS (1985) Dose-related physostigmine-induced ventricular arrhythmia: case report. J Clin Psychiatry 46 (10): 446–447

Ferris SH, Sathananthan G, Gershon S, Clark C, Mashinsky J (1976) Cognitive effects of ACTH 4-10 in the elderly. Pharmacol Biochem Behav 5 [suppl 1]: 73–78

Ferris S, Reisberg B, Crook T, Friedman E, Schneck M, Sherman K, Corwin J, Gershon S, Bartus R (1982) Pharmacologic treatment of senile dementia: choline, L-dopa, piracetam, and choline/piracetam. In: Corkin S, Davis KL, Growdon JH, Usdine E, Wurtman R (eds) Alzheimer's disease: a Report of progress. Raven, New York

Fleischhacker WW, Buchgeher A, Schubert H (1986) Memantine in the treatment of senile dementia of the Alzheimer type. Prog Neuropsychopharmacol Biol Psychiatry 10: 87–93

Gallagher M (1982) Naloxone enhancement of memory. Effects of other opiate antagonists. Behav Neurol Biol 35: 375–382

Gibson GE, Peterson C (1986) Consideration of neurotransmitters and calcium metabolism in therapeutic design. In: Crook T, Bartus R, Ferris S, Gershon S (eds) Treatment development strategies for Alzheimer's disease. Powley, Madison, pp 500–517

Giurgea C (1976) Piracetam: nootropic pharmacology of neurointegrative activity. Curr Dev Psychopharmacol 3: 221–276

Goodnick P, Gershon S (1984) Chemotherapy of cognitive disorders in geriatric subjects. J Clin Psychiatry 45 (5): 196–209

Gottfries CG (1985) Alzheimer's disease and senile dementia: biochemical characteristics and aspects of treatment. Psychopharmacology 86: 245–252

Harbaugh RE (1984) Intercranial drug administration in Alzheimer's disease. Neurosurgery 15: 514–518

Harbaugh RE (1986) Drug delivery to the brain by central infusion: clinical application of a chemical paradigm of brain function. In: Crook T, Bartus R, Ferris S, Gershon S (eds) Treatment development strategies for Alzheimer's disease. Powley, Madison, pp 553–565

Jenike MA, Albert MS, Heller H, LoCastro S, Gunther J (1986) Combination therapy with lecithin and ergoloid mesylates for Alzheimer's disease. J Clin Psychiatry 47 (5): 249–251

Leber P (1986) Establishing the efficacy of drugs with psychogeriatric indications. In: Crook T, Bartus R, Ferris S, Gershon S (eds) Treatment development strategies for Alzheimer's disease. Powley, Madison, pp 1–14

Luft R, Efendic S, Hokfelt T (1978) Somatostatin – both hormone and neurotransmitter? Diabetologia 14: 1–13

Mann DM, Yates PO (1983) Serotonin nerve cells in Alzheimer's disease. J Neurol Neurosurg Psychiatry, 46: 96

McEntee WF, Nair RG (1980) Memory enhancement in Korsakoff's psychosis by clonidine: further evidence for a noradrenergic deficit. Ann Neurol 7: 466–470

McKhann G, Drachman D, Folstein M, Katzman R, Price D, Stadlam EM (1984) Clinical diagnosis of Alzheimer's disease: report of the NINCDS-ADRDA Work Group under the auspices of the Department of Health and Human Services Task Force on Alzheimer's disease. Neurology 34: 939–944

Mohr EM, Bruno G, Foster N, Gillespie M, Cox C, Hare TA, Tamminga C, Fedio P, Chase TN (1986) GABA-antagonist therapy for Alzheimer's disease. Clin Neuropharmacol 9 (3): 257–263

Mohs RC, Davis BM, Greenwald BS, Mathe AA, Johns CA, Horvath TB, Davis KL (1985) Clinical studies of the cholinergic deficit in Alzheimer's disease. II. Psychopharmacologic studies. J Am Geriatr Soc 33 (11): 749–757

Peabody CA, Thiemann S, Pigache R, Miller TP, Berger PA, Yesavage J, Tinklenberg JR (1985) Desglycinamide-9- arginine-8-vasopressin (DGAVP, Organon 5667) in patients with dementia. Neurol Aging 6: 95–100

Peabody CA, Deblois TE, Tinklenberg JR (1986) Thyrotropin-releasing hormone (TRH) and Alzheimer's disease (letter). Am J Psychiatry 143 (2): 262–263

Pirozzolo FJ, Baskin DS, Swihart AA, Appel SH (1987) Oral tetrahydroaminoacridine in the treatment of senile dementia, Alzheimer's type (letter). N Engl J Med 316 (25): 1605

Pomara N, Roberts RR, Rhiew HB, Stanley M, Gershon S (1985) Multiple single-dose naltrexone administrations fail to effect overall cognitive functioning and plasma cortisol in individuals with probable Alzheimer's disease. Neurobiol Aging 6: 233–236

Reisberg B, Ferris S, Anand R, Mir P, Geibel V, DeLeon M, Roberts E (1983) Effects of naloxone in senile dementia: a double-blind trial. N Engl J Med 308: 721–722

Roberts E (1986) A speculative consideration on the neurobiology and treatment of senile dementia. In: Crook T, Gershon S (eds) Strategies for the development of an effective treatment for senile dementia. Powley, Madison, pp 173–219

Rossor MN, Emson PC, Mountjoy CQ, Roth M, Iversen LL (1980) Reduced amounts of immunoreactive somatostatin in the temporal cortex in senile dementia of Alzheimer type. Neurosci Lett 20: 373

Rossor MN, Garrett NJ, Johnson AL, Mountjoy CQ, Roth M, Iverssen LL (1982) A postmortem study of the cholinergic and GABA systems in senile dementia. Brain 105: 313–330

Rotrosen J (1986) Membrane lipids: can modification reduce symptoms or halt progression in Alzheimer's disease? In: Crook T, Bartus R, Ferris S, Gershon S (eds) Treatment strategies for Alzheimer's disease. Powley, Madison, pp 522–537

Saletu B, Grunberger J (1984) Early clinical pharmacological trials with a new anti-epileptic, milacemide, using pharmaco-EEG and psychometry. Methods Find Exp Clin Pharmacol 6 (6): 317–330

SMID Group (1988) Phosphatidylserine in the treatment of Alzheimer's disease: results of a multi-center study. Psychopharmacol Bull (1) 24: 130–134

Soininen H, Koskinen T, Helkala E-L, Pigache R, Riekkinen PJ (1985) Treatment of Alzheimer's disease with synthetic ACTH 4-9 analog. Neurology 35: 1348–1351

Stern Y, Sano M, Mayeux R (1987) Effects of oral physostigmine in Alzheimer's disease. Ann Neurol 22: 306–310

Sudilovsky A, Croog SH, Crook T, Testa MA, Levine S, Klerman G (1988) Differential effects of antihypertensive medications on cognitive functioning. Psychopharmacol Bull. (in press)

Summers WK, Majovski LV, Marsh GM, Tachiki K, Kling A (1986) Oral tetrahydroaminoacridine in long-term treatment of senile dementia, Alzheimer type. N Engl J Med 315 (20): 1241–1245

Tariot PN, Cohen RM, Sunderland T, Newhouse PA, Yount D, Mellow AM, Weingartner H, Mueller EA, Murphy DL (1987) L-Deprenyl in Alzheimer's disease. Arch Gen Psychiatry, 44: 427–433

Tariot PN, Sunderland T, Weingartner H, Murphy DL, Cohen MR, Cohen RM (1986) Naloxone and Alzheimer's disease. Arch Gen Psychiatry 43: 727–732

Wessling H, Agoston S, Van Dam GB, Pasma J, De Wit DJ, Havinga H (1984) Effects of 4-aminopyridine in elderly patients with Alzheimer's disease (letter). N Engl J Med 310 (15): 988–989

Wood PL, Etienne P, Lal S, Gauthier S, Cajal S, Nair NPV (1982) Reduced lumbar CSF somatostatin levels in Alzheimer's disease. Life Sci 31: 2073–2079

Yates C, Allison Y, Simpson J, Maloney AFJ, Gordon A (1979) Dopamine in Alzheimer's disease and senile dementia. Lancet ii: 851–852

Yarbrough GG, Pomara N (1985) The therapeutic potential of thyrotropin releasing hormone (TRH) in Alzheimer's disease (AD). Prog Neuropsychopharmacol Biol Psychiatry 9: 285–289

Zornetzer SF (1986) The noradrenergic locus coeruleus and senescent memory dysfunction. In: Crook T, Bartus R, Ferris S, Gershon S (eds) Treatment development strategies for Alzheimer's disease. Powley, Madison, pp 337–359

The Use of Positron Emission Tomography in the Early Diagnosis of Senile Dementia*

E. Meyer

Summary

This paper first reviews the literature related to the use of positron emission tomography (PET) in the diagnosis of senile dementia. This quantitative functional imaging modality together with its structural counterparts, i. e., computed tomography (CT) and magnetic resonance imaging (MRI), has been used extensively to study senile dementia with the aim of clarifying its pathophysiology and to eventually contribute to an early differential diagnosis of the disease. For that purpose, cerebral functional and metabolic parameters such as cerebral blood flow (CBF) and cerebral metabolic rate of glucose (CMRGlc) and oxygen ($CMRO_2$) have been most frequently studied in the past. After some early enthusiasm, the utility of PET findings in the clinical verification of Alzheimer's disease (AD) is presently undergoing a reassessment (Benson 1988). The value of PET as a research tool in AD, however, remains undisputed, and the use of improved scanning equipment, new radiopharmaceuticals, imaging strategies, and methods of data analysis most likely will help reveal diagnostically useful patterns in the future. At present, efforts are being made to study neurotransmitter function in dementia, and it is expected that the diagnostic capabilities of PET will be greatly increased by information from such studies. The paper then describes some novel approaches to the use of PET in the investigation and possible early diagnosis of AD, including physiological activation studies and imaging of calcium-channel blockers.

Introduction

The need for an early and accurate diagnosis in AD, allowing timely therapeutic intervention and good clinical research, is well recognized. The potential of PET in contributing to this has been explored by many approaches and undergoes continuing investigation.

In the past, functional and metabolic parameters such as CBF, CMRGlc, and $CMRO_2$ have been most frequently studied in AD. The diagnostic utility of such

---

* This work was supported in part by grant SP-5 from the Medical Research Council of Canada and the Isaac Walton Killam Fellowship Fund of the Montreal Neurological Institute.

Bergener, Reisberg (Eds.)
Diagnosis and Treatment
of Senile Dementia
© Springer-Verlag Berlin Heidelberg 1989

studies is still controversial. Recently, efforts have been made to study neurotransmitter function in dementia, which should greatly increase the diagnostic capabilities of PET. Also, cerebral metabolic studies during physiological or cognitive activation have hardly been explored in AD. Several experts in the field are calling for such studies, which will not only increase our basic knowledge of the disease but might also help establish an early diagnostic pattern thereof. The investigation of calcium homeostasis with an appropriate model and imaging agent is another field in which PET studies could hold some promise.

In this paper, we briefly review the PET studies that have been performed to date with particular reference to the capabilities of PET in the diagnosis of AD. We then describe some novel approaches to the use of PET in the investigation and possible early diagnosis of AD, including physiological activation studies and imaging of calcium-channel blockers.

Positron Emission Tomography

Principle

PET is a noninvasive quantitative in vivo imaging technique that provides cross-sectional images of the tissue radioactivity concentration following administration of radiopharmaceuticals labeled with short-lived positron emitting tracers such as ^{11}C, ^{13}N, ^{15}O, and ^{18}F that are produced by an on-site cyclotron. Sophisticated experimental strategies together with appropriate tracer kinetic models allow the regional calculation of a variety of tissue functions, such as CBF, CMRGlc, $CMRO_2$, blood-brain barrier integrity, protein synthesis, drug concentration, and receptor density. Being a noninvasive technique, PET offers the possibility to carry out longitudinal studies documenting the evolution of cerebral functional patterns quantitatively. This makes PET particularly well suited for the study of a progressive disease such as senile dementia. Comprehensive reviews of PET and its various applications have been published recently (Reivich and Alavi 1985; Phelps 1986).

PET-MRI Correlation

PET studies provide primarily functional images with limited or sometimes no structural information. In order to address questions of subtle metabolic changes, particularly in small structures, the precise localization of these structures becomes of critical importance. An exhaustive interpretation of high-quality PET images therefore requires information from a structural imaging modality such as CT, or more recently MRI, that can be used to identify uniquely the anatomy underlying a functional region of interest or vice versa. Several attempts at correlating PET with CT or MRI information have been made in the past (Bajcsy et al. 1983; Mazziotta et al. 1983; Bohm et al. 1983, 1985; Herholz et al. 1985; Fox et al. 1985; Evans et al. 1988). Of these, the approach by Evans et al. (1988) represents the most comprehensive example. For a review of the possibilities and limitations of PET, MRI, and single photon emission computed tomography (SPECT), see the article by Ter-Pogossian (1985).

Correction for Brain Atrophy

Although the results of PET studies in senile dementia patients are usually compared to those obtained in age-matched control subjects, the question has been asked whether the altered metabolic profile found in AD could be merely a reflection of overall brain atrophy and thereby only secondarily reflect the disease process (de Leon et al. 1988). The effect of brain atrophy on the various functional parameters measured with PET must be given due consideration. Various techniques have been proposed to correct for such effects either globally or regionally, using CT or MRI data (Herscovitch et al. 1986; Condon et al. 1986a, b; Clark et al. 1987; Videen et al. 1988). As an example, using a global CT-based correction method, Herscovitch et al. (1986) have shown that the supratentorial cavity occupied by ventricles and sulci was approximately twice as large in six AD patients with mild senile dementia as compared to eight age-matched controls. As a consequence, the difference in decrease in uncorrected $CMRO_2$ seen between the two groups no longer reached statistical significance once the atrophy correction was included. On the other hand, several studies seem to demonstrate the absence of any correlation between the degree of atrophy and the reduction in metabolic function (Alavi and de Leon 1985; McGeer et al. 1986a). It is estimated that with the increased use of PET-MRI or PET-CT correlation for the purpose of anatomical identification, brain atrophy correction procedures will become an integrating part of PET data analysis which will at the same time enhance the truly disease-specific information content of such data.

Cerebral Glucose and Oxygen Metabolic Studies

Normal Aging

The metabolic patterns observed in AD patients are usually evaluated in comparison to results from healthy aging subjects. Cerebral metabolic changes associated with normal aging, therefore, have been studied intensively (Kuhl et al. 1982, 1984a; Metter et al. 1983; Raichle 1982; Riege et al. 1982, 1985a; de Leon et al. 1983, 1986; Duara et al. 1984; Cutler et al. 1985a). There is no uniform conclusion from these studies. Some authors found decreases of global and regional metabolism with age (Kuhl et al. 1984a; Riege et al. 1985a) while others did not observe such changes (de Leon et al. 1983; Duara et al. 1984). Cerebral oxygen consumption does not seem to drop significantly with age (Lammertsma et al. 1981). Hoyer (1986) concludes, based on an extensive literature review, that CBF, $CMRO_2$, and CMRGlc of the normally aged brain are maintained unchanged from the third to the seventh decade of life. Thereafter, these parameters may decrease. Several experts in the field, in their most recent comments, seem to support the age-invariance hypothesis of $CMRO_2$ and CMRGlc (de Leon et al. 1988; Cutler 1988). Improvements in scanning equipment and analysis methods, particularly the inclusion of appropriate corrections for brain atrophy, might lend increased consistency to future aging studies.

Senile Dementia

The glucose and oxygen metabolic findings from PET studies in AD and dementing conditions in general have been described in recent reviews by Leenders and Aquilonius (1987) and Riege and Metter (1988). In this section, we will briefly summarize the major observations with particular reference to those PET results that, in the view of leading experts, appear to have some early diagnostic promise. The use of PET data in the differentiation of AD from other forms of dementia is also included and some of the most recent PET studies are reviewed.

General PET Findings. The observation most frequently reported in probable Alzheimer's disease (pAD) to date is a relative reduction in cortical glucose metabolism (de Leon et al. 1986; Kuhl et al. 1985a) as well as decreases in $CMRO_2$ and CBF (Frackowiak et al. 1981a, b), seen initially in the temporoparietal and later also in the frontal regions. This metabolic decline, confirmed by the pattern of pathology at autopsy, has been associated with reduced FDG phosphorylation rates (Friedland et al. 1983a, Kuhl et al. 1985a, Riege et al. 1985a). The hypometabolic pattern in pAD varies from patient to patient. Compared to age-matched controls, CMRGlc levels in parietal and dorsolateral occipital cortex were reduced by 47%; in frontal, temporal, and calcarine occipital cortices the reduction was 28% (Kuhl et al. 1985a, b) and only 12% in the caudate and thalamus (Kuhl et al. 1985c). In AD, these reductions are, again, most pronounced in temporo parietal structures and least severe in deep nuclei, especially in caudate and thalamus (Brun and Englund 1981), but also in the cerebellum. Metabolic activity in the primary motor-sensory strip is relatively preserved (Benson et al. 1983). The pattern of metabolic reduction is similar to that of choline acetyltransferase (ChAT) concentration (Davies 1979). According to studies by Kuhl et al. (1985b) the parietal to caudate-thalamus CMRGlc ratio of early AD subjects categorized as mild with questionable dementia was significantly lower than that of elderly controls. McNamara et al. (1987) found that focal ratios of regional CMRGlc values where the denominator corresponded to a CMRGlc value from a relatively spared region provided useful measures of metabolic dysfunction in the early stages of AD. There are also suggestions that in mild dementia of the Alzheimer's type, decrements in regional CMRGlc exist despite the absence of measurable cognitive deficits (Foster et al. 1984; Cutler et al. 1985b; Duara et al. 1987).

Intriguing information, although premature for any conclusions to be drawn, comes from a study by Polinsky et al. (1987) in two patients with inherited AD, in which a significantly reduced normalized CMRGlc value was found in the left supramarginal gyrus of an asymptomatic at-risk subject. The need for investigation of the metabolic relationships between multiple brain regions which do not function in isolation but rather in relation to other cerebral structures has been recognized (Metter et al. 1984a; Horowitz et al. 1984). The diagnostic potential of regional glucose utilization values was tested by Alavi and de Leon (1985) and de Leon et al. (1988) via discriminant function classification analyses and found to be accurate to 70%–90% in classifying AD subjects and controls. The reduced glucose utilization pattern observed in AD often shows nonuniformities and asymmetries between the hemispheres. Anteroposterior changes, in general, were found to be more prominent than left-right differences (Friedland et al. 1983a, 1985; Metter et al. 1985a, b). In a recent study, Duara et al. (1988a) found that in their sample of 35 AD patients, 43% showed a predominant left hemispheric glucose hypometabolism while 46% had symmetrical scans. The remaining 11% showed predominantly right hemispheric metabolic depression. In a very recent report, de Leon et al. (1988) describe a unique hippocampal-parahippocampal cerebrospinal fluid accumulation that distinguished AD patients from controls at a level of over 80%. These authors suggest that high-resolution PET imaging with a negative scanning angulation for optimal visualization of the hippocampus might assist in the early detection of AD.

There have been numerous studies trying to correlate brain imaging and cognitive measures. A concise summary of these results is found in the review by Riege and Metter (1988).

The oxygen metabolic findings in AD patients are very similar to the glucose metabolic results. In mild to moderately demented patients, Frackowiak et al. (1981a) observed global and regional decreases in $CMRO_2$ in parallel to changes in CBF (Frachowiak et al. 1981b). The greatest reductions were, again, observed in the parietal and temporal regions. In severely demented patients, the frontal regions were depressed as well.

Bustany et al. (1983, 1985) found a net decrease of the incorporation of $[^{11}C]$methionine into protein, especially in the parietal and frontal cerebral regions. In borderline demented AD patients without CT abnormalities, the reduction was 18% and reached as much as 65% in severely demented patients. It is not quite clear, however, whether their model really measures protein synthesis rate.

Differentiation from Other Forms of Dementia. It has been shown that, although the degree of global and regional reduction may be similar, the regional patterns of metabolic depression in AD and multi-infarct dementia (MID) are significantly different (Benson et al. 1983; Kuhl et al. 1985a, b) and may assist in distinguishing the two forms of dementia from one another. Furthermore, parietal to caudate-thalamus or parietal to cerebellar CMRGlc ratios have been shown to allow distinction between AD, MID, and controls (Kuhl et al. 1985a, 1983) and depression (Riege et al. 1985b). The use of CBF (Perez et al. 1977) and CMRGlc PET data (Riege et al. 1985b, 1984) together with multivariate discriminant analysis has allowed separation of AD patients with a greater than 80% accuracy.

The distinction between the cerebral metabolic changes in pAD and Parkinson's disease (PD) appears to be somewhat more tedious. The global reduction in CBF, $CMRO_2$ (Leenders et al. 1983; Perlmutter and Raichle 1985), and CMRGlc (Kuhl et al. 1985b, 1984b; Rougemont et al. 1983) of approximately 10% observed in PD is smaller than in pAD. The use of ratios between selected regional CMRGlc values has allowed researchers to demonstrate that the number of regional intercorrelations was reduced in PD but increased in pAD (Metter et al. 1985a, 1984b). The PET findings regarding parietal or frontal regional metabolic changes are less consistent in PD than in pAD. Nevertheless, Kuhl et al. (1985d) have found that the parietal-cerebellar ratio was different from controls in both patient groups.

The reliability of the parietal-cerebellar ratio, however, will require a reassessment in light of the recent finding that cerebellar glucose metabolism is elevated in subjects with periventricular white matter lesions which seem to be present in approximately 30% of AD patients (Klinger et al. 1988).

Neurotransmitter Receptor Studies

PET together with the appropriate radiotracer allows measurement of various aspects of neurotransmitter function. Labeled precursors may be used to gather information about neurotransmitter synthesis and receptor densities. Other techniques under development are aimed at the assessment of enzyme activities by means of radiolabeled enzyme inhibitors and PET. Furthermore, current work with monoclonal antibodies (Hyman et al. 1988) in conjunction with PET imaging might be developed into diagnostically useful procedures.

Although there have been several neurochemical studies on neurotransmitter receptor changes in AD (Quirion et al. 1986; Shimohama et al. 1988) involving not only central cholinergic pathways (Perry 1986) but also the serotonin, noradrenaline, dopamine (Gottfries et al. 1983), and somatostatin (Beal et al. 1985) systems, very few PET studies related to this aspect of AD have been conducted thus far. Some preliminary studies and related work are reviewed in the following two sections.

Cholinergic System

In the light of the original cholinergic hypothesis of AD, attempts at in vivo characterization of cholinergic mechanisms are well justified. The markedly reduced concentration of the cholinergic marker enzyme ChAT found postmortem in the cortex and hippocampus of AD patients appears to be accompanied by degeneration of cholinergic neurons projecting from the basal forebrain (Perry 1986). In quest of a primate model for AD, Kiyosawa et al. (in press), in an FDG-PET study on baboons, have found a significant glucose metabolic depression which was most marked in the ipsilateral frontotemporal region 4 days after a stereotactic lesion of the nucleus basalis of Meynert (NbM). This depression, however, slowly recovered to close to normal levels within 6–13 weeks probably due to a postsynaptic plasticity that may be lacking in AD. PET studies with [^{11}C]choline have been performed in anesthetized rhesus monkeys (Friedland et al. 1983b; Eckernäs et al. 1986) and on humans (Gauthier et al. 1985). The ^{11}C-labeled choline analog pyrrolidinocholine has been used on dogs (Redies et al., 1988) and showed that the brain uptake of radiotracer was low. Nevertheless, models for the evaluation of choline brain uptake in relation to functional changes of the cholinergic system are under investigation.

Holman et al. (1985) have used SPECT and ^{123}I-labeled 3-quinuclidinyl-4-iodobenzilate to investigate acetylcholine receptors in one AD patient semiquantitatively. By comparison with an age-matched control subject, the preliminary conclusion was that muscarinic acetylcholine receptor concentrations might be relatively preserved in patients with AD.

Dopaminergic System

Recently, a variety of dopaminergic radioligands suitable for PET studies have become available. The role of this neurotransmitter system in the pathophysiology of dementing conditions such as AD, therefore, may now be assessed in vivo. Whereas presynaptic dopamine metabolism may be assessed by the tracer ^{18}F-labeled dopa (Leenders 1986), postsynaptic dopamine receptors may be investigated with [11C]methyl-spiperone or [11C]raclopride (Farde et al. 1986, 1988). Accumulation of [11C]nomiphensine is an indicator of the dopamine nerve terminal pool (Aquilonius et al. 1987) while monoamine oxidase B (MAO-B), the enzyme that deaminates dopamine, may be locally measured by a combination of the tracers D- and L-[11C]deprenyl (Fowler et al. 1986).

PET studies investigating AD using these, and many other (Halldin et al. 1986; Welch et al. 1988; Blin et al. 1988), tracers should be forthcoming since some of them have already been used to study other conditions associated with dementia such as PD, Huntington's disease (Hägglund et al. 1987), and progressive supranuclear palsy (PSP) (Leenders and Aquilonius 1987).

Finally, PET has already been used together with the selective agent [11C]ketanserin to investigate serotoninergic receptors in normal adults (Baron et al. 1985). Since the 5-HT$_2$ subtype serotoninergic receptor has been shown to be markedly reduced in AD patients (Cross et al. 1984), PET studies with [11C]ketanserin should be most instructive although apparently not easy to perform.

Activation Studies

In a number for recent reviews on the use of PET in the investigation and possible diagnosis of AD, several authors notice the fact that, thus far, most PET dementia studies have only probed the resting brain where possible differences caused by disease might be minimized (Benson 1988; Cutler 1988; de Leon et al. 1988). There is a consensus that activation studies with neuropsychological tasks (Duara et al. 1987) or pharmacological manipulations (Gustafson et al. 1987) are urgently needed and offer considerable promise in the study of dementias in general and in their possible early diagnosis.

To date, there has been only one PET study that has examined glucose metabolic rates during cognitive activation in seven elderly controls and seven pAD patients (Miller et al. 1987). For the temporal lobes, all pAD patients favored the right hemisphere during a verbal recognition memory task, whereas five of the seven control subjects favored the left hemisphere.

The concept of identifying a pathological condition by challenging the organ under study with a specific task (activation) is not new and has been applied in a variety of patient and normal control studies using PET or other functional imaging techniques. For instance, such studies are common practice in conventional nuclear medicine cardiac imaging. Also, Berman (1987) has demonstrated the usefulness of CBF studies during cortical stress tests in schizophrenia. PET methodologies have been recently developed to study blood flow and metabolic changes in the human brain on a regional basis in response to various stimuli, including mental activity (Chang et al.

250   E. Meyer

1987; Roland et al. 1987; Petersen et al. 1988), motor tasks (Roland et al. 1982), and a variety of sensory activations (Ginsberg et al. 1988; Fox et al. 1987a, b). The majority of these studies used the intravenous ^{15}O water bolus CBF method (Herscovitch et al. 1983) which requires a data acquisition time of only 1 min and can be repeated in the same subject up to ten times at intervals of 10–15 min due to the short half-life of ^{15}O (2 min).

In addition to purely physiological applications such as the functional mapping of the human brain in vivo, CBF response activation studies have already been shown to be of some clinical use. For example, they have been used to assess perfusion reserve in patients with cerebrovascular disease (CVD; Gibbs et al. 1984; Norrving et al. 1982; Powers et al. 1987). They might prove equally useful in assessing the hemodynamic status of patients with CVD, since Powers et al. (1987) have found that patients with a history of transient ischemic events and CVD confirmed by angiography had a significantly reduced CBF response to the stimulus in the hemisphere supplied by the diseased vessel.

In an effort to further explore this approach, we are currently evaluating the diagnostic potential of CBF responses to vibrotactile somatosensory stimulation in patients with early AD. We and others have shown that CBF is increased in the primary somatosensory cortex of normal subjects in response to vibrotactile stimulation of the finger tips (Fox et al. 1987b). Given the well-documented depression of CMRGlc, CMRO$_2$, and CBF in both the parietal and frontal cortices of patients with AD, a reduced CBF response from the somatosensory cortex challenged by vibrotactile stimulation might be expected despite the fact that, at rest, the primary motor-sensory strip is relatively spared with regard to metabolic depression. Using the above intravenous ^{15}O water bolus CBF method, we have been able to show that the CBF response to vibrotactile stimulation is influenced by the attentive behavior of the subject. Attention to the stimulus enhances the local CBF response while execution of a distraction task during the stimulation process tends to decrease it. The influence of attentive behavior on neuronal responses to vibrational stimuli in the primary somatosensory cortex of the monkey has been demonstrated before (Hyvaerinen et al. 1980). This finding together with evidence on the involvement of cholinergic neurons in the cerebral cortical blood flow response to somatosensory stimuli (Metherate et al. 1985) might lead to new, hopefully diagnostically useful, results on early AD by means of the CBF activation approach.

Calcium Homeostasis and Calcium-Channel Blockers

Many aspects of calcium homeostasis change with aging (Gibson and Peterson 1987). These changes may be pathophysiologically important in AD. The movement of calcium across membranes is affected, and this may lead to the formation of abnormal proteins in AD. It is now well accepted that cell death due to any cause is preceded by intracellular influx of calcium. To the extent that this occurs in AD, the implied activation of the calcium channels may be measurable with PET. This necessitates labeling of a calcium-channel ligand such as nimodipine, a calcium-channel blocker, with a positron emitter, a goal now actively pursued in a few centers including our own.

Conclusions

The characteristic pathological changes in the metabolic pattern as measured by PET so far may assist in the differentiation of AD, MID, depression, and PSP. Riege and Metter (1988), in their review, state that there are specific dysfunctions both in cognitive and brain-metabolic indices of early pAD, although these are not consistent from patient to patient. Also, while the relationship between cognition and energy metabolism does not seem to be straightforward, Riege and Metter (1988) find that metabolic and cognitive indices were linked already in the early stage of AD, particularly when measures such as parietal hemispheric asymmetry or the parietal to caudate-thalamus ratio were used. In elderly controls, such a correlation was not always found.

Temporal-parietal to cerebellar CMRGlc ratio measures will have to be reassessed in view of the recent finding by Klinger et al. (1988) that cerebellar CMRGlc is elevated in patients with periventricular white matter lesions, which seem to be present in about 30% of the AD patients.

It is recognized that many of the inconsistencies in results from studies on AD can be blamed on the limited diagnostic accuracy and that more stringent classification criteria for AD would improve clinical research in this field. Longitudinal PET studies in families with dominantly inherited AD are therefore of particular value and should be performed wherever possible (Polinsky et al. 1987) since, despite an interesting attempt by Kiyosawa et al. (in press), primate models of AD do not seem to be forthcoming.

As to the diagnostic utility of PET in AD the views diverge, particularly with regard to the early detection of AD. Friedland et al. (1988) agree with Riege and Metter (1988) that presently it is not clear how to detect the earliest symptoms of AD. Although the usefulness of PET as a research tool in dementia is not disputed, Benson (1988) sees a limited future for PET as a diagnostic tool in dementia. On the other hand, Friedland et al. (1988), de Leon et al. (1988), and Cutler (1988) predict an important role for PET in diagnostic decisions even at an early stage of the disease.

Improvements in scanning equipment, particularly an increase in spatial resolution and appropriate correction methods for brain atrophy (Duara et al. 1988b), will enhance the disease-specific content of regional functional parameters and allow investigation of the hippocampal region which, according to de Leon et al. (1988), could potentially assist the early detection of AD. Advanced statistical methods of data analysis, particularly aimed at the evaluation of interregional metabolic correlations, should give PET the potential to contribute considerably to early diagnostic decisions in the future (Cutler 1988; de Leon et al. 1988; Friedland et al. 1988).

A great deal is expected from PET studies with tracers for neurotransmitters and receptors in the near future. Since certain neurotransmitter or receptor changes might precede the known global and focal metabolic depressions, the early diagnostic capabilities of PET in AD should be greatly enlarged by such studies (Leenders and Aquilonius 1987; Cutler 1988). Altered calcium homeostasis observed in AD (Gibson and Peterson 1987) might be investigated with PET by means of labeled calcium-channel blockers such as nimodipine which could lead to valuable diagnostic indices. In the more distant future, imaging with AD-selective monoclonal antibodies (Hyman et al. 1988) might be of considerable early diagnostic use.

There is general agreement that longitudinal studies on carefully selected patients might reveal a more disease-specific metabolic pattern than cross-sectional studies alone and, therefore, should be performed more frequently (Riege and Metter 1988; Cutler 1988; Benson 1988; Polinsky et al. 1987). Equally, the need for an increased number of activation studies has been expressed. Benson (1988) and Cutler (1988) argue that the metabolic response to memory or language tasks, or even more complex cognitive or pharmacological manipulations, in demented patients would most probably be different from that of normal subjects. Such studies, therefore, might provide a more sensitive PET probe for AD (Miller et al. 1987) and could be of value in its early differential diagnosis.

Even though several authors agree that PET is a more sensitive tool than CT or MRI for the detection of cortical involvement and the separation of AD patients from controls or from patients suffering from other forms of dementia (McGeer 1986b; de Leon et al. 1988; Alavi et al. 1988; Kuhl 1988), the idea of using a combined index from various measurements, including structural imaging modalities such as CT and MRI, to identify more uniquely at an early stage individuals with the disease has been put forward repeatedly. Cutler (1988) and Riege and Metter (1988) suggest that PET data combined with measures from specific neuropsychological and cognitive tests might improve the clinical sensitivity for an early diagnosis of AD. Roberts (1988) extends this view and proposes to apply statistical approaches used in pattern recognition to standardized measurements of pertinent physical, psychometric, imaging, biochemical, immunological, and genetic variables obtained from series of carefully selected patients in a multicenter trial. A relatively small selection of those measurements might reveal an AD pattern that could be used to identify with a high degree of certainty individuals with the disease. Such measurements might include data from new promising areas of research in AD such as eye-tracking dysfunctions (Fletcher and Sharpe 1986; Hutton et al. 1984; Jones et al. 1983), olfactory deficits (Eskenazi et al. 1983; Serby 1986; Warner et al. 1986), and abnormal dermatoglyphic patterns (Weinreb 1986). In this manner, as Roberts states (1988), "we may keep narrowing the window of recognition through which, hopefully, eventually only AD will be seen."

Acknowledgements. Special thanks are due to Dr. A. M. Hakim, coordinator of the McConnell Brain Imaging Centre, Montreal Neurological Institute, for his assistance and encouragement during the preparation of this manuscript.

References

Alavi A, de Leon MJ (1985) Studies of the brain in aging and dementia with positron emission tomography and x-ray computed tomography. In: Reivich M, Alavi A (eds) Positron emission tomography. Liss, New York, pp 273–290

Alavi A, Fazekas F, Chawluk JC, Zimmerman RA, Hackney D, Bilaniuk L, Rosen M, Alves WM, Hurtig HI, Jamieson DG, Kushner MJ, Reivich M (1988) A comparison of CT, MR and PET in Alzheimer's dementia and normal aging. J Nucl Med 29: 852

Aquilonius SM, Bergström K, Eckernäs SA, Hartvig P, Leenders KL, Lundquist H, Antoni G, Gee A, Rimland A, Uhlin J, Langström B (1987) In vivo evaluation of striatal dopamine reuptake sites using ^{11}C-nomifensine and positron emission tomography. Acta Neurol Scand 76: 283–287

Bajcsy R, Lieberson R, Reivich M (1983) A computerized system for the elastic matching of deformed radiographic images to idealized atlas images. J Comput Assist Tomogr 7: 618–625

Baron JC, Samson Y, Comar D, Crouzel C, Deniker P, Agid Y (1985) Etude in vivo des récepteurs sérotoninergiques centraux chez l'homme par tomographie à positons. Rev Neurol (Paris) 141: 537–545

Beal MF, Mazurek MF, Tran VT, Chattah G, Bird ED, Martin JB (1985) Reduced numbers of somatostatin receptors in the cerebral cortex in Alzheimer's disease. Science 229: 289–291

Benson FD (1988) PET/dementia: an update. Neurobiol 9: 87–88

Benson DF, Kuhl DE, Hawkins RA, Phelps ME, Cummings JL, Tsai SY (1983) The fluorodeoxy-glucose ^{18}F scan in Alzheimer's disease and multi-infarct dementia. Arch Neurol 40: 711–714

Berman KF (1987) Cortical "stess tests" in schizophrenia: regional cerebral blood flow studies. Biol Psychiatry 22: 1304–1326

Blin J, Pappata S, Kiyosawa M, Crouzel C, Baron JC (1988) [^{18}F]Setoperone: a new high-affinity ligand for positron emission tomography study of serotonin-2 receptors in baboon brain in vivo. Eur J Pharmacol 147: 73–82

Bohm C, Greitz T, Kingsley D, Berggren B, Olsson L (1983) Adjustable computerized stereotaxic brain atlas for transmission and emission tomography. AJNR 4: 731–733

Bohm C, Greitz T, Kingsley D, Berggren BM, Olsson L (1985) A computerized individually variable stereotactic brain atlas. In: Greitz T, Ingvar DH, Widen L (eds) The metabolism of the human brain studied with positron emission tomography. Raven, New York, pp 85–91

Brun A, Englund E (1981) Regional patterns of degeneration in Alzheimer's disease: neuronal loss and histopathological grading. Histopathology 5: 549–564

Bustany P, Henry JF, de Rotrou J, Signoret P, Ziegler M, Zarifian E, Soussaline F, Comar D (1983) Local cerebral metabolic rate of ^{11}C-1-methionine in early stages of dementia, schizophrenia, and Parkinson's disease. J Cereb Blood Flow Metab 3: 492–493

Bustany P, Henry JF, de Rotrou J, Signoret P, Cabanis E, Zarifian E, Ziegler M, Derlon JM, Crouzel C, Soussaline F, Comar D (1985) Correlation between clinical state and positron emission tomography measurement of local brain protein synthesis in Alzheimer's dementia, Parkinson's disease, schizophrenia and gliomas. In: Greitz T, Ingvar DH, Widen L et al. (eds) The metabolism of the human brain studied with positron emission tomography. Raven, New York, pp 241–249

Chang JY, Duara R, Barker W, Apicella A, Finn R (1987) Two behavioral states studied in a single PET/FDG procedure: theory, method and preliminary results. J Nucl Med 28: 852–860

Clark C, Hayden M, Hollenberg S, Li D, Stoessl AJ (1987) Controlling for cerebral atrophy in positron emission tomography data. J Cereb Blood Flow Metab 7: 510–512

Condon B, Patterson J, Wyper D, Hadley D, Teasdale G, Grant R, Jenkins A, Macpherson P, Rowan J (1986a) A quantitative index of ventricular and extraventricular CSF fluid volumes using MR imaging. J Comp Assist Tomogr 10: 784–792

Condon B, Patterson J, Wyper DJ, Hadley DM, Grant R, Teasdale G, Rowan J (1986b) Intracranial CSF volumes determined using magnetic resonance imaging. Lancet I: 1355–1357

Cross AJ, Crow TJ, Ferrier IN, Johnson JA (1984) Serotonin receptor changes in dementia of the Alzheimer type. J Neurochem 43: 1574–1581

Cutler NR (1988) Cognitive and brain imaging measures of Alzheimer's disease. Neurobiol Aging 9: 90–92

Cutler NR, Haxby JV, Duara R, Grady CL, Kay AD, Kessler RM, Sundaram M, Rapoport SI (1985a) Clinical history, brain metabolism, and neuropsychological function in Alzheimer's disease. Ann Neurol 18: 298–309

Cutler NR, Haxby JV, Duara R, Grady CL, Moore AM, Parisi JE, White J, Heton L, Margolin RM, Rapoport SI (1985b) Brain metabolism as measured with positron emission tomography: serial assessment in a patient with familial Alzheimer's disease. Neurology 35: 1556–1561

Davies P (1979) Neurotransmitter-related enzymes in senile dementia of the Alzheimer type. Brain Res 171: 319–327

de Leon MJ, Ferris SH, George AE, Reisberg B, Christman DR, Kricheff II, Wolf AP (1983) Computed tomography and positron emission transaxial tomography evaluations of normal aging and Alzheimer's disease. J Cereb Blood Flow Metab 3: 391–394

de Leon MJ, George AE, Ferris SH (1986) Computed tomography and positron emission tomography correlates of cognitive decline in aging and senile dementia. In: Poon LW (ed) Handbook for clinical memory assessment of older adults. American Psychological Association, Washington DC, pp 367–382 de Leon MJ, George AE, Marcus DL, Miller JD (1988) Positron emission tomography with the deoxyglucose technique and the diagnosis of Alzheimer's disease. Neurobiol Aging 9: 88–90

Duara R, Grady C, Haxby J, Ingvar D, Sokoloff L, Margolin R, Manning RG, Cutler NR, Rapoport SI (1984) Human brain glucose utilization and cognitive function in relation to age. Ann Neurol 16: 702–713

Duara R, Gross-Glenn K, Barker WW, Chang JY, Apicella A, Loewenstein D, Boothe T (1987) Behavioral activation and the variability of cerebral glucose metabolic measurements. J Cereb Blood Flow Metab 7: 268–271

Duara R, Loewenstein DA, Barker WW, Chang JY, Kothari P (1988a) Evidence for predominant left hemisphere dysfunction in FDG/PET scans of patients with Alzheimers' disease (AD) and multi-infarct dementia (MID). J Nucl Med 29: 912

Duara R, Yoshii F, Barker WW, Chang JY, Loewenstein DA, Apicella A, Pascal S, Boothe T (1988b) Sensitivity of cerebral glucose metabolism to age, gender, brain volume, brain atrophy and cerebrovascular risk factors. J Nucl Med 29: 852

Eckernäs SA, Aquilonius SM, Bergström K, Hartvig P, Lilja A, Lindberg B, Lundqvist H, Langström B, Malmborg P, Moström U, Nagren K (1986) The use of positron emission tomography for the evaluation of choline metabolism in the brain of the rhesus monkey. In: Hanin I (ed) Dynamics of cholinergic function. Plenum, New York, pp 303–311

Eskenazi B, Cain WS, Novelly RA, Friend KB (1983) Olfactory functioning in temporal lobectomy patients. Neuropsychologia 21: 365–374

Evans AC, Beil C, Marrett S, Thompson CJ, Hakim A (1988) Anatomical functional correlation using an adjustable MRI-based region of interest atlas with positron emission tomography. J Cereb Blood Flow Metab 8: 513–530

Farde L, Hall H, Ehrin E, Sedval G (1986) Quantitative analysis of dopamine-D-2 receptor binding in the living human brain using positron emission tomography. Science 231: 258–261

Farde L, Pauli S, Hall H, Eriksson L, Halldin C, Högberg T, Nilsson L, Sjögren I, Stone-Elander S (1988) Stereoselective binding of ^{11}C-raclopride in living human brain – a search for extrastriatal central D2-dopamine receptors by PET. Psychopharmacology (Berlin) 94: 471–478

Fletcher WA, Sharpe JA (1986) Saccadic eye movement dysfunction in Alzheimer's disease. Ann Neurol 20: 464–471

Foster NL, Chase TN, Mansi L, Brooks R, Fedio P, Patronas N, Di Chiro G (1984) Cortical abnormalities in Alzheimer's disease. Ann Neurol 16: 649–654

Fowler JS, MacGregor RR, Wolf AP, Arnett CD, Dewey SL, Schlyer D, Christman D, Logan J, Smith M, Sachs H, Aquilonius S-M, Bjurling P, Holldin C, Hartvig P, Leenders KL, Lundqvist H, Oreland L, Stalnacke C-G, Langström B (1986) Mapping human brain monoamine oxidase A and B with ^{11}C-suicide inactivators and positron emission tomography. Science 235: 481–485

Fox PT, Perlmutter JS, Raichle ME (1985) A stereotactic method of anatomical localization for positron emission tomography. J Comput Assist Tomogr 9: 141–153

Fox PT, Miezin FM, Allman JM, Van Essen DC, Raichle ME (1987a) Retinotopic organization of human visual cortex mapped with positron-emission tomography. J Neuroscl; 7: 913–922

Fox PT, Burton H, Raichle ME (1987b) Mapping human somatosensory cortex with positron emission tomography. J Neurosurg 67: 34–43

Frackowiak RSJ, Pozzilli C, Legg NJ, DuBoulay GH, Marshall J, Lenzi GL, Jones T (1981a) Regional cerebral oxygen supply and utilization in dementia: a clinical and physiological study with oxygen-15 and positron tomography. Brain 104: 753–778

Frackowiak RSJ, Pozzilli C, Legg NJ, DuBoulay GH, Marshall J, Lenzi GL, Jones T (1981b) A prospective study of regional cerebral blood Glow and oxygen utilization in dementia using positron emission tomography and oxygen-15. J Cereb Blood Flow Metab 1: S453–S454

Friedland RP, Budinger TF, Ganz E, Yano Y, Mathis CA, Koss B, Ober BA, Huesman RH, Derenzo SE (1983a) Regional cerebral alterations in dementia of the Alzheimer type: positron emission tomography with ^{18}F-fluorodeoxyglucose. J Comput Assist Tomogr 7: 590–598

Friedland RP, Mathis CA, Budinger TF, Moyer BR, Rosen M (1983b) Labeled choline and phosphorylcholine: body distribution and brain autoradiography. Concise communication. J Nucl Med 24: 812–815

Friedland RP, Budinger TF, Koss B, Ober BA (1985) Alzheimer's disease: anterior-posterior and lateral hemispheric alterations in cortical glucose utilization. Neurosci Lett 53: 235–240

Friedland RP, Horwitz B, Koss E (1988) Measurement of disease progression in Alzheimer's disease. Neurobiol Aging 9: 95–97

Gauthier S, Diksic M, Yamamoto L, Tyler J, Feindel W (1985) Positron emission tomography with ^{11}C-choline in human subjects. Can J Neurol Sci 12: 214

Gibbs JM, Wise RJS, Leenders KL, Jones T (1984) Evaluation of cerebral perfusion reserve in patients with carotid-artery occlusion. Lancet 1: 310–314

Gibson GE, Peterson C (1987) Calcium and the aging nervous system. Neurobiol Aging 8: 329–343

Ginsberg MD, Chang JY, Kelley RE, Yoshii F, Barker WW, Ingenito G, Boothe TE (1988) Increases in both cerebral glucose utilization and blood flow during execution of a somatosensory task. Ann Neurol 23: 152–160

Gottfries CG, Adolfsson R, Aquilonius SM, Carlsson A, Eckernäs SA, Nordberg A, Oreland L, Svennerholm L, Wiberg A, Winblad B (1983) Biochemical changes in dementia disorders of Alzheimer type (AD/SDAT). Neurobiol Aging 4: 261–271

Gustafson L, Edvinsson L, Dahlgreen N, Hagberg J, Risberg J, Rosen I, Ferno H (1987) Intravenous physostigmine treatment of Alzheimer's disease evaluated by psychometric testing, regional cerebral blood flow (rCBFF) measurement, and EEG. Psychopharmacology (Berlin) 93: 31–35

Hägglund J, Aquilonius S-M, Eckernäs S-A, Hartvig P, Lundquist H, Gullberg P, Langström B (1987) Dopamine receptor properties in Parkinson's disease and Huntington's chorea evaluated by positron emission tomography using ^{11}C-N-methyl-spiperone. Acta Neurol Scand 75: 87–94

Halldin C, Stone-Elander S, Farde L, Ehrin E, Fasth KJ, Langström B, Sedvall G (1986) Preparation of ^{11}C-labelled SCH 23390 for the in vivo study of dopamine D-1 receptors using positron emission tomography. Int J Rad Appl Instrum [A] 37: 1039–1043

Herholz K, Pawlik G, Weinhard K, Heiss W-D (1985) Computer assisted mapping in quantitative analysis of cerebral positron emission tomograms. J Comput Assist Tomogr 9: 154–161

Herscovitch P, Raichle ME (1985) What is the correct value for the brain-blood partition coefficient for water? J Cereb Blood Flow Metabol 5: 65–69

Herscovitch P, Markham J, Raichle ME (1983) Brain blood flow measured with intravenous 0–15 H$_2$O. 1. Theory and error analysis. J Nucl Med 24: 782–789

Herscovitch P, Auchus AP, Gado M, Chi D, Raichle ME (1986) Correction of positron emission tomography data for cerebral atrophy. J Cereb Blood Flow Metab 6: 120–124

Holman BL, Gibson RE, Hill TC, Eckelman WC, Albert M, Reba RC (1985) Muscarinic acetylcholine receptors in Alzheimer's disease. In vivo imaging with iodine 123-labeled 3-quinuclidinyl-4-iodobenzilate and emission tomography. JAMA 254: 3063–3066

Horowitz B, Duara R, Rapoport SI (1984) Intercorrelations of glucose metabolic rates between brain regions: applications to healthy males in a state of reduced sensory input. J Cereb Blood Flow Metab 4: 484–499

Hoyer S (1986) Senile dementia and Alzheimer's disease. Brain blood flow and metabolism. Prog Neuropsychopharmacol Biol Psychiatry 10: 447–478

Hutton JT, Nagel JA, Loewenson B (1984) Eye tracking dysfunction in Alzheimer-type dementia. Neurology 34: 99–102

Hyman BT, Van Hoesen GW, Wolozin BL, Davies P, Kromer LJ, Damasio AR (1988) Alz-50 antibody recognizes Alzheimer-related neuronal changes. Ann Neurol 23: 371–379

Hyvaerinen J, Poranen A, Jokinen Y (1980) Influence of attentive behavior on neuronal responses to vibration in somatosensory cortex of the monkey. J Neurophysiol 43: 870–882

Jagust WJ, Friedland RP, Budinger TF, Koss E, Ober B (1988) Longitudinal studies of regional cerebral metabolism in Alzheimer's disease. Neurology 38: 909–912

Jones A, Friedland RP, Koss B, Stark L, Thompkins-Ober BA (1983) Saccadic intrusions in Alzheimer-type dementia. J Neurol 229: 189–194

Kanno I, Iida H, Miura S et al. (1987) A system for cerebral blood flow measurement using an O-15 H$_2$O autoradiographic method and positron emission tomography. J Cereb Blood Flow Metab 7: 143–153

Kiyosawa M, Baron JC, Hamel E, Pappata S, Duverger D, Riche D, Mazoyer B, Naguet R, MacKenzie ET (in press) Time-course of effects of unilateral lesions of the nucleus basalis of Meynert on glucose utilization of the cerebral cortex: positron tomography in baboons. Brain

Klinger A, de Leon MJ, George AE, Miller JD, Wolf AP (1988) Elevated cerebellar glucose metabolism in microvascular white matter disease: normal aging and Alzheimer's disease. J Cereb Blood Flow Metab 8: 433–435

Kuhl DE (1988) Dementia: clinical application of positron emission tomography. Am J Physiol Imaging 3: 59–60

Kuhl DE, Metter EJ, Riege WH, Phelps ME (1982) Effects of human aging on patterns of local cerebral glucose utilization determined by ^{18}F fluorodeoxyglucose method. J Cereb Blood Flow Metab 2: 163–171

Kuhl DE, Metter EJ, Riege WH, Hawkins RA, Mazziotta JC, Phelps ME, Kling AS (1983) Local cerebral glucose utilization in elderly patients with depression, multi-infarct dementia and Alzheimer's disease. J Cereb Blood Flow Metab 3: S494–S495

Kuhl DE, Metter EJ, Riege WH, Hawkins RA (1984a) The effect of normal aging on patterns of local cerebral glucose utilization. Ann Neurol 15: S133–S137

Kuhl DE, Metter EJ, Riege WH, Markham CH (1984b) Patterns of cerebral glucose utilization in Parkinson's disease and Huntington's disease. Ann Neurol 15: S119–S125

Kuhl DE, Metter EJ, Riege WH (1985a) Patterns of cerebral glucose utilization in depression, multiple infarct dementia, and Alzheimer's disease. In: Sokoloff L (ed) Brain imaging and brain functions. Raven, New York, pp 211–226

Kuhl DE, Metter EJ, Riege WH, Hawkins RA (1985b) Determinations of cerebral glucose utilization in dementia using positron emission tomography. Dan Med Bull 32: 51–55

Kuhl DE, Metter EJ, Riege WH, Hawkins RA (1985c) Patterns of cerebral glucose utilization in dementia. In: Greitz T, Ingvar DH, Widen L (eds) The metabolism of the human brain studied with positron emission tomography. Raven, New York, pp 419–431

Kuhl DE, Metter EJ, Benson DF, Ashford JW, Riege WH, Fujikawa DG, Markham CH, Maltese A, Dorsey DA (1985d) Similarities of cerebral glucose metabolism in Alzheimer's and Parkinsonian dementia. J Cereb Blood Flow Metab 5: S169–S170

Lammertsma AA, Frackowiak RSJ, Lenzi GL, Heather JD, Pozzilli C, Jones T (1981) Accuracy of the oxygen-15 steady state technique for measuring CBF and CMRO$_2$. J Cereb Blood Flow Metab 1: S3–S4

Leenders KL (1986) Movement disorders: a study with positron emission tomography. Thesis, Rodopi, Amsterdam

Leenders K, Aquilonius SM (1987) Dementing conditions studied with PET. J Neural Transm [Suppl] 24: 31–41

Leenders K, Wolfson L, Gibbs J, Wise R, Jones T, Legg NJ (1983) Regional cerebral blood flow and oxygen metabolism in Parkinson disease and their response to L-dopa. J Cereb Blood Flow Metab 3: S488–S489

Mazziotta JC, Phelps ME, Plummer D, Schwab R, Halgren E (1983) Optimization and standardization of anatomical data in neurobehavioral investigations. J Cereb Blood Flow Metab 3 (Suppl 1): S266

McGeer PL, Kamo H, Li DKB, Tuokko H, McGeer EG, Adam MJ, Ammann W, Beattie BL, Calne DB, Martin WRW, Pate BD, Rogers JG, Ruth TJ, Sayre CI, Stoessl AJ (1986a) Positron emission tomography in patients with clinically diagnosed Alzheimer's disease. Can Med Assoc J 134: 597–607

McGeer PL, Kamo H, Harrop R, McGeer EG, Martin WRW, Pate BD, Li DKB (1986b) Comparison of PET, MRI, and CT with pathology in a proven case of Alzheimer's disease. Neurology 36: 1569–1574

McNamara D, Horwitz B, Grady CL, Rapoport SI (1987) Topographical analysis of glucose metabolism, as measured with positron emission tomography, in dementia of the Alzheimer type: use of linear histograms. Int J Neurosci 36: 89–97

Metherate R, Tremblay N, Dykes RW (1985) Changes in neuronal function produced in cat primary somatosensory cortex by iontophoretic application of acetylcholine. Soc Neurosci Abstr 11: 753

Metter EJ, Riege WH, Kuhl DE, Phelps ME (1983) Differences in regional glucose metabolic intercorrelations with aging. J Cereb Blood Flow Metab 3 (Suppl 1): 482–483

Metter EJ, Riege WH, Kuhl DE, Phelps ME (1984a) Cerebral metabolic relationships for selected brain regions in healthy adults. J Cereb Blood Flow Metab 4: 1–7

Metter EJ, Riege WH, Kameyama M, Kuhl DE, Phelps ME (1984b) Cerebral metabolic relationships for selected brain regions in Alzheimer's, Huntington's, and Parkinson's disease. J Cereb Blood Flow Metab 4: 500–506

Metter EJ, Riege WH, Benson D, Kuhl DE, Phelps ME (1985a) Patterns of regional cerebral metabolism in Alzheimer's disease patients. In: Hutton JT, Kenny AD (eds) Senile dementia of the Alzheimer's type. Liss, New York

Metter EJ, Riege WH, Benson D, Kuhl DE, Phelps ME (1985b) Variability of regional cerebral glucose metabolism in Alzheimer's disease patients as compared to normal subjects. J Cereb Blood Flow Metab 5: S127–S128

Miller JD, de Leon MJ, Ferris SH, Kluger A, George AE, Reisberg B, Sachs HJ, Wolf AP (1987) Abnormal temporal lobe response in Alzheimer's disease during cognitive processing as measured by ^{11}C-2-deoxy-D-glucose and PET. J Cereb Blood Flow Metab 7: 248–251

Norrving B, Nilsson B, Risberg J (1982) RCBF in patients with carotid occlusions. Resting and hypercapnic flow related to collateral pattern. Stroke 13: 155–162

Perez FI, Mathew NT, Stump DA, Meyer JS (1977) Regional cerebral blood flow statistical patterns and psychological performance in multi-infarct dementia and Alzheimer's disease. Can J Neurol Sci 4: 53–62

Perlmutter JS, Raichle ME (1985) Reduced blood flow in the frontal mesocortex in parkinsonian patients. J Cereb Blood Flow Metab 5: S171–S172

Perry EK (1986) The cholinergic hypothesis – ten years on. Br Med Bull 42: 63–69

Petersen SE, Fox PT, Posner MI, Mintun M, Raichle ME (1988) Positron emission tomographic studies of the cortical anatomy of single-word processing. Nature 331: 585–589

Phelps ME, Mazziotta JC, Schelbert HR (eds) (1986) Positron emission tomography and autoradiography. Raven, New York, pp 237–580

Polinsky RJ, Noble H, Di Chiro G, Nee LE, Feldman RG, Brown RT (1987) Dominantly inherited Alzheimer's disease: cerebral glucose metabolism. J Neurol Neurosurg Psychiatry 50: 752–757

Powers WJ, Press GA, Grubb RL, Gado M, Raichle ME (1987) The effect of hemodynamically significant carotid artery disease on the hemodynamic status of the cerebral circulation. Ann Intern Med 106: 27–35

Quirion R, Martel JC, Robitaille Y, Etienne P, Wood P, Nair NPV, Gauthier S (1986) Neurotransmitter and receptor deficit in senile dementia of the Alzheimer type. Can J Neurol Sci 13 (Suppl): 503–510

Raichle ME (1982) Positron emission tomography. In: Thompson RA, Green JR (eds) New perspectives in cerebral localization. Raven, New York

Redies C, Diksic M, Collier B, Gjedde A, Thompson CJ, Gauthier S, Feindel W (1988) Influx of a choline analog to dog brain measured by PET. Synapse 2: 406–411

Reivich M, Alavi A (eds) (1985) Positron emission tomography. Liss, New York

Riege WH, Metter EJ (1988) Cognitive and brain imaging measures of Alzheimer's disease. Neurobiol Aging 9: 69–86

Riege WH, Metter EJ, Kuhl DE, Hawkins RA, Phelps ME (1982) Multivariate memory and local cerebral glucose metabolism in human aging. Gerontologist 22: 131

Riege WH, Metter EJ, Kuhl DE, Phelps ME, Kling A (1984) Differences in asymmetry of memory and brain glucose metabolism in schizophrenic, depressed, and Alzheimer's patients. Soc Neurosci Abstr 10: 541

Riege WH, Metter EJ, Kuhl DE, Phelps ME (1985a) Brain glucose metabolism and memory functions: age decrease in factor scores. J Gerontol 40: 459–467

Riege WH, Metter EJ, Kuhl DE (1985b) Correlation of memory and brain glucose metabolism in depression and probable Alzheimer's disease. J Cereb Blood Flow Metab 5: S125–S126

Roberts E (1988) Beyond measurement: the pattern is the thing. Neurobiol Aging 9: 97–100

Roland PE, Meyer E, Shibasaki T, Yamamoto YL, Thompson CJ (1982) Regional cerebral blood flow changes in cortex and basal ganglia during voluntary movements in normal human volunteers. J Neurophysiol 48: 467–480

Roland PE, Eriksson L, Stone-Elander S, Widen L (1987) Does mental activity change the oxidative metabolism of the brain? J Neurosci 7: 2373–2389

Rougemont D, Baron JC, Collard P, Bustany P, Comar D, Agid Y (1983) Local cerebral metabolic rate of glucose (lCMRGLc) in treated and untreated patients with Parkinson's disease. J Cereb Blood Flow Metab 3: S504–S505

Serby M (1986) Olfaction and Alzheimer's disease. Prog Neuropsychopharmacol Biol Psychiatry 10: 579–586

Shimohama S, Taniguchi T, Fujiwara M, Kameyama M (1988) Changes in benzodiazepine receptors in Alzheimer-type dementia. Ann Neurol 23: 404–406

Ter-Pogossian MM (1985) PET, SECT, and NMRI: competing or complementary disciplines. J Nucl Med 26: 1487–1498

Videen TO, Perlmutter JS, Mintun MA, Raichle ME (1988) Regional correction for the effects of brain atrophy in positron emission tomography. J Nucl Med 29: 773

Warner MD, Peabody CA, Flattery JJ, Tinklenberg JR (1986) Olfactory deficits and Alzheimer's disease. Biol Psychiatry 21: 116–118

Weinreb HJ (1986) Dermatoglyphic patterns in Alzheimer's disease. J Neurogenet 3: 233–246

Welch MJ, Katzenellenbogen JA, Mathias CJ, Brodack JW, Carlson KE, Chi DY,, Dence CS, Kilbourn MR, Perlmutter JS, Raichle ME, Ter-Pogossian MM (1988) N-(3-[^{18}F]Fluoropropyl)-spiperone: the preferred ^{18}F labeled spiperone analog for positron emission tomographic studies of the dopamine receptor. Nucl Med Biol 15: 83–97

An Approach to the Treatment of Senile Dementia: Calcium Channel Modulation

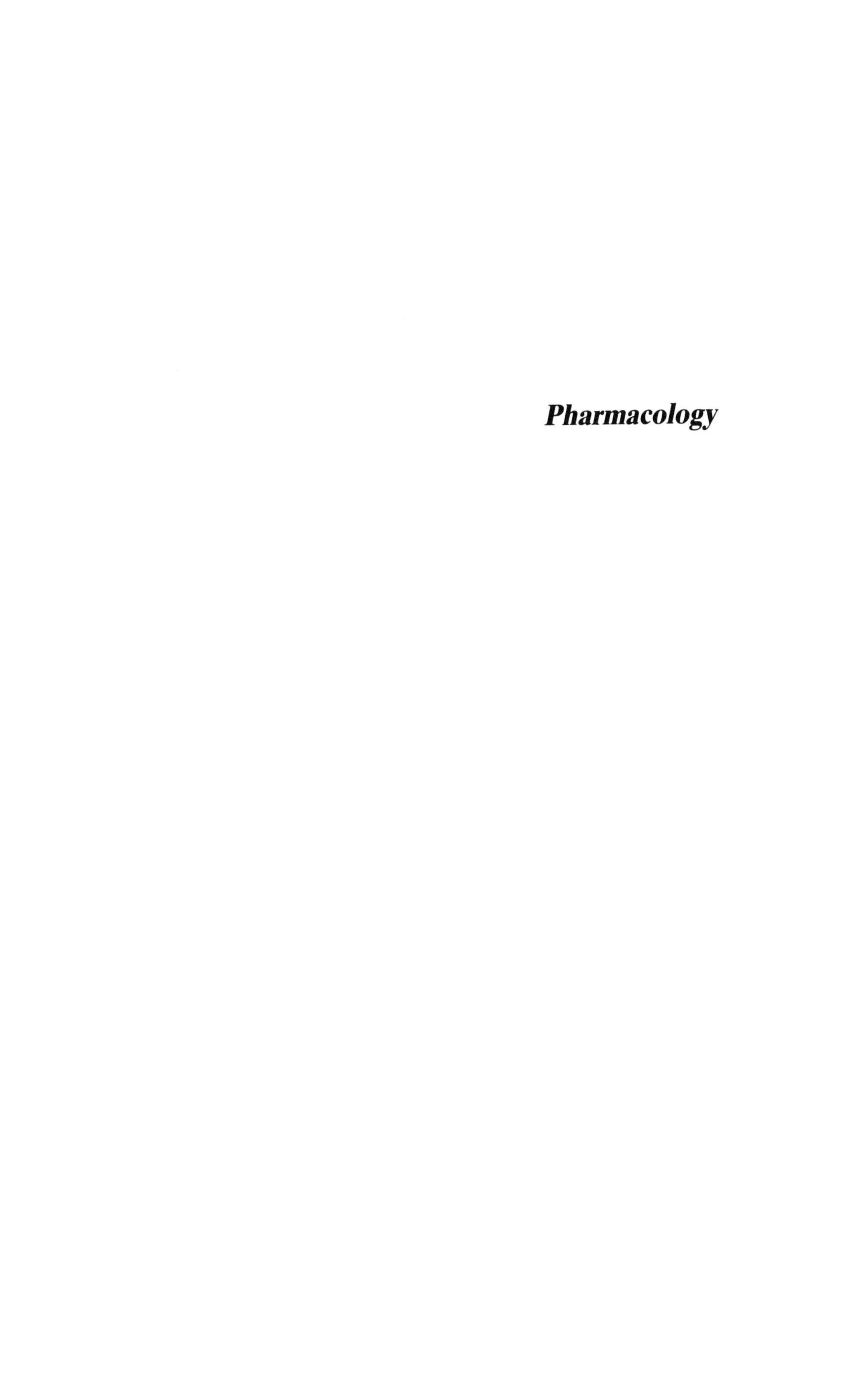

Pharmacology

Molecular Pharmacology of Calcium Channel Modulation

H. Glossmann, J. Striessnig, H. G. Knaus, A. Grassegger, C. Zech, and G. Zernig

Calcium is the most important intracellular messenger for many signal-transducing pathways. In electrically excitable cells, especially in neurons, one way to raise the cytosolic free calcium concentration is by means of Ca^{2+}-selective voltage-regulated plasma membrane channels. These channels convert electrical signals into the chemical signal calcium. Other ionic pores exist which are not primarily designed to pass calcium, but can play a role in calcium homeostasis especially under pathological conditions. An example is a subtype of the glutamate receptor activated channel family, the NMDA channel. This channel is of clinical interest as it may participate in ischemic brain damage and can be blocked by a variety of drugs, including MK 801 (Choi 1985, 1988).

Table 1 gives an overview on the different types of voltage-regulated calcium channels found on neurons. The different types, designated N, T and L, are distinguished by their electrophysiological behaviour, ion selectivity, drug and toxin sensitivity and last but not least by their subcellular location and functional role (Miller 1987). The N type, which only occurs on central and peripheral neurons, is important for neurotransmitter release (Hirning et al. 1988; Miller et al. 1988; Thayer et al. 1987). The channel activity is regulated by receptors, most likely via GTP binding proteins. $GABA_B$ and (subtypes of) opioid receptors are among the neurotransmitter receptors which regulate N channel activity mainly in an inhibitory fashion (Glossmann and Striessnig 1988).

There is very little known about the T-type channel, which also occurs in heart and other tissue (Nilius et al. 1985; Nowycky et al. 1985; Tsien et al. 1987, 1988). One of the reasons is that there is no toxin or drug known affecting the channels in a highly specific manner. Flunarizine and amiloride (Tang et al. 1988) block T channels in heart and presumably do so in neurons as well, but these drugs – in comparison to the 1,4-dihydropyridines for example – are not very selective.

The L-type channel is the only calcium channel which has been purified and from which two subunits (alpha$_1$, alpha$_2$) have been cloned (Tanabe et al. 1987; Ellis et al. 1988). Interestingly, this scientific breakthrough was achieved not from the study of brain, but of skeletal muscle tissue. Here the transverse tubule channel (together with the ryanodine receptor Ca^{2+} release channel in the sarcoplasmatic reticulum) serves as an essential component in the process of excitation-contraction coupling (Rios and Brum 1987; Rios et al. 1989; Saito et al. 1988; Imagawa et al. 1987; Hymel et al. 1988; Leung et al. 1988). In transverse tubule membranes the L-type channel drug receptors are present in very high density. The role of the alpha$_1$ subunit was recently proven by

Bergener, Reisberg (Eds.)
Diagnosis and Treatment
of Senile Dementia
© Springer-Verlag Berlin Heidelberg 1989

Table 1. Calcium channel types and subtypes

Type	Electrophysiological criteria	Location/function	Pharmacology
T	Low-threshold, rapidly inactivating, single-channel conductance (100 mM Ba^{2+}): 8–9 pS	Pacemaker current Rhythmic activity Found in sinus node cells, heart, skeletal muscle	Gallopamil, verapamil, amiloride, flunarizine block High concentrations required for Cd^{2+} block, Ni^{2+} is more effective
			MVIIA blocks weakly and is reversible (frog atria and chick dorsal root ganglion cells) 1,4-dihydropyridines have no effect
L	Long-lasting, high-threshold, single-channel conductance: 25 pS		Phenylalkylamines, Benzothiazepines, 1,4-dihydropyridines, Ca^{2+} antagonists and diphenylbutyl-piperidines block – 1,4-dihydropyridine Ca^{2+} agonists activate low concentrations required for Cd^{2+} block, Ni^{2+} is not as effective
L$_n$ (neuronal)		Cell soma, metabolic control?	GVIA blocks irreversibly
L$_m$ (muscular)		Contraction in heart and smooth muscle; secretion of hormones	GVIA has no effect
L$_{sk}$ (skeletal)	Different gating kinetics than L$_n$ or L$_m$	Excitation-contraction coupling	GVIA has no effect (?)
N	Activates like the L-type, but inactivates like the T-channel Single-channel conductance: 13 pS	In general presynaptic location Neurotransmitter release	Low concentrations are required for Cd^{2+} block: Cd^{2+} is more effective than Ni^{2+}
N$_A$		Presynaptic (i.e. in peripheral mammalian neurons)	Aminoglycoside block, but no GVIA block
N$_B$		Presynaptic (i.e. in central mammalian neurons)	Both aminoglycoside and GVIA block

Table 1 gives an overview of the different types of Ca^{2+} channels found in neurons and – as a comparison – in other tissues. The neuronal N-type channels have been subdivided into the N$_A$ and the N$_B$ type (for further details see Suzkiw et al. 1987; Gray and Olivera 1988).

micro-injection experiments with the cDNA of alpha$_1$ in the (mutant) muscular dysgenesis mouse muscle cell system (Tanabe et al. 1988).

L-type channel regulation is extremely complex. Phosphorylation mainly by cAMP-dependent protein kinase and activation by G$_s$ via receptors are some of the key features. In contrast to the N-type channel, the L channel plays only a facilitatory role for neurotransmitter release in many systems (Miller, 1987), is located at the membrane of the cell soma, and it is speculated that L channels in neurons play a role in controlling metabolism. R. Miller (1987) has suggested a specific arrangement of the N- and L-type channels in adult neurons.

The N channels are concentrated on the presynaptic membrane at the transmitter release zones. The toxins and drugs which alter channel function are indicated in Fig. 1.

Nature did not regard the L-type channel on neurons and in the periphery as an important target for toxins, although there is some evidence that the N-type channel toxin, omega conotoxin GVIA, may block L-type channels in neuronal systems (McCleskey et al. 1987).

In Table 2 we give an overview of the drugs or toxins which alter L- and N-type channel activity in a highly specific manner. The L-type channel, very similar to the voltage-dependent sodium channel or the GABA$_A$ receptor-operated chloride channel, has different and distinct domains for drugs which communicate with each other allosterically.

Binding and action of these drugs are voltage- and/or use-dependent. The dissociation binding constants of the radiolabelled drugs for depolarized membranes are listed

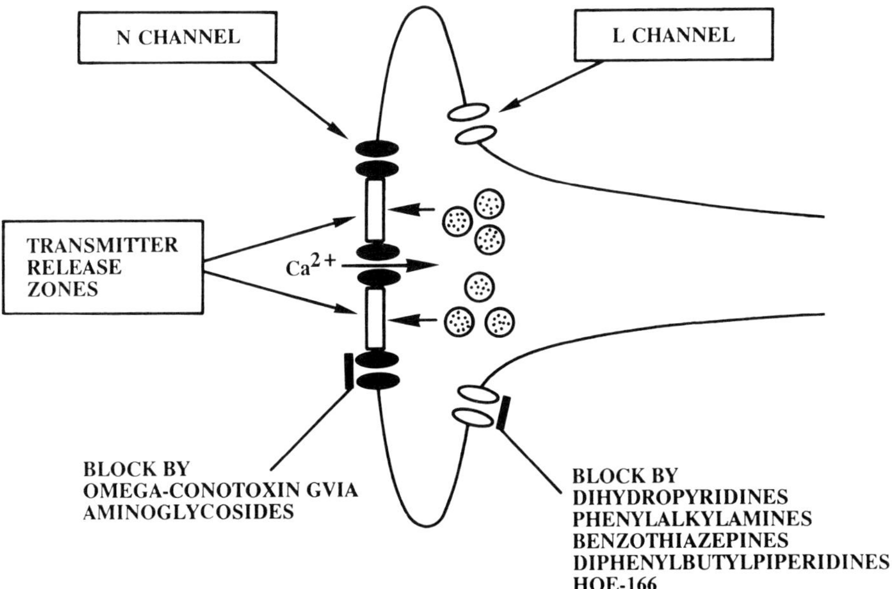

Fig. 1. Location of N- and L-type channels on neurons. The action of drugs is also indicated. It has been suggested that the N-type channel directly delivers calcium ions to the neurotransmitter release zones. L-type channels have only a facilitatory role in this process in most (but not all) neuronal systems and may possibly regulate metabolic functions. (From Miller 1987)

in Table 2. In the first and most important class of drugs, the 1,4-dihydropyridines, compounds exist which activate L-type calcium channels. These are termed "calcium channel agonists". Bay K 8644 is the best studied example. The activators are important tools to study neuronal L-type channel functions.

L-type channels in neurons also have receptors for verapamil and for diltiazem. These two drugs belong to the phenylalkylamine and benzothiazepine class, respectively. Of great interest are the diphenylbutylpiperidines, e. g. fluspirilene (Qar et al. 1987). These calcium-channel blockers also have dopamine-antagonistic properties and are useful in certain types of schizophrenia. HOE-166 is a representative of still another class of compounds, the benzothiazinones, which also block the calcium channel in nanomolar concentrations (Striessnig et al. 1988a; Qar et al. 1988) and

Table 2. Ca^{2+} channel drugs used for structural and functional characterization

L-type channels Class	Label	Name(s)	Dissociation constants [nmol/l]		
			Skeletal muscle	Heart	Brain
1,4-Dihydropyridines	^{3}H	(+)-Isradipine (PN 200-110) (reversible ligand)	0.29–0.7	0.051	0.075
		(−)-Azidopine (±)-Azidopine (photoaffinity ligand)	0.35	0.030	0.096
	^{125}I	(−)-Iodipine (±)-Iodipine	0.4	N.D.	0.06
	^{35}S	(−)-Sadopine (+)-Sadopine	0.51 0.4	N.D. N.D.	N.D. N.D.
Phenylalkylamines	^{3}H	(−)-Desmethoxyapamil (reversible ligand)	1.5 −2.2	1.4–2.5	1.6
		[N-methyl^{3}H]LU 49888 (photoaffinity ligand)	2.0	N.D.	1.4
Benzothiazepines	^{3}H	(+)-cis Diltiazem	39–50	40–80	37–50
		(+)-cis Azidodiltiazem (photoaffinity ligand)	100	N.D.	N.D.
Diphenylbutyl- piperidines	^{3}H	Fluspirilene	0.100	0.070	N.D.
Benzothiazinones	^{3}H	HOE-166	0.100	N.D.	N.D.
N-type channels					
Peptide toxins	^{125}I	Mono[^{125}I]omega-conotoxin GVIA	apparent K_d in the pM range (irreversibel label)		
	^{3}H	Mono[^{3}H]proprionyl omega-conotoxin GVIA			
Aminoglycosides		E. g. neomycin, streptomycin	in the mM range		

Table 2 summarizes the different classes of drugs which are employed for functional and structural characterization of the different types of Ca^{2+} channels. For further details and references consult Glossmann and Striessnig (1988a, 1989). N.D., not determined bind to a distinct domain which is different from the 1,4-dihydropyridine-selective domain.

Certain calcium channels in *Drosophila melanogaster* (head) neuronal membranes have only high affinity receptors for phenylalkylamines and lack high-affinity drug receptors for diltiazem, 1,4-dihydropyridines and benzothiazinones (Pauron et al. 1987).

It is interesting that the *Drosophila* neuronal calcium channel is approximately half of the size (135 kDa) of the L-type channel polypeptide in skeletal muscle (210 kDa) (for reviews see Glossmann and Striessnig 1988, 1989) according to cDNA analysis (Tanabe et al. 1987; Ellis et al. 1988).

Specific probes for the N-type channels exist, whereby omega-conotoxin (GVIA (Kerr and Yoshikami 1984) is the one most well known (Cruz and Olivera 1986; Knaus et al., 1987; Abe and Saisu 1987; Rivier et al. 1987; McCleskey et al. 1987; Yamaguchi et al. 1988). Aminoglycosides are now known to block N-type channels selectively, and they also interact in a specific manner with the omega-conotoxin GVIA binding sites (Knaus et al. 1987; Wagner et al. 1987). The distribution of L-type channels in mammalian brain can be visualized by autoradiographic examination of their specific receptor sites. We have developed several novel tools for this purpose, including an ^{35}S-labelled 1,4-dihydropyridine, which has been named sadopine. These novel labels (which have two chiral centers) have specific activities of >1000 Ci/mmol and bind with very high affinity to the L-type channel in brain, heart and skeletal muscle (Knaus et al. 1988).

Compared with the first generation 1,4-dihydropyridines (such as nifedipine and nimodipine) the sadopine diastereomers have bulky side chains, but fit very well into the 1,4-dihydropyridine binding domain on the alpha$_1$ subunits of the L-type channels. The highest density of 1,4-dihydropyridine receptors is in discrete regions of the brain cortex and especially in the molecular layer of the dentate gyrus (Fig. 2).

The distribution of N-type channels, labelled with [^{125}I]omega-conotoxin GVIA is clearly different in the hippocampal formation (Fig. 2). It is also evident that the cortex has a relatively high density of N-type channels – compared with L-type channel-associated 1,4-dihydropyridine receptors.

Figure 3 shows the primary amino acid sequence of omega-conotoxin GVIA, a 27 amino acid peptide isolated from the venom of the fish hunting sea snail *Conus geographus* (Kerr and Yoshikami 1984). In comparison MVIIA is shown, which helps to subdivide N-type channels (Gray and Olivera 1988; Suszkiw et al. 1987). The GVIA toxin can be [^{125}I]mono-iodinated at 22 and is an (irreversible) radiolabel for N-type channels. The iodinated toxin can be chemically modified to yield a high-affinity arylazide photolabel (Abe et al. 1987; Glossmann and Striessnig 1988a and b; Glossmann and Striessnig 1989; Barhanin et al. 1988), which is termed "[^{125}I]azido-omega-conotoxin GVIA". The in vitro pharmacology of the N-type channels in guinea-pig brain membranes (labelled with [^{125}-I]omega-conotoxin GVIA) is shown in Fig. 4. Here we illustrate the ability of several drugs and cations to inhibit the irreversible interaction of the radiolabeled toxin with its receptor sites.

The apparent very high affinity of the unlabelled and labelled toxin is remarkable. The reported dissociation constants are in the range of 1 to 10 pM, but these numbers are not very meaningful as the toxin is fixed irreversibly and the density of receptor sites in the test tube determines the $K_{0.5}$ value (for inhibition) of the unlabelled (or

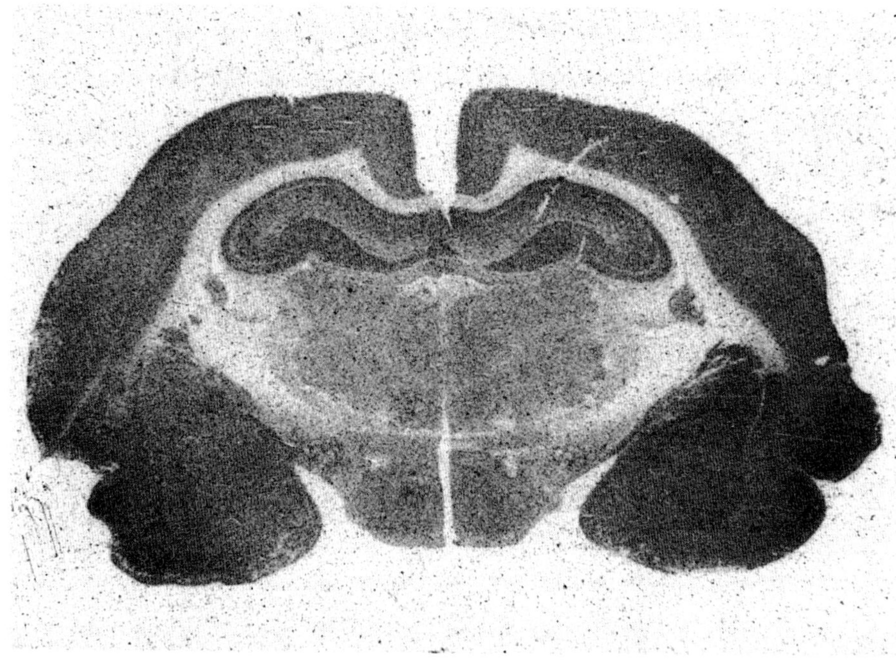

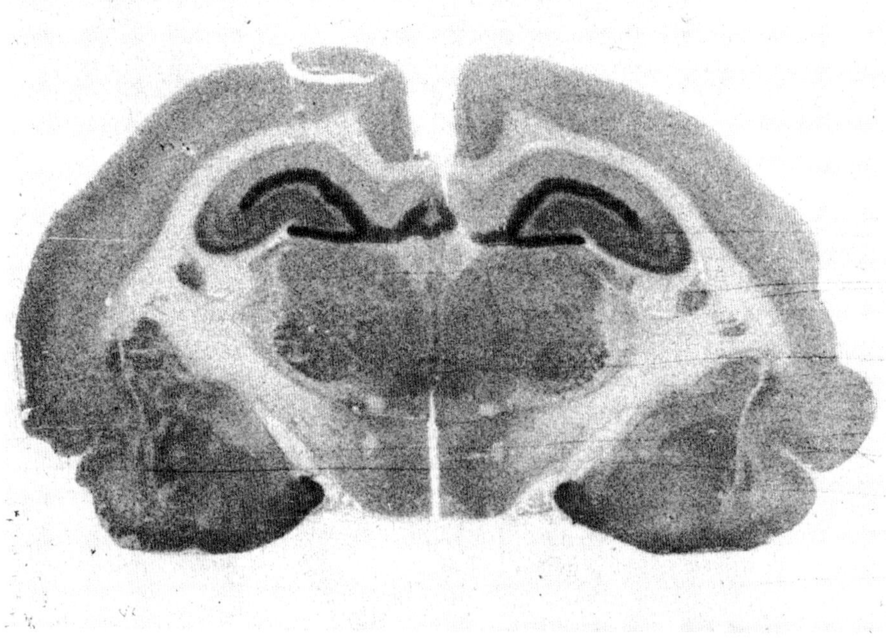

Fig. 2. Autoradiographic visualization of [^{125}I]omega-conotoxin GVIA sites (*upper panel*) and (+)-[^{3}H]isradipine (*lower panel*) sites in (adjacent) frontal sections (10 μm slices) of the guinea-pig brain. Note the differences especially in the dentate gyrus

C K S P̲ G S S C S P̲ T S Y N C C R + S C N P̲ Y T K R C Y ⋆ GVIA

C K G K G A K C S R L M Y D C C T G S C R + + S G K C ⋆   MVIIA

Fig. 3. Structure of the omega-conotoxins GVIA and MVIIA (one-letter code). GVIA is from *Conus geographus*, whereas MVIIA is from *Conus majus*. Disulfide bridges exist between the Cys residues 1 and 16, 8 and 19, 15 and 26. ⋆, amidated carboxyl terminals; *P*, hydroxyproline; +, alignement gap. (From Gray and Olivera 1988)

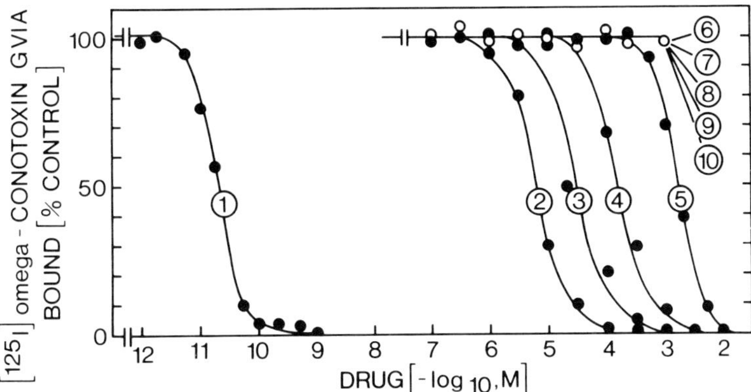

Fig. 4. Inhibition profile of [^{125}I]omega-conotoxin GVIA (2000 Ci/mmol) binding to guinea pig cerebral cortex membranes. Amounts of 0.01 to 0.02 mg of membrane protein per ml were labelled with 15 to 30 pmol of [^{125}I]omega-conotoxin GVIA in the absence or presence of unlabelled [^{125}I]omega-conotoxin GVIA (*curve 1*), different antibiotics (*curves 2–4* and *6–10*) or CaCl$_2$ (*curve 5*). The following apparent IC$_{50}$ values were calculated: [^{125}I]omega-conotoxin GVIA (1), 21 pM; neomycin (2), 5.2 µM; streptomycin (3), 28 µM; kanamycin (4), 161 µM; CaCl$_2$ (5), 2 mM; benzyl-penicillin, erythromycin, tetracycline, chloramphenicol and lincomycin (6–10) were ineffective at 1 mM (open symbols) (From Glossmann and Striessnig 1988b)

binding of labelled) toxin, whereas the time of incubation is the main factor for the K$_{0.5}$ value of the aminoglycosides or the cations.

Figure 5 shows photoaffinity labelling experiments of the N-type channel polypep-tides. After ultraviolet irradiation the membranes are separated by sodium dodecyl phosphate polycrylamide gel electrophoresis (SDS-PAGE) and photolabelled bands are visualized by autoradiography. With [^{125}I]azido-omega-conotoxin GVIA we have consistently found three specifically labelled polypeptides. The molecular sizes are: 245, 195 and 40 KDa. These polypeptides do not change their mobility upon reduction in contrast to cross-linking experiments which identify alpha$_2$-like polypeptides (Cruz et al. 1987; Barhanin et al. 1988). Alpha$_2$-delta (see legend Table 3) is a L-type Ca^{2+} channel-associated glycoprotein in the skeletal muscle transverse tubule membrane which reduces its molecular size by 30–35 kDa upon reduction of disulfide bridges.

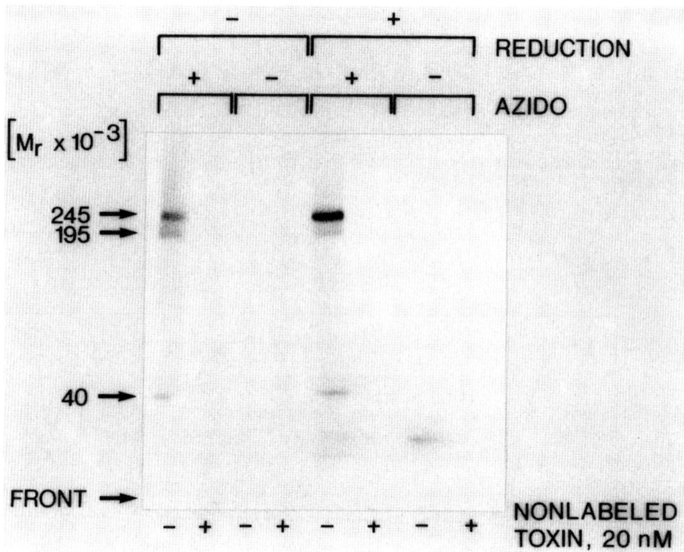

Fig. 5. Identification of omega conotoxin GVIA (Cg-Tx) binding sites in guinea-pig cerebral cortex membranes by photoaffinity labelling. [^{125}I]azido omega-conotoxin was synthesized by incubating [^{125}I]omega-conotoxin GVIA with an excess of N-hydroxysuccinimidyl-azidobenzoate for 60 min on ice. An aliquot of the photolabel (AZIDO +) was then incubated with 0.5 mg of guinea-pig cerebral cortex membranes in the absence (indicated by '−') and presence (indicated by '+') of 20 nM unlabelled -CgTx at 25 °C. Nonderivatized [^{125}I]-CgTx (AZIDO −) was employed as a control. After 25 min the membranes were irradiated with UV light and collected by centrifugation. The pellets were solubilized in electrophoresis sample buffer in the absence (reduction −) or presence (reduction +) of 10 mM dithiothreitol. The samples were electrophoresed on a 5%–15% SDS polyacrylamide gel, stained with Coomassie blue, dried and the radioactive bands visualized by autoradiography. The apparent molecular weights of the radioactive bands were obtained from the relative mobility of standard proteins on the same gel

Table 3 gives an overview of the sizes of the receptor polypeptides which can be photolabelled in guinea-pig brain membranes with different arylazide probes.

With a phenylalkylamine photolabel, [N-methyl^{3}H]LU49888, we find two polypeptides, but with the 1,4-dihydropyridine photolabel (−)-[^{3}H]azidopine only one with 195 KDa (Striessnig et al. 1988b). Three polypeptides (as mentioned above) are identified with the N-type channel photoligand. The very similar sizes (e. g. around 195 KDa) could indicate that essential components of the different types of calcium channels are close structural relatives. The N-type channel has a very large component (245 KDa) nearly identical to the alpha subunit of the voltage-dependent sodium channel in size. It is not known whether the smaller photolabelled components are fragments of the 245-kDa band, represent (e. g. the 195-kDa polypeptide) neuronal L-type channels or are all subunits of the same ionic pore.

For several years the L-type channel drug receptors in brain, e. g. for 1,4-dihydropyridines, were regarded as silent binding sites. There is, however, increasing evidence that 1,4-dihydropyridine agonists and antagonists have actions on the central nervous system and on neurons which are clearly not mediated by vasodilation

Table 3. Ca^{2+} channel-associated drug or toxin receptors – identification by photoaffinity labeling

Receptor	Channel type	Brain	Skeletal muscle	Heart	Photolabel
1,4-Dihydropyridine	L	195	155–170	165	$(-)$-[^{3}H]Azidopine
Phenylalkylamine	L	195 and 265	155–170	N.D.	[N-methyl^{3}H]LU 49888
Benzothiazepine	L	–	170	–	$(+)$-*cis*[^{3}H]Azidodiltiazem
Omega-conotoxin GVIA	N	210–310 195–230 33– 40	–	–	Azido[^{135}I]omega-conotoxin GVIA

Table 3 shows the molecular sizes of the specifically photolabelled polypeptides by arylazide ligands in brain. As a comparison the data on L-type channel-associated drug receptors in other tissues are shown. With the phenylalkylamine photoligand (N-methyl^{3}H]LU 49888 a 265-kDa band in guinea-pig brain membranes (but not in skeletal muscle) is irreversibly labelled which could be a T-type channel component, whereas with [^{3}H]azidopine in skeletal muscle, heart and brain polypeptides of 155–195 kDa are identified. The benzothiazepine-selective receptor domain has been specifically photolabelled with $(+)$-*cis* [^{3}H]azidodiltiazem in purified skeletal muscle L-type channels. The L-type channel drug receptor domains are located on the alpha$_1$ subunit of the channel complex which consists of alpha$_1$, alpha$_2$-delta, beta and gamma subunits (in skeletal muscle) with a $1:1:1:1$ stoichiometry. Alpha$_2$-delta is a heavily glycosilated protein where alpha$_2$ is disulfide linked to delta subunits. The functional role of the non-alpha$_1$ subunits is, at present, unknown. N.D., not determined.

(Table 4). Apart from the action of diphenylbutylpiperidines (which is most likely by a combination of dopamine receptor and calcium channel blockade) a number of clinical and experimental observations indicate very interesting effects, especially of the 1,4-dihydropyridines.

In one experimental system L-type calcium channels have a role which is distinct from that of the N-type channels. Inositolphosphates (especially IP$_3$) and diacylglycerol are intracellular messengers for hormones or neurotransmitters. Hydrolysis of the membrane inositol phospholipids can be also initiated by depolarization-induced Ca^{2+} influx (Kendall and Nahorski 1985; Rooney and Nahorski 1986).

Table 4. Effects of L-type channel drugs

1. Prevention of symptoms of alcohol (heroin?) withdrawal
2. Improvement of symptoms of tardive dyskinesia
3. Augmentation of analgesic and antinociceptive effects of opioids
4. Alterations of mood
5. Attenuation of seizures
6. Effects on migraine
7. Effects on symptoms of aging
8. Effects on neuronal regeneration

Table 4 summarizes some reported effects, especially for 1,4-dihydropyridines (i.e. nimodipine) on patients (1–6) or in animal experiments (7, 8). Improvement of symptoms of tardive dyskinesia was reported after treatment with diltiazem only, whereas flunarizine (not included) induces parkinsonism, most likely by dopamine receptor blockade.

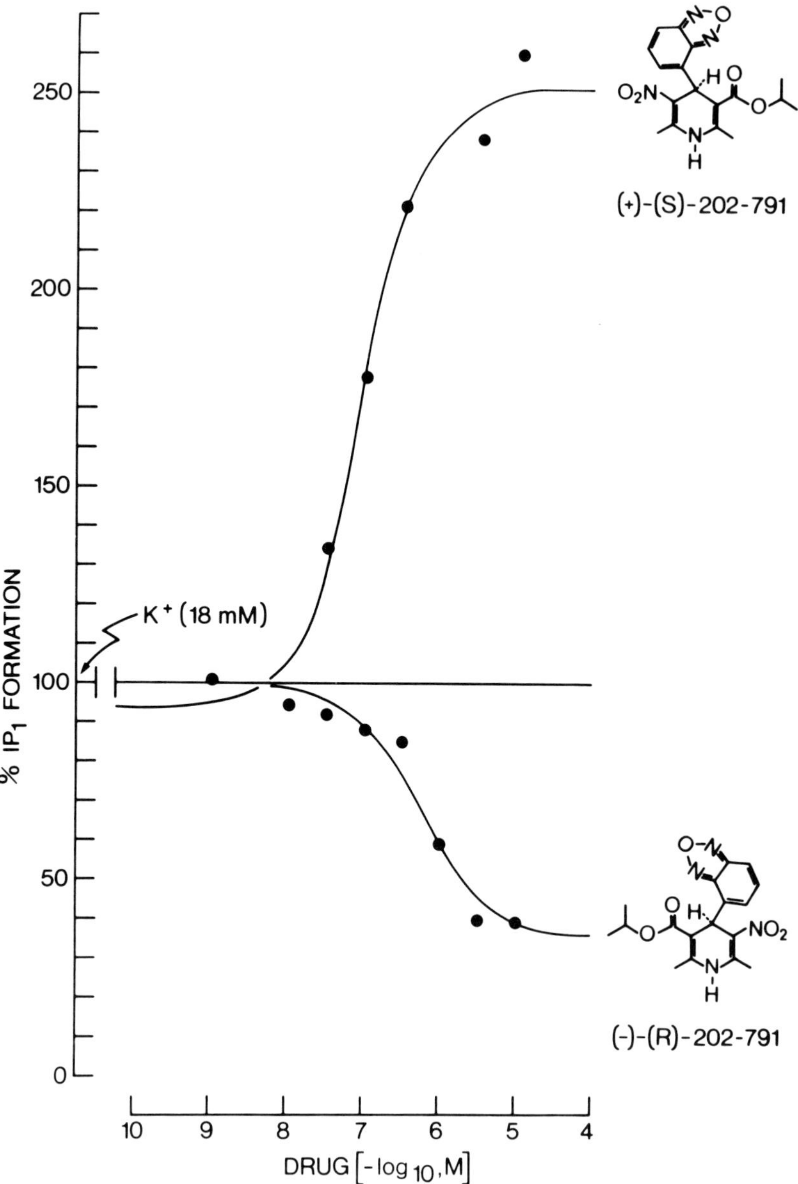

Fig. 6. Stereospecific regulation of depolarization-induced [³H]inositolmonophosphate ([³H]IP₁) formation in rat brain slices by the enantiomers of R 202–791. Rat brain slices (2.2 ± 0.2 mg protein) were incubated in a final assay volume of 300 ul of Krebs-Ringer buffer (KRB) with 0.25 uM [³H]inositol. R 202–791 (if present) was added after 15 min. After a total preincubation time of 35 min, depolarization was induced by addition of KRB in which Na⁺ had been iso-osmotically replaced by K⁺. The reaction was terminated after 90 min and inositol phosphates determined as described (Zernig et al. 1986). Values are given as percent of 18 mM K⁺-induced [³H]IP₁ formation (basal [³H]IP₁ levels subtracted) and represent means from 3 experiments performed in duplicate

In Fig. 6 we have measured one product of Ca^{2+} induced phosphatidylinositol breakdown, inositol-l-phosphate, in [^{3}H]inositol prelabelled adult rat brain slices (Zernig et al. 1986). In this experimental system we employed the benzoxadiazol 1,4-dihydropyridine 202–791. This compound is chiral and the (−)-S-enantiomer acts as an agonist, whereas the (+)-R-enantiomer ia a specific L-type channel blocker.

The stereoselective stimulation and inhibition of K^+ depolarization-induced (Ca^{2+}-dependent) inositolphosphate release by the optical isomers of 202–791 clearly proves that the L-type channels in neurons have a functional role. The N-type channel blocker omega-conotoxin GVIA had no effect on the inositolphosphate release (not shown). Thus, L-type channel drugs may have their effects on neuronal functions by modulation of the second messenger systems, perhaps also on the protein kinase C system. We have not directly measured activity of the kinase, but diacylglycerol is released when phosphatidylinositolbisphosphate is cleaved by activation of phospholipase C.

Acknowledgement: Research of the authors was funded by FWF, OFG, Dr. Legerlotz. Foundation and by Bundesministerium für Wissenschaft und Forschung.

References

Abe T, Saisu H (1987) Identification of the receptor for omega-conotoxin in brain. Probable components of the calcium channel. J Biol Chem 262: 9877–9882

Barhanin J, Schmid A, Lazdunski M (1988) Properties of structure and interaction of the receptor for omega-conotoxin, a polypeptide active on Ca^{2+} channels. Biochem Biophys Res Commun 150: 1051–1062

Choi DW (1985) Glutamate neurotoxicity in cortical cell culture is calcium dependent. Neurosci Lett 58: 293–297

Choi DW (1988) Calcium-mediated neurotoxicity: relationship to specific channel types and role in ischemic damage. Tends Neurosci 11: 465–469

Cruz LJ, Olivera BM (1986) Calcium channel antagonists. Omega-conotoxin defines a new high affinity site. J Biol Chem 261: 6230–6233

Cruz LJ, Johnson DS, Olivera BM (1987) Characterization of the omega-conotoxin target. Evidence for tissue-specific heterogeneity in calcium channel types. Biochemistry 26: 820–824

Ellis SB, Williams ME, Ways NR, Brenner R, Sharp AH, Leung AT, Campbell KP, McKenna E, Koch WJ, Hui A, Schwartz A, Harpold MM (1988) Structure and expression of mRNAs encoding the alpha 1 and alpha 2 subunits of a DHP-sensitive calcium channel. Science 241: 1661–1664

Glossmann H, Striessnig J (1988a) Calcium channels. Vitam Horm 44: 155–328

Glossmann H, Striessnig J (1988b) Structure and pharmacology of voltage-dependent calcium channels. ISI Atlas Pharmacol 2: 202–210

Glossmann H, Striessnig J (1989) Molecular properties of calcium channels. Rev Physiol Biochem Pharmacol (in press)

Glossmann H, Striessnig J, Hymel L, Zernig G, Knaus HG, Schindler H (1988) The structure of the calcium channel: photoaffinity labeling and tissue distribution. In: Calcium channels: structure, function and implications. Morad M, Naylor WG, Kazda S, Schramm M (eds) Springer Berlin Heidelberg New York, pp 168–192

Gray WR, Olivera BM (1988) Peptide toxins from venomous conus snails. Annu Rev Biochem 57: 665–700

Hirning LD, Fox AP, McCleskey EW, Olivera BM, Thayer SA, Miller, RJ, Tsien RW (1988) Dominant role of N-type Ca^{2+} channels in evoked release of norepinephrine from sympathetic neurons. Science 239: 57–61

Hymel L. Inui M, Fleischer S, Schindler H (1988) Purified ryanodine receptor of skeletal muscle sarcoplasmic reticulum forms Ca^{2+}-activated oligomeric Ca^{2+} channels in planar bilayers. Proc Natl Acad Sci USA 85: 441–445

Imagawa T, Smith JS, Coronado R, Campbell KP (1987) Purified ryanodine receptor from skeletal muscle sarcoplasmic reticulum is the Ca^{2+}-permeable pore of the calcium release channel. J Biol Chem 262: 16636–16643

Kendall DA, Nahorski SR (1985) Dihydropyridine calcium channel activators and antagonists influence depolarization-evoked inositol phospholipid hydrolysis in brain. Eur J Pharmacol 115: 31–36

Kerr LM, Yoshikami D (1984) A venom peptide with a novel presynaptic blocking action. Nature 308: 282–284

Knaus HG, Striessnig J, Koza A, Glossmann H (1987) Neurotoxic aminoglycoside antibiotics are potent inhibitors of [^{125}I]-Omega-Conotoxin GVIA binding to guinea-pig cerebral cortex membranes. Naunyn Schmiedebergs Arch Pharmacol 336: 583–586

Knaus H, Striessnig J, Glossmann H, Hering S, Schwenner E, Kinast G, Grosser R, Marsmann M (1988) [^{35}S]Sadopine, a novel high specific activity, high affinity calcium channel probe (abstract). Naunyn Schmiedebergs Arch Pharmacol 338: R36

Leung AT, Imagawa T, Block B, Franzini-Armstrong C, Campbell KP (1988) Biochemical and ultrastructural characterization of the 1,4-dihydropyridine receptor from rabbit skeletal muscle. Evidence for a 52000 Da subunit. J Biol Chem 263: 994–1001

McCleskey EW, Fox AP, Feldman DH, Cruz LJ, Olivera BM, Tsien RW, Yoshikami D (1987) Omega-conotoxin: direct and persistent blockade of specific types of calcium channels in neurons but not muscle. Proc Natl Acad Sci USA 84: 4327–4331

Miller RJ (1987) Multiple calcium channels and neuronal function. Science 235: 46–52

Nilius B, Hess P, Lansman JB, Tsien RW (1985) A novel type of cardiac calcium channel in ventricular cells. Nature 316: 443–446

Nowycky MC, Fox AP, Tsien RW (1985) Three types of neuronal calcium channel with different calcium agonist sensitivity. Nature 316: 440–443

Pauron D, Qar J, Barhanin J, Fournier D, Cuany A, Pralavorio M, Berge JB, Lazdunski M (1987) Identification and affinity labeling of very high affinity binding sites for the phenylalkylamine series of Ca^+ channel blockers in the *Drosophila* nervous system. Biochemistry 26: 6311–6315

Qar J, Galizzi JP, Fosset M, Lazdunski M (1987) Receptors for diphenylbutylpiperidine neuroleptics in brain, cardiac, and smooth muscle membranes. Relationship with receptors for 1,4-dihydropyridines and phenylalkylamines and with Ca^{2+} channel blockade. Eur J Pharmacol 141: 261–268

Qar J, Barhanin J, Romey G, Henning R, Lerch U, Oekonomopulos R, Urbach H, Lazdunski M (1988) A novel high affinity class of Ca^{2+} channel blockers. Mol Pharmacol 33: 363–369

Rios E, Brum G (1987) Involvement of dihydropyridine receptors in excitation-contraction coupling in skeletal muscle. Nature 325: 717–720

Rios E, Fitts R, Uribe I, Pizarro G, Brum G (1989) A third role for calcium in excitation-contraction coupling. In: Bacigalupo J (ed) Transduction in biological systems. Plenum, New York (in press)

Rivier J, Galyean R, Gray WR, Azimi-Zonooz A, McIntosh JM, Cruz LJ, Olivera BM (1987) Neuronal calcium channel inhibitors. Synthesis of omega-conotoxin GVIA and effects on 45Ca uptake by synaptosomes. J Biol Chem 262: 1194–1198

Rooney TA, Nahorski SR (1986) Regional characterization of agonist and depolarization-induced phosphoinositide hydrolysis in rat brain. J Pharmacol Exp Ther 239: 873–880

Saito A, Inui M, Radermacher M, Frank J, Fleischer S (1988) Ultrastructure of the calcium release channel of sarcoplasmic reticulum. J Cell Biol 107: 211–219

Striessnig J, Meusburger E, Grabner M, Knaus HG, Glossmann H, Kaiser J, Schölkens B, Becker R, Linz W, Henning R (1988a) Evidence for a distinct Ca^{2+} antagonist receptor for a novel benzothiazinone compound HOE 166. Naunyn Schmidebergs Arch Pharmacol 337: 331–340

Striessnig J, Knaus HG, Glossmann H (1988b) Photoaffinity labelling of the calcium-channel-associated 1,4-dihydropyridine and phenylalkylamine receptor in guinea-pig hippocampus. Biochem J 253: 37–46

Suszkiw JB, Murawsky MM, Fortner RC (1987) Heterogeneity of presynaptic calcium channels revealed by species differences in the sensitivity of synaptosomal 45Ca entry to omega-conotoxin. Biochem Biophys Res Commun 145: 1283–1286

Tanabe T, Takeshima H, Mikami A, Flockerzi V, Takahashi H, Kangawa K, Kojima M, Matsuo H, Hirose T, Numa S (1987) Primary structure of the receptor for calcium channel blockers from skeletal muscle. Natur 328: 313–318

Tanabe T, Beam KG, Powell JA, Numa S (1988) Restoration of excitation-contraction coupling and slow calcium current in dysgenic muscle by dihydropyridine receptor cDNA. Nature 336: 134–138

Tang CM, Presser F, Morad M (1988) Amiloride selectively blocks the low threshold (T) calcium channel. Science 240: 213–215

Thayer SA, Hirning LD, Miller RJ (1987) Distribution of multiple types of Ca2+ channels in rat sympathetic neurons in vitro. Mol Pharmacol 32: 579–586

Tsien RW, Hess P, McCleskey EW, Rosenberg RL (1987) Calcium channels: mechanisms of selectivity, permeation, and block. Annu Rev Biophys Chem 16: 265–290

Tsien RW, Lipscombe DV, Madison KR, Bley KR, Fox AP (1988) Multiple types of neuronal calcium channels and their selective modulation. Trends Neurosci 11: 431–438

Wagner JA, Snowman AM, Olivera BM, Snyder SH (1987) Aminoglycoside effects on voltage-sensitive calcium channels and neurotoxicity [letter]. N Engl J Med 317: 1669–1669

Yamaguchi T, Saisu H, Mitsui H, Abe T (1988) Solubilization of the omega-conotoxin receptor associated with voltage-sensitive calcium channels from bovine brain. J Biol Chem 263: 9491–9498

Zernig G, Moshammer T, Glossmann H (1986) Stereospecific regulation of [^{3}H]inositol monophosphate accumulation by calcium channel drugs from all three main chemical classes. Eur J Pharmacol 128: 221–229

Calcium Homeostasis in Brain Aging and Alzheimer's Disease

P. W. Landfield

Altered Calcium Homeostasis and Aging: Conflicting Evidence

The nature of the role of altered calcium (Ca) homeostasis in mammalian aging is far from clear. Although there is growing evidence that age-related changes in Ca homeostasis occur, and may be present in key physiological processes in excitable tissues, the experimental evidence on the nature of these changes appears somewhat contradictory. In addition, it still remains to be shown that altered Ca homeostasis is a primary causal factor of some aspects of aging, rather than a secondary response to more basic changes.

Two apparently conflicting lines of evidence on age-dependent alterations in Ca homeostasis have developed in the past several years. One of these indicates that Ca availability or flux into excitable cells may be decreased in aged animals; conversely, the other suggests that Ca influx may be increased in aged brain cells.

It is not yet clear whether these lines of evidence are mutually exclusive in terms of functional implications, or whether the discrepancies are only apparent, and that both types of evidence are reflections of a common underlying deficit. That is, depending on the method of measuring Ca influx or availability in aging, it seems conceivable that one might find either an increase or a decrease resulting from the same underlying change. This is because, as discussed furhter below, Ca influx occurs through several kinds of voltage- and receptor-dependent channels, each of which exhibit very different time courses and activation patterns. Moreover, Ca influx is subject to a variety of inactivation processes, and it is therefore critical to define the activation/inactivation state of the Ca mechanism under investigation.

Evidence of Decreased Ca Availability or Influx with Aging

The main evidence in support of the possibility that Ca availability or influx is deficient with aging derives from a number of studies (reviewed in [10, 36]) in which impaired Ca-dependent physiological processes have been partially or fully restored in aged animals by experimentally increasing Ca influx. These processes include beta adrenergic-stimulated myocardial contraction, α-adrenergic-activated processes in parotid cells, serotonergic-stimulated aortic contraction, lectin-stimulated thymic lymphocyte mitogenesis, and releasing factor-activated gonadotropin release from pituitary cells. In studies in which impaired catecholamine-dependent processes in the

Bergener, Reisberg (Eds.)
Diagnosis and Treatment
of Senile Dementia
© Springer-Verlag Berlin Heidelberg 1989

rodent cardiovascular system and parotid glands were found with aging, the capacity of these cells to respond to elevated Ca was not diminished. In addition, agents which stimulated Ca influx were able to restore these Ca-dependent functions to levels similar to those found in young animals [36].

Other studies have shown that a variety of Ca-dependent neurobiological phenomena, including learning and motor functions, brain oxidative metabolism, and specific enzyme activities, are altered with aging and/or can be improved in aged animals treated with agents that are thought to increase Ca influx. Studies of synaptosomal preparations have also indicated that less voltage-dependent Ca influx and, consequently, less Ca-dependent transmitter release occurs in brain synaptosomes from aged animals (see review in [10]). Using cultured fibroblasts from human donors, moreover, it was recently found that Ca was taken up to a lesser degree in cell cultures from aged humans, and particularly from those with Alzheimer's disease [32]!

The considerable evidence on altered Ca homeostasis and reduced Ca availability in neural tissues was recently reviewed by Gibson and Peterson [10]. However, it is important to recognize that much of the evidence on Ca homeostasis is, of necessity, based on indirect measures, and that most of the agents and drugs used in these studies exert effects on processes other than Ca flux. Further, as noted below, the nature of some of the preparations (e. g., synaptosomes, tissue cultures) may alter the states of internal Ca buffering and inactivation mechanisms.

Evidence of Increased Ca Influx or Availability with Aging

The findings in support of the view that Ca availability or influx into brain neurons increases with aging are less extensive than the results outlined above in support of a decrease. However, the evidence of an increase includes electrophysiological measures of millisecond-duration Ca currents in nondisrupted brain cells (see below), and therefore provides information on Ca mechanisms with somewhat different time scales.

Although the likelihood that elevated intracellular Ca concentrations are cytotoxic to excitable cells has been recognized for some time [28, 37, 38, 41], the possibility that a similar mechanism might contribute to normal brain aging or Alzheimer's disease was discussed in detail only relatively recently in a review by Khachaturian [13]. Based on several preliminary and/or emerging lines of evidence that were beginning to link Ca and aging, it was suggested that altered buffering, extrusion, or sequestering of intracellular Ca, for example by changes in mitochondrial pyruvate dehydrogenase or calmodulin, could result in elevated intracellular Ca and, consequently, in nerve cell deterioration during aging or Alzheimer's disease [13]. Among the few preliminary studies supporting these concepts were experiments indicating the possible relevance to brain aging of alterations in pyruvate dehydrogenase [5, 31], membrane extrusion mechanisms [26], and Ca-dependent electrophysiological processes [15, 20, 24]. In addition, Ca had been found to accumulate in brain neurons containing neurofibrillary tangles [30]. (More recent studies indicate that Ca also accumulates in fibroblasts from subjects with Alzheimer's disease; see [33]).

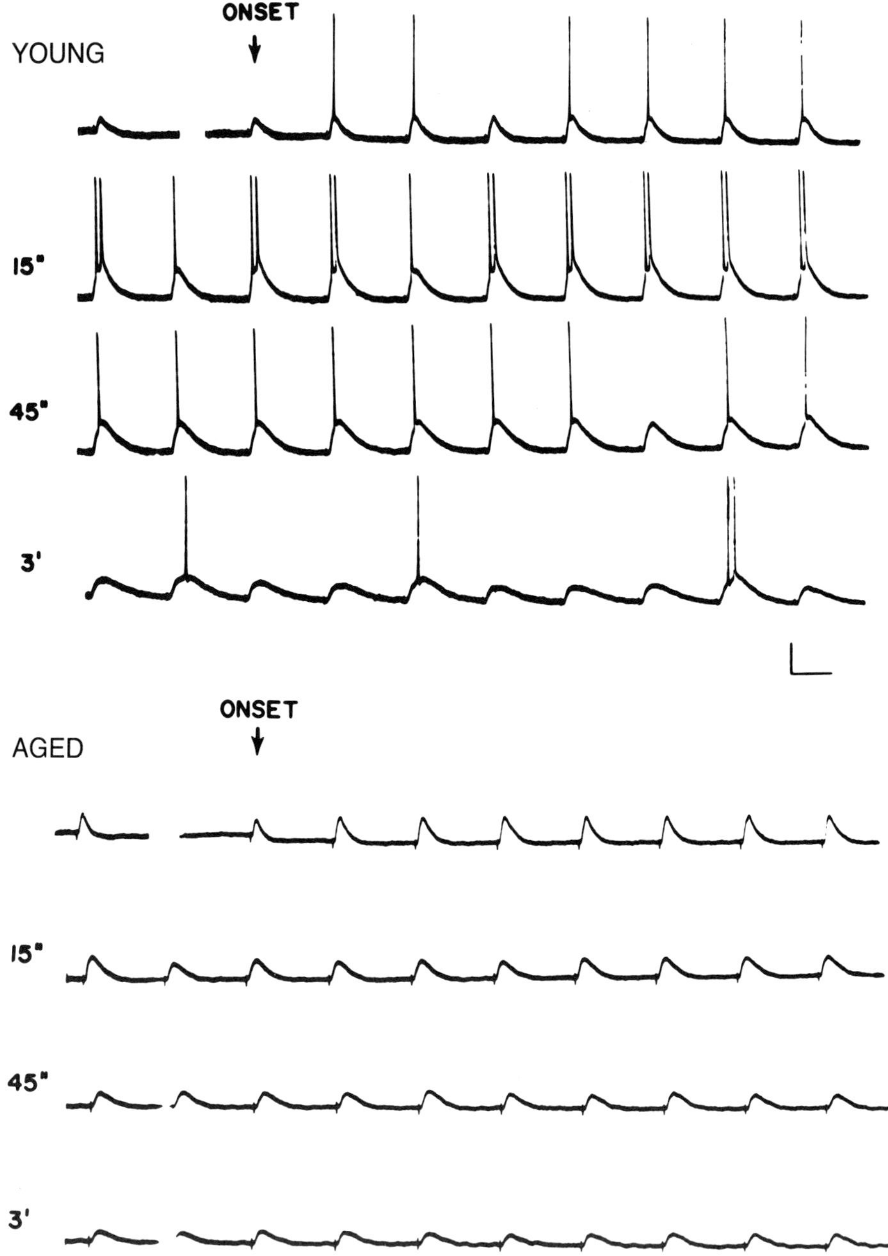

Fig. 1. Intracellular recordings from CA1 cells in hippocampal slices of young and aged rats. The excitatory postsynaptic potential (EPSP) is shown before and after the onset *(arrow)* of 10-Hz synaptic stimulation. *15"*, EPSPs during the 15th second of 10-Hz stimulation. *45"*, EPSPs during the 45th second of 10-Hz stimulation. *3'*, EPSPs at the third minute of 10-Hz stimulation. During repetitive stimulation, the EPSP was usually potentiated substantially more in young rat cells. In the examples shown, the EPSP reached threshold for triggering an action potential only in the young rat cell, although control EPSPs were set at 75% of spike threshold in both instances. *Calibration:* 20 mV, 50 ms. (From [24])

With regard to the electrophysiological studies, experiments on hippocampal synaptic function in both in vivo [19] and in vitro [18] rat preparations had indicated that one of the key synaptic deficits exhibited in aged rats was an impairment of Ca-dependent synaptic plasticity, in particular, of a process termed frequency potentiation (the growth of the monosynaptic EPSP during repetitive synaptic activation; for descriptions of this process see [1, 35]; (Fig. 1). A number of findings and considerations suggest that synaptic frequency potentiation (FP) may be a key mechanism for amplifying biologically significant information (i. e., information carried at higher frequencies) and might be important in learning and memory, perhaps by acting as a "trigger" for long-lasting changes such as long-term potentiation [19, 20, 23, 35] (see review in [24]).

One of the first clues that the age-related impairment of FP might be due to elevated Ca was the finding that high magnesium (Mg), a Ca antagonist, could strengthen synaptic FP, particularly in hippocampal slices of aged rats; conversely, high Ca impaired FP [15, 23] (Fig. 2). Moreover, high Mg in the diet strengthened FP in intact aged animals, and improved the age-related impairment in maze learning as well [20]. Since Ca-dependent synaptic and postsynaptic physiological responses to repetitive stimulation appeared to be depressed by high Ca, it seemed possible that the aged brain might be characterized by elevated Ca influx [15, 23, 24].

However, synaptic function is influenced by factors other than Ca influx, and a process more exclusively dependent on Ca influx was needed to directly test this hypothesis of an age-dependent increase in Ca influx. The slow, Ca-dependent, K-mediated afterhyperpolarization ($AHP_{(Ca)}$), which is elicited by depolarization of hippocampal cells, is a well defined Ca-dependent process that appears to vary primarily in relation to intracellular levels of Ca [2, 14, 44].

We used this $AHP_{(Ca)}$ as an index of Ca influx into hippocampal slice neurons following a regulated amount of depolarization (e. g., either two or three Na spikes, elicited by intracellular current injection). In aged rat neurons, the $AHP_{(Ca)}$ was significantly longer [21] (Fig. 3). In addition, this effect was recently replicated, and it was found that amplitude as well as the duration of the $AHP_{(Ca)}$ also increased significantly with age (Kerr and Landfield, in preparation). Thus, a key prediction of the increased Ca hypothesis was tested, and the results were fully consistent with the hypothesis. Nevertheless, an increased duration and amplitude of the Ca-dependent AHP could result from a number of Ca-related mechanisms other than Ca influx per se, including reduced buffering/extrusion of Ca [13, 26] or changes in the regulatory sites of the K channels.

Therefore, we recently measured Ca influx more directly, by measuring Ca spikes and Ca currents isolated from K and Na currents by cesium injection and the application of tetrodotoxin (TTX) and tetraethylammonium (TEA). In these studies, we found that isolated Ca spikes and inward Ca currents are increased in aged rat brain neurons [22]. Thus, in the rat hippocampal slice preparation, neuronal voltage-dependent Ca influx and at least some Ca-dependent processes are increased with aging. Since elevated Ca is also able to impair synaptic function [23], it seems very possible that this change in voltage-dependent Ca regulation is the basis of the impaired synaptic FP found in aged rats [18–20, 23, 24]. Further, if the hypothesis that FP is an important mechanism for learning and memory [24] is correct, then increased

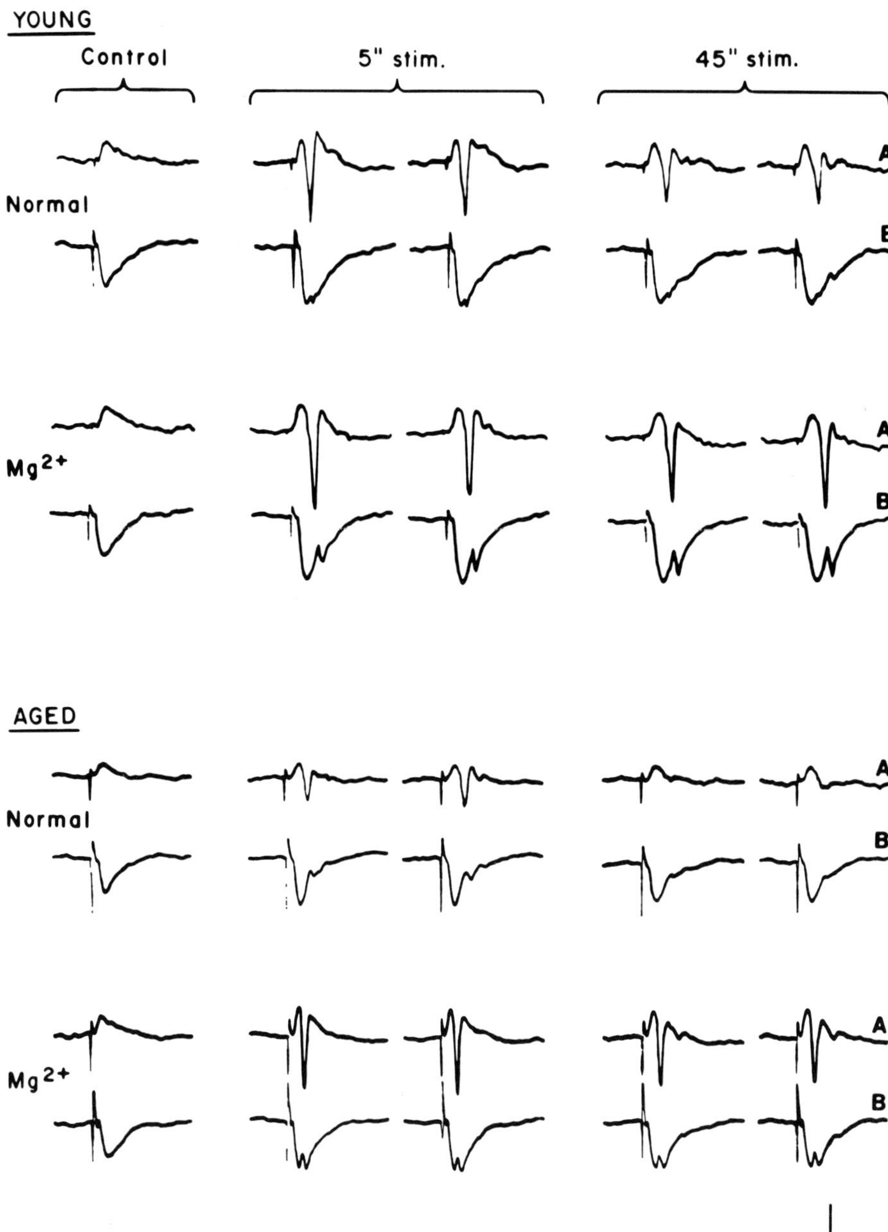

Fig. 2. Effects of a high-Mg incubating medium on frequency potentiation (FP) of the extracellular field EPSP (*B* traces) and population spike (*A* traces) in hippocampal slices from young and aged rats. *Normal,* Slices incubated in medium with equal Mg and Ca concentrations. Mg^{2+}, Slices incubated in medium with a 2:1 ratio of Mg to Ca. *Control,* Responses obtained at 0.2-Hz synaptic stimulation, before the onset of a 7-Hz stimulation train. *5" stim.:* Responses obtained in the 5th second of 7-Hz stimulation. *45" stim.:* Responses obtained in the 45th second of 7-Hz stimulation. *Calibration:* 2 mV, 10 ms. During 7-Hz stimulation, slices in high Mg exhibited greater potentiation and less depression than slices in normal medium. The effect was greater in aged rat slices. (From [23])

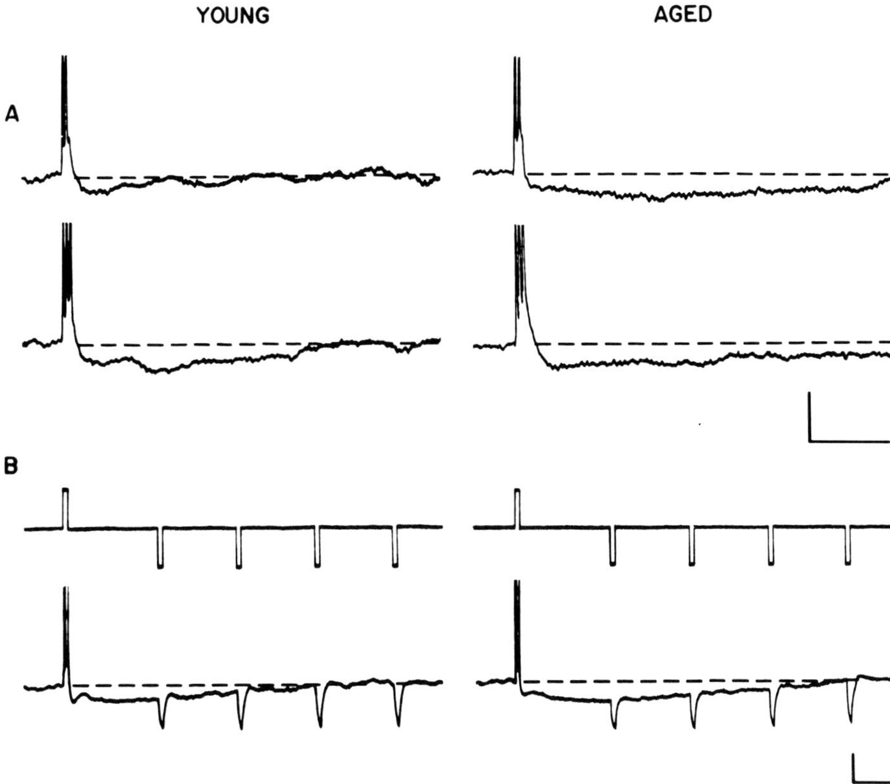

Fig. 3A, B. Intracellular current-induced bursts of action potentials and subsequent afterhyperpolarizations (AHPs) in CA1 neurons of hippocampal slices from young and aged rats. **A** AHPs following a current-induced burst of two spikes *(upper traces)* or three spikes *(lower traces)*, in slices from young or aged rats. **B** AHPs and concomitant conductance increases following a 0.4-nA current-induced burst of three spikes. *Dashed lines* show resting potentials befor the burst. In the *upper trace* of **B** are shown the initial intracellular depolarizing current pulse used to induce a spike burst and the subsequent 2-Hz train of 0.4-nA hyperpolarizing pulses used to assess input conductance during the AHP, for cells shown in the *lower trace* of **B**. (From [21])

voltage-dependent Ca influx could well be a key factor in age-related memory impairment.

Significance of Ca Inactivation Mechanisms

The evidence summarized above does not provide much insight into how to resolve the two apparently contradictory lines of evidence on the direction of changes in Ca availability during aging. That is, although our data point consistently to age-dependent increases in Ca currents, it remains unclear why numerous other studies have found evidence of age-related decreases in Ca availability or influx.

Some clues to this paradox may be found in recent evidence of Ca inactivation mechanisms in mammalian brain neurons. It had been thought for some years that Ca currents (I_{Ca}) in brain neurons were relatively inactivating [7], and did not exhibit the Ca-dependent inactivation of Ca currents found in invertebrate neurons or some muscle cells [9].

However, studies in our laboratory have indicated that hippocampal neurons are characterized by a powerful form of Ca-dependent inactivation of I_{Ca}. Utilizing experimental designs in which most potentially confounding Ca-dependent outward currents (e.g., K, Cl) were blocked or controlled for, we found that there was pronounced inactivation of the Ca spike or isolated Ca current during repetitive depolarizations. This inactivation was accelerated in high-Ca media, reduced by nimodipine (a Ca channel antagonist; see [40]; Fig. 4) and was blocked in media in which barium was substituted for calcium [8, 34].

The relevance of I_{Ca} inactivation processes to attempts to evaluate the role of Ca homeostasis in aging is suggested by the observation that Ca-dependent inactivation of I_{Ca} in the hippocampus appears to be pronounced and rapid in onset. A single Ca spike can induce inactivation that is measurable for several seconds following the spike [34]. In addition to Ca-dependent inactivation, moreover, many cell types exhibit strong voltage-dependent inactivation of Ca channels [27, 29]. Further, Ca channels are highly sensitive to "rundown" and irreversible inactivation. That is, there appear to be both short-term, reversible and long-term, irreversible forms of Ca channel inactivation; the latter lead to steady rundown of Ca channel function in many in vitro preparations. As a consequence of rundown, it has proven difficult to study Ca channels in dissociated neuronal preparations (for a review see [27]).

Thus, unless considerable precautions are taken to control rundown, it seems certain that synaptosomal, tissue culture, and some slice preparations will be characterized by rundown of Ca channel function. Moreover, methods of depolarization which require seconds to minutes (e. g., high-K-induced depolarization) will certainly elicit pronounced inactivation by both voltage- and Ca-dependent mechanisms.

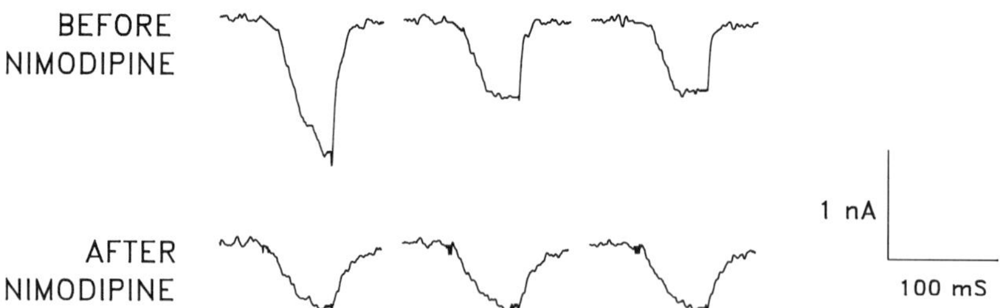

Fig. 4. Single-electrode voltage-clamp measures of inward Ca currents during a 2-Hz train of depolarizing command steps in Cs-loaded, TTX- and TEA-treated CA1 pyramidal cells of hippocampal slices. Holding potential of approximately −60 mV. *Upper trace*, the first three current responses to train of depolarizing command steps are shown, prior to nimodipine. Substantial inactivation of current is seen during the train. *Lower trace*, following application of nimodipine to the same cell, the initial Ca current is reduced in response to the first command step, and there is reduced inactivation during the train. Current traces are corrected for leak current and capacitance by adding the current trace induced by an equal hyperpolarizing voltage step. (Data from [8])

For these reasons, it seems clear that in many studies of Ca and aging Ca influx has been able to occur only through a limited class of Ca channels (e. g., the noninactivating channels). Paradoxically, the presence of strong inactivating mechanisms raises the possibility that either reduced or increased Ca influx through voltage-dependent channels could, under different experimental conditions, result from the same aging mechanism. For example, if voltage-dependent Ca influx were measured electrophysiologically during brief depolarizations (e. g., less than 1 s), one might find increased Ca influx with age. Conversely, if Ca influx into these same cells were measured after dissociation or after several seconds of depolarization, one might find decreased Ca with age, due to greater inactivation of Ca channels elicited by the initially greater Ca influx.

These considerations indicate that the apparent contradictions in the literature may not be as mutually exclusive as they appear, and may in fact represent different phases or manifestations of a similar underlying process. However, it is clear that resolving this issue in future studies will require careful assessment of the experimental conditions and the activation/inactivation states of various Ca mechanisms.

There is another reason why Ca-dependent inactivation may prove of particular relevance to the study of age-related changes in membrane Ca conductance. Namely, our finding of increased voltage-dependent Ca conductance in aged rat hippocampal neurons [21, 22] could clearly be due in part to an impairment of this inactivation mechanism. This possibility is currently under active investigation in our laboratory.

A Mechanistic Hypothesis on the Role of Altered Membrane Ca Conductance in Alzheimer's Disease

As noted some years ago [43], there is an important conceptional similarity between Alzheimer's disease and cancer, in that the development of each becomes increasingly likely with aging, yet neither is universal among the aged. This observation implies that something in the normal aging process increases the susceptibility to these destructive conditions, but that these conditions are not simply extreme examples of universal aging processes. Aging is a very gradual phenomenon, yet cancer and Alzheimer's disease progress relatively rapidly once they begin. In turn, this implies that some threshold of susceptibility may be reached, after which these conditions begin to accelerate by self-regenerative processes.

Several years ago [16], it was suggested that the pattern of interrelations between aging and Alzheimer's disease might be indicative of a gradual decline in some nerve cell "defense" mechanism that ordinarily controls a normal function. As in cancer, which entails loss of control over normal cell division functions, the failure of control in Alzheimer's disease appears to permit a "runaway" condition that is rapidly destructive. The research findings in our laboratory and others outlined above seem to raise the possibility that the defense mechanism altered by aging and Alzheimer's disease [16] might be one which controls the influx of Ca into brain neurons. Thus, it seems conceivable that aging could gradually impair neuronal regulatory mechanisms involved in the control of Ca influx and intracellular Ca concentrations, thereby permitting intracellular Ca influx to increase following a depolarization. In turn, this could result in greater feedback inactivation of Ca-dependent increases in transmitter release during frequency potentiation [23], and perhaps, in some aspects of impaired memory [20, 24]. Ca-dependent inactivation of presynaptic Ca channels has previously been seen in some invertebrate preparations [3].

In addition, however, elevations of intracellular Ca are now well known to be cytotoxic, due at least in part to the activation of Ca-dependent proteases and the alteration of the cytoskeleton [28, 37, 38, 41]. It therefore seems possible that increases in Ca influx and, consequently, the duration of intracellular elevation, could gradually induce the accumulation of small increments of irreversible cellular damage. Over time, this might lead to the gradual loss of some nerve cells during aging [5, 13, 17, 21].

Alzheimer's disease, it is suggested here, reflects a runaway condition of this gradual deterioration of membrane Ca-regulation mechanisms, in which some genetic or extraneous factor (e. g., exposure to viruses, aluminum, endocrine factors) greatly accelerates the rate of deterioration of membrane Ca defense mechanisms. Because Alzheimer's disease and normal human brain aging share nearly every overt qualitative manifestation of pathology (e. g., plaques, tangles, neocortical and hippocampal cell loss, glial cell reactivity, recent memory impairment) and differ primarily in the quantitative incidence of these markers (e. g., these pathological signs may be an order or magnitude greater in Alzheimer's disease) [4, 42, 43], it seems possible that Alzheimer's disease is an accelerated, uncontrolled form of changes already underway in the normal brain [43]. Thus, this pattern implies that in some individuals there may be a threshold beyond which these defense mechanisms fail almost completely.

It may be no coincidence that the neurons of the hippocampus, which are among the most devastated of all brain cells in Alzheimer's disease [4, 6, 42, 43], are also characterized by highly pronounced Ca currents and regenerative Ca spikes [11, 12, 39, 44]. Moreover, cerebellar Purkinje cells are also among the cell populations that have been found most consistently to decline with aging [6], and Purkinje neurons, like hippocampal pyramidal cells, exhibit large calcium spikes [25]. Again, as noted by Khachaturian [13] and Gibson and Peterson [10], it may be no coincidence that, on the one hand, elevated Ca appears to influence Ca-dependent enzymes which act on the cytoskeleton [38], and, on the other, a hallmark of Alzheimer's disease is disruption of the neuronal cytoskeleton, as manifested in neurofibrillary tangles [43].

Much work remains to be done to test this hypothesis. In addition, even if altered Ca regulation is pinpointed as a key factor in brain aging and Alzheimer's disease, a great deal of work will be needed to define the specific Ca regulatory processes that are most affected by aging, as well as to define initial causes of changes in these mechanisms. That is, as has been reviewed extensively [10,13, 27], Ca homeostasis is regulated by a large array of processes (Fig. 5) that (A) maintain Ca channel selectivity and sensitivity, (B) modulate both voltage- and Ca-dependent inactivation mechanisms, (C) terminate Ca influx by Ca-dependent repolarization (deactivation) mechanisms, (D) buffer and sequester intracellular Ca, and (E) extrude Ca (e. g., the Na-Ca exchange).

Moreover, most of these general categories of mechanism include several subtypes. If the capacity to regulate Ca of one – or – more of these mechanisms were impaired, then intracellular concentrations of Ca would likely reach levels that would disrupt physiological function and induce abnormal and destructive activity in Ca-dependent enzymes (5F). Under some conditions, near complete breakdown of a regulatory

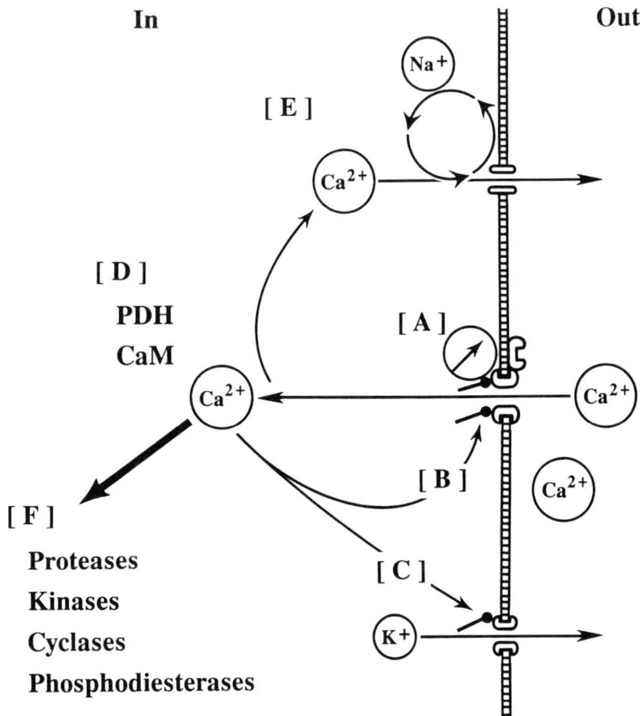

Fig. 5A-F. Illustration of the general types of Ca regulatory mechanisms found in brain cells, in relation to the hypothesis of Ca-induced brain cellular dysfunction during aging. **A**, Voltage- and receptor-sensitive mechanisms regulating Ca influx. **B**, Ca-dependent Ca channel inactivation mechanisms **C**, Ca-dependent K currents that repolarize the cell. **D**, Ca binding proteins that act as buffers and modulators; *PDH*, mitochondrial pyruvate dehydrogenase; *CaM*, calmodulin. **E**, Ca extrusion mechanisms (e. g., the Na-Ca exchange process). **F**, in the case of regulatory impairment and abnormally elevated Ca *(large arrow)*, Ca-dependent enzymes reach levels of activity that disrupt cellular function and induce structural degeneration. It is suggested that age-related alterations at **A** and **B** may be key factors in neuronal decline in brain aging and Alzheimer's disease [17]

mechanism could account for the widespread cellular degeneration found in Alzheimer's disease. At present, our data implicate mechanisms which regulate voltage-dependent Ca influx (e. g., A and B, Fig. 5), but it is not yet clear whether this is the only or the essential aspect of altered Ca homeostasis.

Thus, although there are new and interesting data on the possible age-related alteration of a key Ca regulatory mechanism, much remains to be done in defining the specific putative mechanism that underlies this alteration and in definitively testing the degree of its contribution to brain aging.

References

1. Andersen P, Lomo T (1967) Control of hippocampal output by afferent volley frequency. Prog Brain Res 27: 400–412

2. Alger BE, Nicoll RA (1980) Epileptiform burst afterhyperpolarization: calcium-dependent potassium potential in hippocampal CA1 pyramidal cells. Science 210: 1122–1144
3. Augustine GJ, Eckert R (1984) Calcium-dependent inactivation of presynaptic calcium channels. Soc Neurosci Abstr 10: 194
4. Ball MJ (1977) Neuronal loss, neurofibrillary tangles and granulovascular degeneration in the hippocampus with aging and dementia: a quantitative study. Acta Neuropathol 37: 11–118
5. Baudry M, Fuchs J, Kessler M, Arst D, Lynch G (1982) Entorhinal cortex lesions induce a decreased calcium transport in hippocampal mitochondria. Science 216: 411–413
6. Brody H (1973) Aging of the vertebrate brain. In: Rockstein M, Sussman M (eds) Development and aging in the central nervous system. Academic, New York, pp 121–133
7. Brown DA, Griffith WH (1983) Persistent slow inward calcium current in voltage-clamped hippocampal neurones of the guinea pig. J Physiol (Lond) 337: 303–320
8. Campbell LW, Hao SY, Landfield PW (1988) Calcium-dependent inactivation of calcium currents in hippocampal neurons: Effects of tetraethylammonium and nimodipine. Soc Neurosci Abstr 14: 138
9. Eckert R, Ewald D (1983) Inactivation of calcium conductance characterized by tail current measurements in neurones of *Aplysia californica*. J Physiol (Lond) 345: 549–565
10. Gibson GE, Peterson C (1987) Calcium and the aging nervous system. Neurobiol Aging 8: 329–344
11. Halliwell JW (1983) Caesium loading reveals two distinct Ca-currents in voltage-clamped guinea-pig hippocampal neurones in vitro. J Physiol (Lond) 341: 10–11
12. Johnston D, Hablitz JJ, Wilson WA (1980) Voltage clamp discloses slow inward current in hippocampal burst firing neurones. Nature 286: 391–393
13. Khachaturian ZS (1984) Towards theories of brain aging. In: Kay D, Burrows GD (eds) Handbook of studies on psychiatry and old age. Elsevier, Amsterdam
14. Lancaster B, Adams PR (1986) Calcium-dependent current generating the afterhyperpolarization of hippocampal neurons. J Neurophysiol 55: 1268–1282
15. Landfield PW (1981) Age-related impairment of hippocampal frequency potentiation: evidence of an underlying deficit in transmitter release from studies of Mg^{2+}-bathed hippocampal slices. Soc Neurosci Abstr 7: 371
16. Landfield PW (1983) Mechanisms of altered neural function during aging. In: Gipsen WH, Traber J (eds) Aging of the brain. Elsevier, New York, pp 51–71
17. Landfield PW (1987) "Increased calcium current" hypothesis of brain aging. Neurobiol Aging 8: 346–347
18. Landfield PW, Lynch G (1977) Impaired monosynaptic potentiation in *in vitro* hippocampal slices from aged, memory-deficient rats. J Gerontol 32: 523–533
19. Landfield PW, McGaugh JL, Lynch G (1978) Impaired synaptic potentiation processes in the hippocampus of aged, memory-deficient rats. Brain Res 150: 85–101
20. Landfield PW, Morgan G (1984) Chronically elevating plasma Mg^{2+} improves hippocampal frequency potentiation and reversal learning in aged and young rats. Brain Res 322: 167–171
21. Landfield PW, Pitler TA (1984) Prolonged Ca^{2+}-dependent afterhyperpolarizations in hippocampal neurons of aged rats. Science 226: 1089–1092
22. Landfield PW, Pitler TA (1987) Calcium spike duration: prolongation in hippocampal neurons of aged rats. Soc Neurosci Abstr 13: 718
23. Landfield PW, Pitler TA, Applegate MD (1986) The effects of high Mg^{2+} to Ca^{2+} ratios on frequency potentiation in hippocampal slices of young and aged rats. J Neurophysiol 56: 797–811
24. Landfield PW, Pitler TA, Applegate MD (1986) The aged hippocampus: a model system for studies on mechanisms of behavioral plasticity and brain aging. In: Isaacson RL, Pribram KH (eds) The hippocampus, vol. 3. Plenum, New York, pp 323–367
25. Llinas R, Hess R (1976) Tetrodotoxin resistant dendritic spikes in avian Purkinje cells. Proc Natl Acad Sci USA 73: 2520–2523
26. Michaelis ML, Johe K, Kitos TE (1984) Age-dependent alterations in synaptic membrane systems for Ca^{2+} regulation. Mech Ageing Dev 25: 215–225
27. Miller RJ (1987) Calcium channels in neurones. In: Venter JC, Triggle D (eds) Structure and physiology of the slow inward calcium channel. Liss, New York, p 161
28. Nayler WG, Poole-Wilson PA, Williams A (1979) Hypoxia and calcium. J Mol Cell Cardiol 11: 683–706

29. Nowycky MC, Fox AP, Tsien RW (1985) Three types of neuronal calcium channel with different agonist sensitivity. Nature 316: 440–443
30. Perl DP, Gajdusek DC, Garruto RM, Yanagihara RT, Gibbs CJ (1982) Aluminum accumulation in amyotropic lateral sclerosis and Parkinsonism-dementia of Guam. Science 217: 1053–1055
31. Perry EK, Perry RH, Gibson P, Tomlinson BE, Blessed G, Gibson PH (1980) Coenzyme-A-acetylating enzymes in Alzheimer's disease: possible cholinergic "compartment" of pyruvate dehydrogenase. Neurosci Lett 18: 105–110
32. Peterson C, Gibson GE, Blass JP (1985) Altered calcium uptake in cultured skin fibroblasts from patients with Alzheimer's disease. N Engl J Med 312: 1063–1065
33. Peterson C, Goldman J (1986) Alterations in calcium content and biochemical processes during aging and Alzheimer's disease. Proc Natl Acad Sci USA 83: 2758–2761
34. Pitler TA, Landfield PW (1987) Probable Ca^{2+}-mediated inactivation of Ca^{2+} currents in mammalian brain neurons. Brain Res 410: 147–153
35. Pitler TA, Landfield PW (1987) Postsynaptic membrane shifts during frequency potentiation of the hippocampal EPSP. J Neurophysiol 58: 866–882
36. Roth GS (1988) Mechanisms of altered hormone and neurotransmitter action during aging: the role of impaired calcium mobilization. Ann NY Acad Sci 521: 170–176
37. Rothman S, Olney JW (1986) Glutamate and the pathophysiology of hypoxic-ischemic brain damage. Ann Neurol 19: 105–111
38. Schlaepfer WW, Hasler MB (1979) Characterization of the calcium-induced disruption of neurofilaments in rat peripheral nerve. Brain Res 168: 299–309
39. Schwartzkroin DA, Slawsky MA (1977) Probable calcium spikes in hippocampal neurones. Brain Res 135: 157–161
40. Scriabine A (1987) Ca^{2+} channel ligands: Comparative pharmacology. In: Venter JC, Triggle D (eds) Structure and physiology of the slow inward calcium channel. Liss, New York, p 51
41. Siesjo BK (1981) Cell damage in the brain: a speculative synthesis. J Cereb Blood Flow Metab 1: 155–185
42. Tomlinson BE, Henderson G (1976) Some quantitative cerebral findings in normal and demented old people. In: Terry RD, Gershon S (eds) Neurobiology of aging. Raven, New York, pp 183–204
43. Wisniewski HM, Terry RD (1973) Morphology of the aging brain, human and animal. Prog Brain Res 40: 167–186
44. Wong RKS, Prince DA (1981) After potential generation in hippocampal pyramidal cells. J Neurophysiol 45: 87–97

Nimodipine and Neural Plasticity

R. Gerritsen van der Hoop, C. E. E. M. van der Zee, and W. H. Gispen

Introduction

Brain aging is often considered in terms of a reduced neural plasticity. Commonly, the term neural plasticity is used to describe the adaptive capacity of the nervous system. It is now recognized that this adaptive capacity plays a key role in the development of specific neuronal networks and in the response to trauma or intoxication. Furthermore, it has been shown that dynamic adaptive changes at the synapse may lead to totally different communication patterns, resulting in an altered output of the brain. Neural plasticity can be studied at the molecular, morphological, neurophysiological, and the behavioral level and at all these levels specific age-related decreases in the adaptive capacity of the nervous system have been described (Swaab et al. 1986).

As outlined elsewhere (Gelijns et al. 1987), nervous system plasticity is of great significance in relation to a number of health-associated problems such as injury to peripheral nerves, spinal cord, and brain and also developmental disorders, learning disabilities, and age-related diseases such as Parkinson's disease and senile dementia. Profound insight into the mechanism of neural plasticity is a prerequisite for eventual advances in the therapy of these pathologies.

The existence of an animal model is a major step forward in the analysis of disease processes. Unfortunately, for senile dementia of the Alzheimer type (SDAT) there seem to be very few relevant animal models, which are often only of selected aspects of the disease (Bick 1984). In some of these models, the animals bearing lesions are tested for their cognitive capacity in various behavioral tasks. Such studies further our insight into the functional organization of the brain with respect to cognitive abilities that are impaired in patients with senile dementia. Furthermore, they provide the possibility to check the efficacy of potential pharmacotherapy aimed at ameliorating the lesion-related loss of cognitive function (Pepeu et al. 1985; Leventer and Hanin 1985). Clearly, this model of SDAT in part relates to aspects of the disease such as cell loss and neuronal degeneration – signs of diminished plasticity – which are present in brain structures that are presumably involved in cognition.

In this paper we shall emphasize the importance of postlesion repair mechanisms and briefly highlight our recent data on the neurotrophic effect of the calcium-entry blocker nimodipine in this animal model.

Bergener, Reisberg (Eds.)
Diagnosis and Treatment
of Senile Dementia
© Springer-Verlag Berlin Heidelberg 1989

Postlesion Plasticity

The neuron is an extremely specialized and differentiated cell and has proven to be the most vulnerable cell in the mammalian central and peripheral nervous system. In general, it is assumed that damage to cell bodies of neurons results in irreversible degeneration and cell death. On the other hand, if the damage is restricted to the neuronal processes (dendrites and axons) regeneration with resulting reinnervation of the target is, in principle, possible. For reasons still not completely understood, it appears that neurons in the peripheral nervous system show better regeneration than neurons in the central nervous system. The milieu surrounding the damaged axon is important in this respect. If a motor axon is damaged within the vertebral column, hardly any outgrowth of newly formed sprouts is seen, as is typical of central nervous system neurons. If the same sort of lesion is more distal, outside the vertebral column, axonal regeneration and eventual target muscle reinnervation is evident. Similarities in many aspects make postlesion neuronal plasticity a fast replay of processes that take place during neuronal development. In other words, cellular or network repair is very much determined by factors that also govern the development and maturation of the cell or network. It is well known that development, elongation, and repair of axons is guided by a variety of humoral and structural factors which are of neuronal, glial, and target cell origin (Varon 1985).

Indeed the notion has been put forward that in SDAT brain trophic factors are out of balance, and this may cause specific cell loss and neural degeneration in regions involved in cognition (Appel et al. 1985).

Calcium and Neural Plasticity

It is evident that neural Ca^{2+} homeostasis is a key factor in the control of neuronal development and plasticity. The tip of an outgrowing nerve is known as the growth cone and is a specialized motile axonal terminal which in situ appears to have a variety of shapes. The "classical" image of a growth cone as a broad flattened lamellipodium with numerous spike-like filopodia is obtained when neurites are studied in culture (Kater et al. 1988). Evidence is accumulating to suggest that intracellular Ca^{2+} is a major factor in the regulation of growth cone motility. Intracellular levels of free Ca^{2+} were always lower in spontaneously inactive growth cones than in those that were active. In fact, different growth cone behaviors such as protrusion, retraction, and elongation seem to have different Ca^{2+} dependencies (Kater et al. 1988). Apparently the balance between influx, efflux, and Ca^{2+}-buffering systems such as pumps, Ca^{2+}-binding proteins, and organelle sequestering systems play a crucial part in the regulation of growth cone behavior (Kater et al. 1988). Both too large increases and too large decreases in intracellular Ca^{2+} impair growth cone function and thus the ability of the axon to reach its proper target.

As growth cones form the presynaptic terminal, these structures share a number of important features, i.e., voltage-sensitive ion channels, transmitter release, and receptors. Indeed, also at the synaptic level, neural plasticity in the form of long-term potentiation of monosynaptic connections is highly dependent on Ca^{2+} influx (Lynch et al. 1983), and involves activation of Ca^{2+}-sensitive processes such as proteolysis

(Lynch and Baudry 1984), phosphatidylinositol-4,5-biphosphate breakdown (Bär et al. 1984), and protein kinase C-mediated phosphorylation of a specific presynaptic membrane protein B50/F1 (Akers et al. 1986; De Graan et al. 1986). This protein is identical to growth-associated protein GAP43 (Karns et al. 1987) and P57 (Cimler et al. 1987). It is present in presynaptic terminals and in growth cones. B50-GAP43 is considered to play a crucial role in the capacity of axons to grow since the protein is expressed in injured nerves that do regenerate and not in nerves that do not sucessfully reform their axons (Willard and Skene 1982). Furthermore, the protein is an atypical neuron-specific binder of intracellular calmodulin. The degree of phosphorylation of this protein affects its calmodulin binding capacity (Cimler et al. 1985) and regulates the activity of a lipid kinase involved in the so-called polyphosphoinositide response (Van Dongen et al. 1985).

In line with the notion that brain aging is related to diminished neural plasticity, numerous studies suggest a severe disturbance of Ca^{2+} homeostasis in the aged brain (Katchaturian 1984; Gibson et al. 1984; Landfield, this volume). However, there is still some debate whether a reduced or increased level of intracellular Ca^{2+}, in both instances influencing the coupling between calcium-dependent neurophysiological and neurochemical processes, is responsible for the age-related pathological and behavioral changes.

Nimodipine and Peripheral Nerve Plasticity

The peripheral nerve is an excellent model to study the plasticity of nervous tissue. When this part of the nervous system is damaged by mechanical trauma (cut or crush injury) to its neurites, remarkable regenerative powers are mobilized, resulting in the formation of new sprouts that grow in the direction of the target at approximately the speed of the slow component of axonal transport. In the rat, recovery of both sensory and motor function of the foot following a transection in the mid-thigh region ensues within 36 days (Edwards et al. 1986) and within a mere 23 days after a crush lesion (Bijlsma et al. 1983), as assessed by foot withdrawal reflex. In humans this process can take years and complete return of all modalities is seldom achieved (Sunderland 1978). An additional advantage of using this type of lesion as a model, as compared to central lesions, is that the plasticity of neurons can be easily examined at a number of different levels, ranging from molecular to functional.

The effects of nimodipine on plasticity of the peripheral nerve have been studied in rats using a crush lesion model. Return of both sensory and motor function can be easily monitored in a reproducible way applying techniques described by De Koning et al. (1986). Aspects of speed can be assessed by using foot flick withdrawal, while quality of recovery can be monitored with an analysis of the free walking pattern (Fig. 1). Orally administered nimodipine was shown to enhance recovery of both sensory and motor function in this model, reducing the number of days needed for recovery by 2–3 days (Fig. 2), and to improve the walking pattern (Van der Zee et al. 1987). The exact mechanism underlying this effect is not known at present, but it is unlikely that nimodipine acts through a reduction of secondary cell loss. Presumably the Ca^{2+}-entry blocking agent affects lesion induced sprouting (Van der Zee et al. 1987).

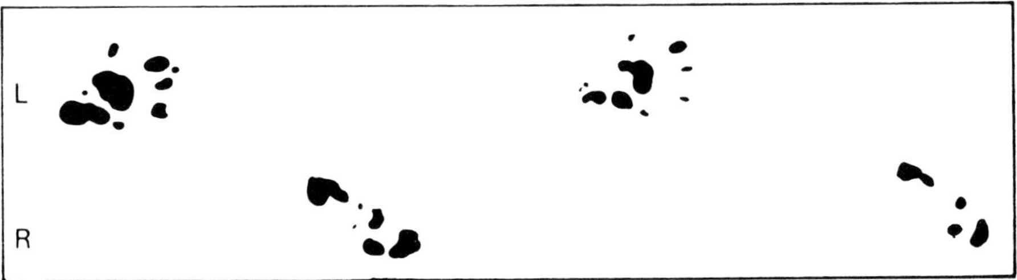

Fig. 1. Footprint pattern of a rat bearing a crush lesion in the right sciatic nerve 12 days following injury. Such prints allow the assessment of the quality of the use of the paw in an unforced manner. Note for instance difference in toe spreading and exo-rotation between the two paws

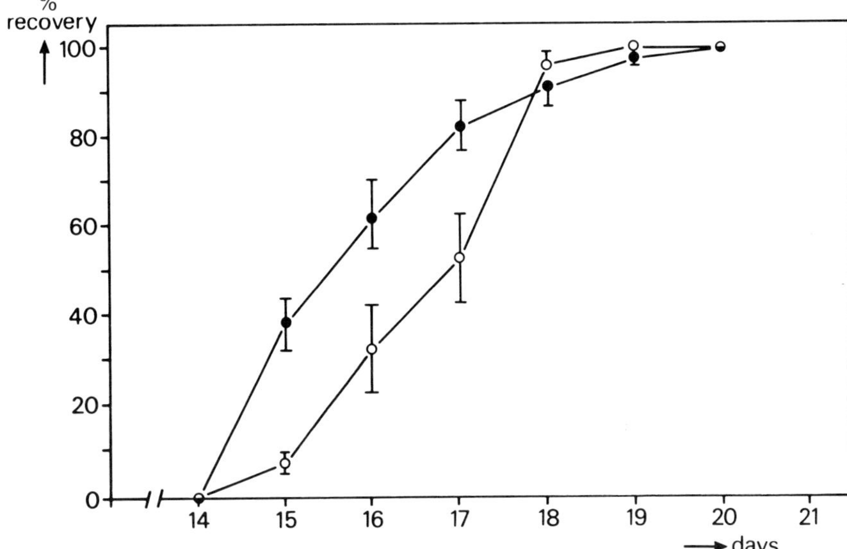

Fig. 2. Effect of oral nimodipine treatment on recovery of sensorimotor function following a crush lesion in the sciatic nerve, as assessed by a foot reflex withdrawal test. ●— ●, nimodipine 860 ppm, $n = 10$; ○ — ○, control food, $n = 10$

It is well-known that aging in the rat is accompanied by a gradual impairment of locomotion. This decline in motor performance seems to appear independently from other age-related deficits and therefore cannot solely be attributed to the malfunctioning of the peripheral neuromuscular systems. Also, a loss of coordination (diminished proprioceptive feedback) and a general slowing down of central control mechanisms seem to be involved (Coper et al. 1986). A number of parameters can be studied to establish the quality of motor performance, ranging from balance tests to detailed walking pattern analyses. Using these different tests major deficits were seen in rats of more than 2 years of age (Schuurman et al. 1987). In view of the beneficial effect of nimodipine on postlesion plasticity in the peripheral (PNS, see above) and

292   R. Gerritsen van der Hoop et al.

central nervous system (CNS; Betz et al. 1985), it was decided to investigate the efficacy of chronic nimodipine treatment in the PNS in old rats.

Results of an experiment with rats, 24 months of age, receiving oral treatment with nimodipine (860 ppm; Bayer, Leverkusen, FRG) in food pellets showed that the drug was capable of delaying and/or suppressing the occurrence of the above-mentioned motor deficits (Schuurman et al. 1987).

In a second experiment only rats were used that were already troubled by a considerable amount of motor deficit. The animals were matched for severity of motor function disturbances and randomly selected to either receive treatment with nimodipine (860 ppm) or placebo food pellets. In addition to the standard walking pattern analysis, both sensory and motor conduction velocities in the sciatic nerve were measured at the end of the treatment period of 20 weeks, using the technique described by De Koning and Gispen (1988). Finally, a number of animals from each group was randomly selected for histological follow-up. After killing these animals the sciatic nerves were quickly dissected and fixed with glutaraldehyde and osmium tetroxide. Following dehydration and embedding in epoxy resin, semithin cross sections were made at a distance of 1 cm from the sciatic notch and stained for myelin. The number of myelinated fibers was assessed by means of an image analysis system. The experiment was performed in a blind fashion.

During the treatment period of 20 weeks, a considerable improvement was seen in the walking pattern of nimodipine-treated rats, while deterioration proceeded rapidly in control animals (Schuurman et al., this volume). Only at the end of the treatment period did a decrease in motor function also become apparent in nimodipine-treated rats. However, on electrophysiological examination higher nerve conduction velocities were registered in the sciatic nerve in rats that received nimodipine (Fig. 3). Histological analysis showed that fiber density in the aged, control rats was much lower than that seen in young animals. The compact aspect of the sciatic nerve had been replaced by an image of nerve fibers situated in a generous amount of connective tissue. Thick amyloid-like deposits were seen around vascular structures, comparable

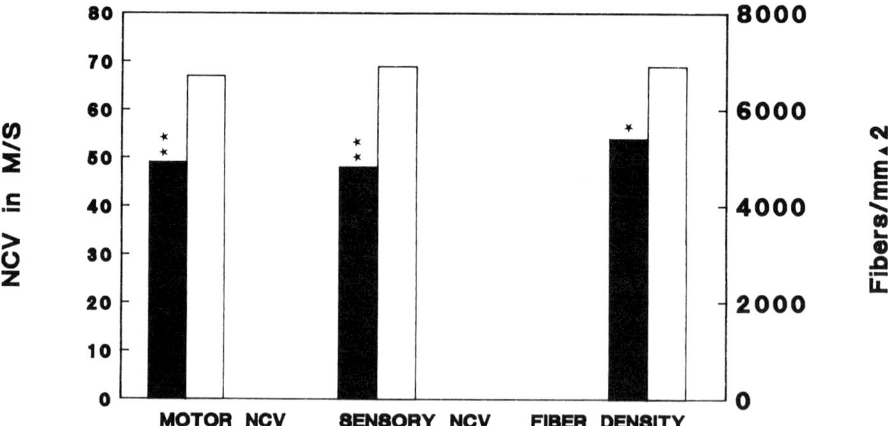

Fig. 3. Nerve conduction velocities (*NCV, n* = 12) and fiber density (*n* = 6) in sciatic nerves of aged rats treated with nimodipine food pellets (□) or control food pellets (■; *p* < 0.05, **p* < 0.001, Student's *t*t test)

to those reported for blood vessels in the aged rat brain (Luiten, personal communication). In contrast, in nimodipine-treated rats the total number of fibers was higher and the fiber density was larger than in control animals (Fig. 3), while deposits around blood vessels were rarely seen (Van de Zee et al., in preparation).

These data support the suggestion that nimodipine improves the condition of peripheral nerve tissue in older rats, at the functional, electrophysiological, and histomorphological level.

Concluding Remarks

In this paper aspects of nerve regeneration and Ca^{2+} homeostasis were discussed in the context of brain aging. The calcium-entry blocker nimodipine was shown to exert a beneficial effect on regeneration following traumatic injury to the peripheral nervous system. This observation, combined with the data pointing to a possible anti-ischemic effect of the drug, prompted investigation of nimodipine in aspects of brain and or nerve function in the aged rat, because the presumed age-related diminishment in neural plasticity suggests that the aged nervous system is in need of trophic support. Indeed, in the aged rat, a number of functional and morphological parameters could be positively influenced by chronic oral treatment with nimodipine.

At present more detailed information is required to allow proper speculation on the precise mechanism of action of nimodipine in this respect. It is tempting, however, to suggest that the drug directly affects parameters involved in the trophic response to trauma and aging. Whether the improvement of calcium homeostasis by entry blocking is part of the mechanism of action of the drug remains to be shown. Nonetheless, the present data further support the potential significance of nimodipine pharmacotherapy of neuronal repair and age-related deficits in nervous system function.

References

Akers RF, Lovinger DM, Colley PA, Linden DJ, Routtenberg A (1986) Translocation of protein kinase C activity may mediate hippocampal long-term potentiation. Science 231: 587–589

Appel SH, Ojika K, Tomozawa Y, Bostwick R (1985) Trophic factors in brain aging and disease. In: Traber J, Gispen WH (eds) Senile dementia of the Alzheimer type. Springer, Berlin Heidelberg New York, pp 218–230

Bär PR, Wiegant F, Lopes da Silva FH, Gispen WH (1984) Tetanic stimulation affects the metabolism of phosphoinositides in hippocampal slices. Brain Res 321: 381–385

Betz E, Deck K, Hoffmeister F (1985) Nimodipine: pharmacological and clinical properties. Schattauer, Stuttgart

Bick L (1984) Research in Alzheimer's disease: an American perspective. In: Knook DL, Calderine B, Amaducci L (eds) Aging of the brain and senile dementia. Eurage, Rijswijk, pp 171–182

Bijlsma WA, Jennekens FGI, Schotman P, Gispen WH (1983) Stimulation by ACTH (4–10) of nerve fiber regeneration following sciatic nerve crush. Muscle Nerve 6: 104–112

Cimler BM, Andreasen TJ, Andreasen KI, Storm DR (1985) The P57 is a neuron specific calmodulin binding protein. Biochem J 260: 10784–10788

Cimler BM, Giebelhaus DH, Wakim BT, Storm DR, Moon RT (1987) Characterization of murine cDNA's encoding P57, a neuron specific calmodulin binding protein. Biochem J 262: 1258–1263

Coper H, Jänicke B, Schulze G (1986) Biopsychological research on adaptivity across the life-span of animals. In: Baltes PD, Featherman DL, Lerner RM (eds) live-span development and behavior. Erlbaum, Hillsdale, NJ, pp 207–232

De Graan PNE, Oestreicher AB, Schrama LH, Gispen WH (1986) Phosphoprotein B-50: localization and function. Prog Brain Res 69: 37–50

De Koning P, Gispen WH (1988) A rationale for the use of melanocortins in the treatment of nervous tissue damage. In: Stein DG, Sabel B (eds) Pharmacological approaches to the treatment of brain and spinal cord injuries. Plenum, New York, pp 233–258

De Koning P, Brakkee JH, Gispen WH (1986) Methods for producing a reproducible crush in the sciatic and tibial nerve of the rat and rapid and precise testing of return of sensory function. J Neurol Sci 74: 237–241

Edwards PM, Kuiters RRF, Boer GJ, Gispen WH (1986) Recovery from peripheral nerve transection is accelerated by local application of alpha-MSH by means of microporous Accurel propylene tubes. J Neurol Sci 74: 171–176

Gelijns AC, Graaff PJ, Lopes da Silva FH, Gispen WH (1987) Future health care applications resulting from progress in the neurosciences: the significance of neural plasticity research. Health Policy 8: 265–276.

Gibson GE, Perrino P, Dienel G (1984) Alterations of in vivo brain calcium homeostasis with aging. J Am Aging Assoc 14: 62

Karns LR, NG SC, Freeman JA, Fishman MC (1987) Cloning of complementary DNA for GAP43, a neuronal growth related protein. Science 236: 597–599

Katchaturian Z (1984) Towards theories of brain aging. In: Kay DW, Burrows GD (eds), Handbook of studies in psychiatry and old age. Elsevier, New York, pp 7–30

Kater SB, Mattson MP, Cohan C, Connor J (1988) Calcium regulation of the neuronal growth cone. TINS 11: 315–320

Leventer SM, Hanin I (1985) AF64A cholinotoxicity: functional aspects. In: Traber J, Gispen WH (eds) Senile dementia of the Alzheimer type. Springer, Berlin Heidelberg New York, pp 316–324

Lynch G, Baudry M (1984) The biochemistry of memory: a new and specific hypothesis. Science 224: 1057–1063

Lynch G, Larson J, Kelso S, Barrionuevo G, Schottler F (1983) Intracellular injections of EGTA block induction of hippocampal long-term potentiation. Nature 305: 719–721.

Pepeu G, Casamenti F, Bracco L, Ladinsky H, Consolo S (1985) Lesions of the nucleus basalis in the rat: Functional changes. In: Traber J, Gispen WH (eds) Senile dementia of the Alzheimer type, Springer, Berlin Heidelberg New York, pp 305–315

Schuurman T, Klein H, Beneke M, Traber J (1987) Nimodipine and motor deficits in the aged rat. Neurosci Res Commun 1: 9–15

Sunderland S (1978) Nerves and nerve injuries. Churchill Livingstone, New York

Swaab DF, Fliers E, Mirmiran M, Van Gool WA, Van Haaren F (1986) Aging of the brain and Alzheimer's disease. Progr Brain Res 70: 413–428

Van der Zee CEEM, Schuurman T, Traber J, Gispen WH (1987) Oral administration of nimodipine accelerates functional recovery following peripheral nerve damage in the rat. Neurosci Lett 83: 143–148

Van Dongen CJ, Zwiers H, de Graan PNE, Gispen WH (1985) Modulation of the activity of purified phosphatidylinositol 4-phosphate kinase by phosphorylated and dephosphorylated B-50 protein. Biochem Biophys Res Commun 8: 1219–1227

Varon S (1985) Factors promoting the growth of the nervous system. Neurosciences 3: 62

Willard M, Skene JHP (1982) Molecular events in axonal regeneration. In: Nicholls A (ed) Repair and regeneration of the nervous system. Springer, Berlin Heidelberg New York, pp 71–89

Old Rats as an Animal Model for Senile Dementia: Behavioural Effects of Nimodipine

T. SCHUURMAN, and J. TRABER

Behavioural Differences Between Old and Young Rats

One of the goals in behavioural pharmacology is the development and validation of useful animal models for psychiatric diseases and other disorders of the central nervous system (CNS). For some of these pathological conditions, e. g. anxiety and depression, a number of animal models already exist and have been shown to have reasonable predictive value for the clinical situation as far as drug effects are concerned. For many other CNS diseases, however, such models have not yet been developed. This is especially true for diseases related to brain aging, such as senile dementia, senile dementia of the Alzheimer type (SDAT) and other diseases characterized by a severe impairment of cognitive functions. One of the reasons for the lack of valid models for age-related disorders of the CNS is the difficulty in mimicking the complex and multiform symptoms of these diseases in animals. The main symptom of dementias is impaired learning and memory capability, however, other behavioural alterations, such as reduction of social behaviour and adaptability, increase in aggressiveness, changes in personality, disturbances in diurnal rhythms and in motor functions are also present. Whereas e. g. by lesioning the hippocampus, the nucleus basalis or other areas of the rat brain, one is able to induce learning and memory deficits, until now no animal model has been shown to mimic all the behavioural deficits of dementia mentioned above. Another problem in using brain-lesioned rats as a dementia model is the spontaneous behavioural recovery after surgery. Senile dementia has, however, a progressive course which makes a comparison with lesion models difficult.

Dementia is certainly a disease confined to human beings. However, if one assumes that there are fluent transitions from normal aging to dementia, then the use of aged animals as a model to study age-related disorders might be a useful approach.

The aim of the present study was to investigate whether the old rat can be used as such a model. Therefore we compared the behaviour of old rats (male Wistar rats, up to 30 months of age) with that of young ones (age 2–3 months). The behavioural testing was not limited to learning and memory paradigms, but behaviour of old and young rats was also compared in a social interaction test and in different sensorimotor function tests. Furthermore, grooming, diurnal rhythms, adaptability and walking patterns were studied. A part of the results of these behavioural studies is discussed in the following sections. Moreover, effects of a proposed geriatric drug, nimodipine, on behaviour of old rats are presented.

Bergener, Reisberg (Eds.)
Diagnosis and Treatment
of Senile Dementia
© Springer-Verlag Berlin Heidelberg 1989

One-Trial Passive Avoidance Learning

In this test it was investigated whether rats learn to avoid a place in which they previously received a painful stimulus. Rats aged 2, 13, 19 or 25 months (20 rats per age group) were placed singly on a brightly illuminated platform facing the entrance of a dark compartment (Ader et al. 1972). During four consecutive trials we measured how much time elapsed before they entered the dark compartment. After the fourth trial each rat received an electric shock to the feet (175 µA, 3 s) in the dark box. The rats were put again on the lit platform 24 h after the shock (learning) trial, and latent periods before entry were measured. Rats with long post-shock latencies were regarded as having learned the task.

Table 1 shows that 2-month-old rats learned the task perfectly, their median latency period was more than 300 s. In contrast, 25-month-old rats had a median latency period of only 40 s; 13- and 19-month-old rats showed intermediate latencies. Pre-shock latencies did not differ significantly between age groups.

In a separate experiment it was shown that the impaired passive avoidance response of old rats could not be attributed to a decreased sensitivity to painful stimulation. Thus the age-related impaired passive avoidance response is most likely due to a reduction of the ability of old rats to learn this response. Interestingly, 24-month-old rats which were subjected repeatedly to avoidance tests did learn to avoid electric shocks. Apparently, repetition of the task is a prerequisite for avoidance learning in senescent rats.

Table 1. Age-dependent impairment of passive avoidance learning in the rat

Age	Median time (s) before entering the dark box	
(months)	Before shock	24 h after shock
2	10	> 300
13	8	240
19	8	160*
25	10	40**

* $P < 0.05$ (Mann-Whitney U test), compared with 2-month-old rats
** $P < 0.01$ (Mann-Whitney U test), compared with 2-month-old rats

Learning in a Water Labyrinth

Learning and memory ability of old and young rats was further compared in a more complex test situation, a water labyrinth. This maze, originally described by Giurgea and Mouravieff-Lesuisse (1972), consisted of a tank (120 × 50 × 40 cm) filled halfway with cold (15°C) water (Fig. 1). Single rats (3 and 25 months of age, 20 per group) were put gently into the water at the entrance of the maze and had to swim around a series of barriers in order to find the escape ladder at the opposite end of the labyrinth. Rats were trained once a day for 11 consecutive days. The number of errors the rats made (swimming in the wrong direction) and the time needed were measured.

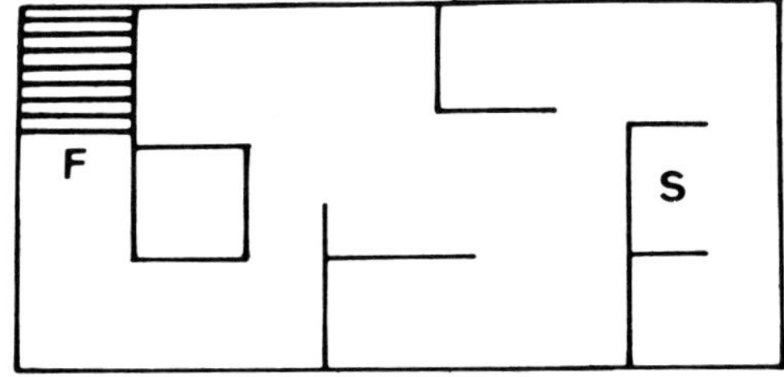

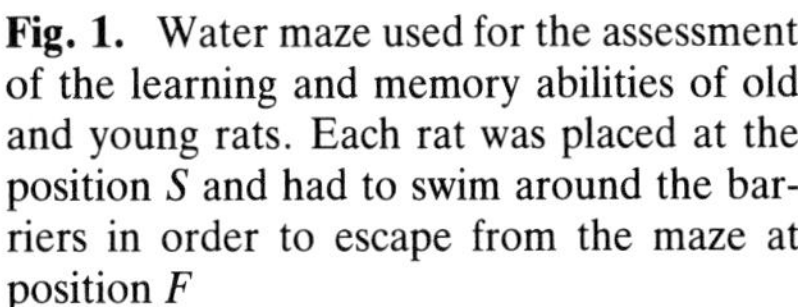

Fig. 1. Water maze used for the assessment of the learning and memory abilities of old and young rats. Each rat was placed at the position *S* and had to swim around the barriers in order to escape from the maze at position *F*

Table 2. Difference in learning rate between old (aged 25 months) and young rats (aged 3 months) as assessed in a watermaze task

Trial	Mean number of errors	
	3 months	25 months
1	17	18
2	16	16
3	11	14
4	6	14
5	3	13
6	2	13
7	2	9
8	1	11
9	1	8
10	1	7
11	1	6
Total	61	129

Table 2 shows that both old and young animals made fewer errors in the course of the training procedure. However, the decrease was much faster in the young rats than in the old ones. A difference in rate of learning was also expressed in the swimming times (data not shown). These and other data (e. g. Gage et al. 1984; Schuurman et al. 1986) show that the old rat has a reduced capacity to learn complex spatial tasks.

Social Behaviour

Social behaviour of rats is characterized by a rich repertoire of different acts and postures which can easily be distinguished by experienced observers. When two male Wistar rats (a relatively non-aggressive strain) which do not know each other are paired in an unfamiliar observation cage many social activities such as approaching, anogenital inspection, oral inspection, sniffing or nibbling at the fur of the conspecific, following, crawling over and under can be observed. Frequencies and durations of these social and of nonsocial behavioural elements can be recorded with the help of a personal computer. We paired male rats of the same age and body weight for 5 min in an observation cage (60 × 60 × 40 cm) which was only illuminated by a 15 Watt bulb

Table 3. Age-dependent decrease of social behaviour in male rats

Age (months)	Social interaction (s/5 min)
2	116
4	135
6	88
12	82
18	65
24	52
28	40

to decrease the novelty stress and measured the amount of social interaction as described above. Pairs of rats of the following age categories were studied: 2, 4, 6, 12, 18, 24 and 28 months (6–12 pairs per age group).

In Table 3 it can be seen that 2- and 4-month-old rats spent 2 out of 5 min in social activities. The remaining time was spent on exploration of the cage (sniffing, rearing, locomotion). At the age of 6 months a significant (Mann-Whitney U test) reduction of social interaction was observed. In the course of the aging process social behaviour further decreased.

The low level of social interaction in aged rats was not only expressed in the duration of social behaviours, but also in the frequency (data not shown).

Sensorimotor Functions

A battery of simple tests described in essence by Gage et al. (1984) was applied to investigate sensorimotor functions of old, middle aged and young male Wistar rats. Among these tests were three balance rod tests varying in difficulty, a traction test for the forepaws and a pole climbing test. Individual animals were placed in the middle of the balance rods ("bridges"). The time it took to reach one of the safety platforms at the ends of the bridge or before falling off was measured. The rats subjected to these tests were 3, 4, 6, 9, 12, 18 or 24 months old. Each age group consisted of 12 rats. In the easiest balance test (keeping balance on a bridge 5 cm in width), only 24-month-old animals performed significantly worse than their younger conspecifics. Using a bridge 2.5 cm wide, 9-month-old rats scored worse than younger ones. From that age on performance declined further with age (Fig. 2). Also with the third bridge, which was round, an age-dependent decline of performance was measured.

Middle-aged and old rats subjected to the suspended hanging test (hanging by the forepaws) and the pole climbing test, also performed in these tests worse than the young ones (Schuurman et al. 1986). In all of these tests bodyweight of the animals plays a role in the outcome of the experiments. Heavy animals have a disadvantage as compared with lean ones, and one could argue that this might explain the age-related decrease of motor performance. However, male individuals of the Wistar strain used in these experiments hardly gain weight after the age of 6 months. From 24 months on many of them even lose weight. Thus the impaired motorfunction of aging rats is not due to gradually increasing bodyweights. The sensorimotor deficits of old rats are most probably caused by the aging process of the nervous system (see also Coper et al.

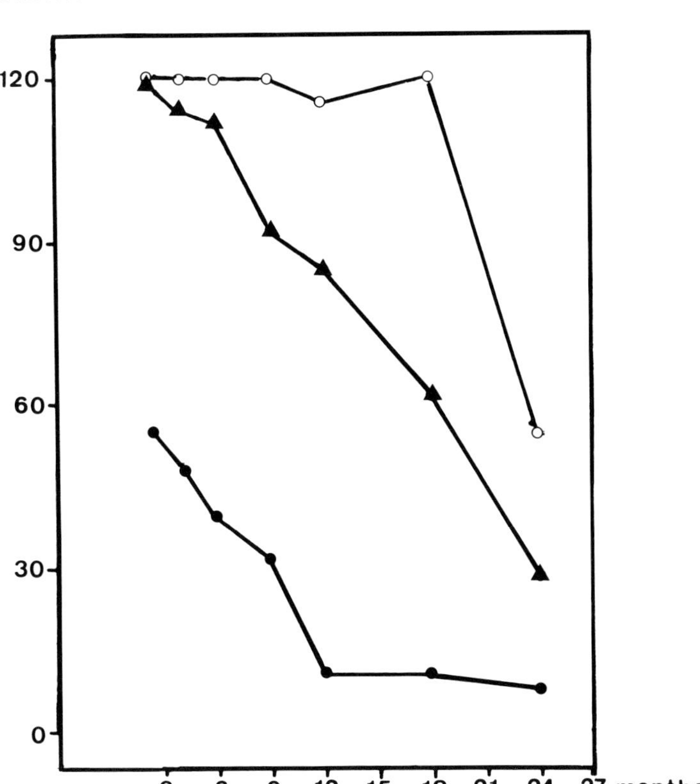

Fig. 2. Age-related decrease of the ability of rats to keep their balance on small horizontal rods. *Open circles,* bridge width 5 cm; *Triangles,* bridge width 2.5 cm; *Solid circles,* round bridge, diameter 2.5 cm. Latency period before falling off is presented

1986). The neurobiological mechanisms underlying this process, however, are hardly understood.

Walking Patterns

When carefully observing old rats as they walk it can be seen that their gait is uncertain. This abnormal walking becomes evident at the age of about 26–28 months and gets worse with increasing age. To study the motor coordination of the hindpaws during walking in more detail we applied a walking pattern test originally described by De Medicanelli et al. (1982). In short, the hindpaws of a rat were dipped into photographic developer. Thereafter the rat had to walk through a corridor giving access to a darkened goalbox. The bottom of the corridor had been covered with a sheet of photographic paper. After walking through the corridor the footprints of the hindpaws of the rat appeared on the paper. Detailed analysis of footprints of young (3 months of age) and 24 to 30 month-old rats revealed that young rats walk on their toes, whereas old rats place also their heels on the surface. Furthermore, the majority of rats aged over 27 months produced prints with abnormal signs which could be regarded as pathological. These abnormal features were:

a) fuzzy footprints as a consequence of lateral rotation of one or both hindfeet after placement on the floor (exorotation),
b) fuzzy prints due to the lack of elevation of the feet at the onset of a new step (dragging feet) and
c) small additional footprints between steps (Fig. 3).

The time of onset of these latter pathological signs varied between animals, but in the course of aging the occurrence and severity of these symptoms increased (Schuurman et al. 1987). The abnormal prints were not related to the bodyweight of the rats, both lean (300 g) and heavy (400–500 g) old rats showed this pathology.

The age-related loss of hindfeet coordination was related to a reduction of the nerve conduction velocity in the sciatic nerve of senescent rats. Histological examination of sciatic nerves of the same rats revealed that fiber density was decreased in aged rats (Gispen et al., this volume). Thus it is tempting to speculate that degenerative processes in the nervous system underly the age-related abnormal walking patterns and the loss of other sensorimotor functions in senescent rats.

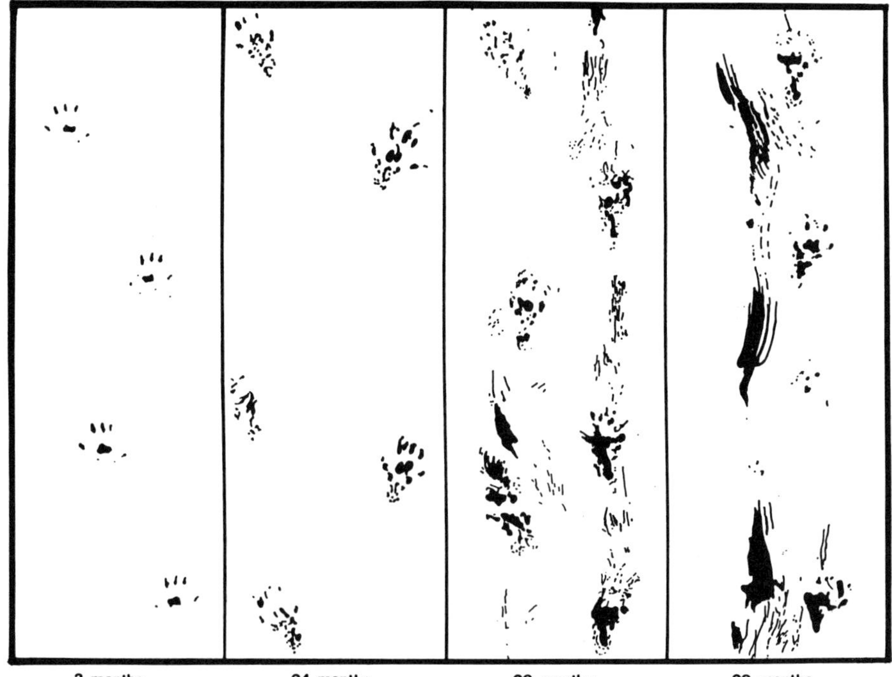

Fig. 3. Footprints of the hindfeet of 3, 24 and 29-month-old rats

Effects of Nimodipine in Old Rats

In the previous sections data have been presented which show that old rats have different behavioural deficits. Besides learning and memory capabilities, social behaviour, the ability to keep balance, other sensorimotor functions and locomotion are affected by aging. The resemblence between these multivariate deficits in the aged rat and the diverse symptoms of demented patients make the old rat a promising model for the study of behavioural aspects of normal and pathological brain aging in humans and for the preclinical evaluation of drugs for the treatment of dementias.

In the following, effects of the centrally active Ca^{2+} entry blocker nimodipine on behaviours of old rats are described.

Effects on Learning in a Water Labyrinth

To study the effects of nimodipine on learning and memory 23 rats, aged 16 months, were subjected to two water maze trials using the maze described above. Thereafter the rats were divided into two groups. The mean number of errors made during the two initial trials and the swimming times did not differ between these groups. After these two drug-free trials one group of animals ($n = 12$) was treated with a daily nimodipine dose of 10 mg/kg (po) for 6 days, whereas the other group ($n = 11$)

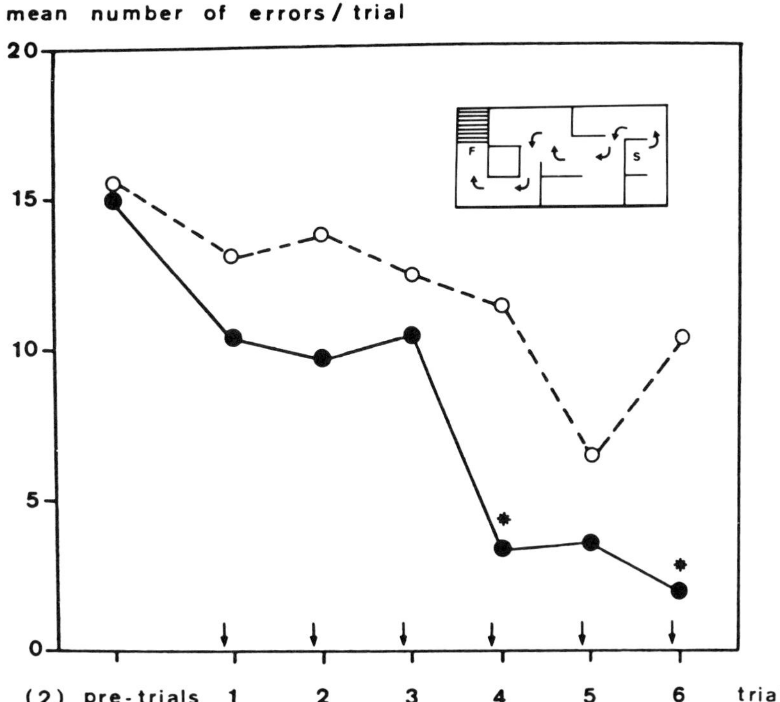

Fig. 4. Learning curves of nimodipine-treated *(solid circles)* and vehicle-treated *(open circles)* 16-month-old rats subjected daily to a water maze test. *Arrows,* nimodipine/vehicle administration

received the nimodipine vehicle. All rats were subjected to a daily trial in the water labyrinth half an hour after administration of nimodipine or its vehicle. The number of errors and swimming times of individual rats were measured, group means were calculated and compared with each other. Fig. 4 shows that both groups of rats made fewer errors in the course of the training procedure. The number of errors of the nimodipine-treated animals, however, decreased faster than that of the vehicle controls. The total number of errors made during the 6 test days differed significantly between the groups ($P < 0.05$, Mann-Whitney U test). The faster learning rate of the rats treated with nimodipine was also expressed in shorter swimming times (data not shown). Also in 27-month-old rats daily treatment with the same dose of nimodipine resulted in improved learning.

In another experiment using a water maze with movable barriers the complexity of the task could be increased during the course of the experiment by changing the maze configuration. Previous experiments showed that the difference between young and old rats in the variable maze are even bigger than in the simple maze with a fixed configuration. The behaviour of 10 rats, aged 26 months, fed for 7 weeks with food containing nimodipine (275 ppm) was compared with that of rats which had been fed with normal food. Figure 5 shows that the nimodipine-treated rats needed less time (P

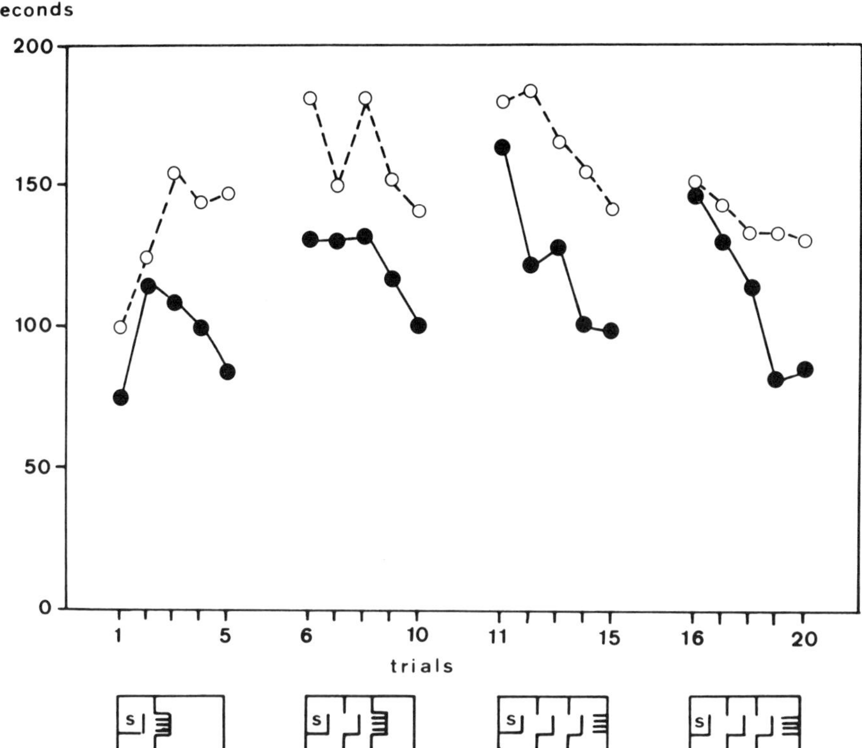

Fig. 5. Mean swimming times of nimodipine-fed old rats *(solid circles)* and normally fed old controls *(open circles)* in a water maze with different degrees of complexity. Rats were subjected to 5 trials per day

< 0.05, Mann-Whitney U test) to escape from the variable maze than normally fed rats. The difference in swimming times was not only found in the beginning of the experiment using the more simple configuration of the maze, but also at the end with the most complex maze configuration. The number of errors, however, was not significantly different between the groups.

The above results and recent data from learning and memory experiments with young, brain-lesioned rats (Le Vere et al. 1988) show that nimodipine may have beneficial effects in animals with impaired learning and memory function. The role of the dose of nimodipine, treatment schedule, age of the animals, test situation and complexity of the task have to be investigated further.

The finding that old rats treated for 7 weeks with food containing nimodipine escaped significantly faster from a complex maze, though making as many errors, than the age-matched controls suggests that nimodipine might improve the ability of the senescent rats to swim. Future studies should anwer the question whether the performance-enhancing effects of nimodipine are a consequence of a drug effect on arousal state, motivation, physical condition or on processes in the CNS more directly involved in learning and memory.

Effects on Exploratory Behaviour

A behavioural characteristic of old rats not mentioned in the previous sections is their reduced exploratory activity in a new environment. This was measured by comparing the behaviour of 3-month-old rats with that of 24–25-month-old rats put into an open field consisting of an observation cage ($60 \times 60 \times 40$ cm) from which the bottom was divided into 16 equal squares. Locomotion of individual rats was measured by counting the number of squares crossed by a rat during a 5-min observation period. Frequency and duration of rearings (vertical movements) were further measurements of exploratory activity. Young, 3-month-old rats ($n = 20$) crossed an average number of 103 ± 7 (SEM) squares, whereas 25-month-old rats ($n = 20$) made 72 ± 10 crossings. We investigated whether nimodipine could reverse this age-related decrease of exploration. Therefore open field behaviour of 20 rats (aged 25 months) fed for 4 weeks with food containing nimodipine (275 ppm) was compared with that of age-matched controls receiving drug-free food. In Table 4 it can be seen that nimodipine-treated old rats were significantly more active than controls. Locomotion and rearing increased, whereas immobility decreased.

One can only speculate about the way in which nimodipine increases exploration in senescent rats. Is it by increasing arousal state or by a reduction of fatigue or fear?

Table 4. Exploratory behaviour of nimodipine-treated 25-month-old rats and nontreated rats in an open field test

Parameter	Vehicle	Nimodipine
Mean ($\pm$ SD) number of crossings	95 ± 10	$112 \pm 8^*$
Mean ($\pm$ SD) number of rearings	15 ± 5	$25 \pm 6^*$
Mean ($\pm$ SD) duration of immobility (s)	108 ± 12	$90 \pm 13^*$

* Significantly different ($P < 0.025$) from vehicle controls (Mann-Whitney U test)

Interestingly, acute oral treatment with 15 mg/kg nimodipine did not stimulate exploratory behaviour of old rats. Thus an amphetamine-like or stimulant-like effect of nimodipine on behaviour can be excluded (see also Hoffmeister et al. 1982).

Effects on Sensorimotor Function

It was suggested above that old rats treated for one or more months with nimodipine (feeding experiment) were in better physical condition than untreated controls. To study this in more detail we applied the sensorimotor tests described. Nimodipine-fed (275 ppm in the food) and normally fed old rats (30 per group) were subjected to balance rod and other tests 4, 6, 12 and 24 weeks after initiation of the drug treatment. Drug treatment was started at the age of 24 and continued till the age of 30 months. After 4 weeks of nimodipine treatment the first sensorimotor tests were conducted. It was found that nimodipine-fed rats remained on the balance rods longer than their controls (Table 5). Also, after 6 and 12 weeks, performance of the drug group was better than that of controls. However, after 24 weeks of treatment, at the age of 30 months, the difference was not significant anymore. A positive effect of chronic nimodipine treatment on sensorimotor function was also observed in other balance tests and in climbing and traction tests (Schuurman et al. 1987). Long-term nimodipine treatment could not prevent, however, senile decay at very old age (28 months) in our Wistar strain.

Table 5. Performance on a balance rod (square, width 5 cm) of nimodipine-treated senescent rats and age-matched controls

Weeks of treatment	Median latency (s) to fall off		P^*
	Control	Nimodipine	
4	56	84	0.01
6	68	90	0.01
12	56	96	0.001
24	44	58	NS

* Mann-Whitney U test

Effects on Walking Patterns

Old rats develop abnormal walking patterns in the course of aging as has been assessed in the footprint test. It was investigated whether long-term treatment with nimodipine could delay or prevent the occurrence of this pathology. A group of 26 senescent rats was fed with nimodipine-containing food (860 ppm), whereas a second group ($n = 26$) received normal food. Treatment was started at 24 and continued until 28 months of age. The rats were subjected to footprint tests at 4-week intervals. In the control rats the percentage of rats with pathological signs increased from 25% to 100% in the course of the experiment, whereas the number of rats with abnormal prints in the nimodipine group increased from 20% to only 40% (Schuurman et al. 1987). Thus, nimodipine treatment delayed the onset of abnormal walking in old age.

In a second experiment we investigated whether nimodipine has beneficial effects in rats already showing the pathology. Ten footprints each of 50 animals, aged 24 months, were analysed. Thereafter the rats were divided into two equal groups. In both groups 50% of the prints showed the pathology described above. One group of rats was fed with food containing nimodipine (850 ppm) for 5 months, whereas the other group was still fed with normal food. Footprint analyses were performed at 4–6-week intervals. In the 6th week of the experiment, the percentage of abnormal footprints had decreased from 47% to 22% in the nimodipine group, whereas in the control group no improvement was measured (Fig. 6). The difference between nimodipine-treated and control rats was maintained during the further course of the experiment.

Between week 16 and 20 a rapid increase of the number of abnormal footprints was observed in both groups. Footprints of nimodipine-treated and nontreated rats were still qualitatively different, however (see Fig. 7).

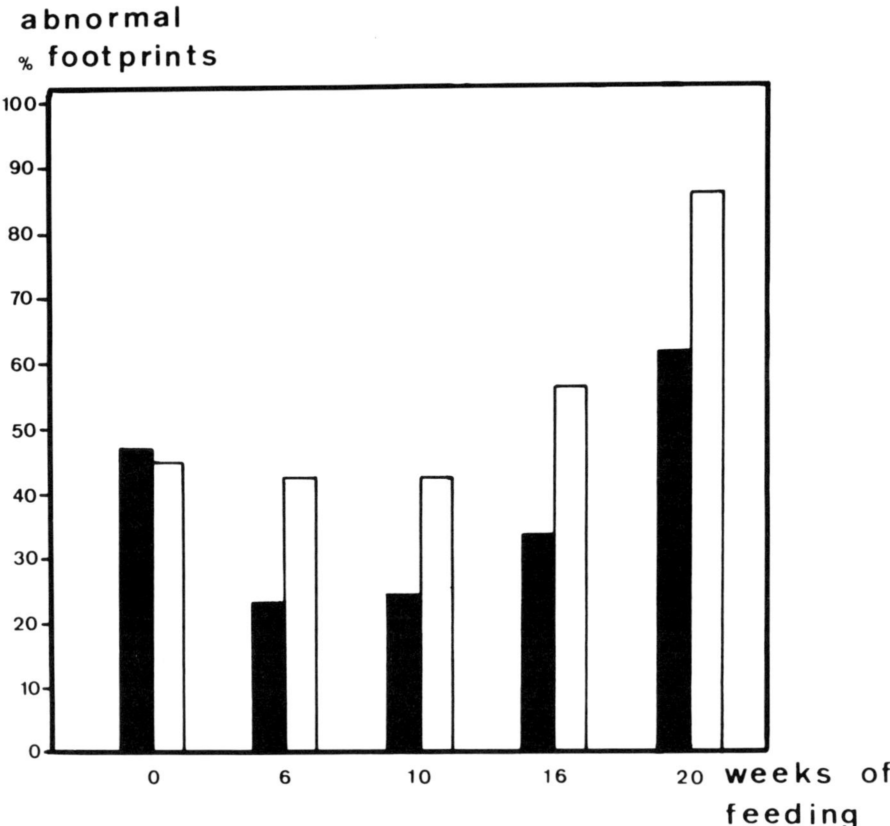

Fig. 6. Abnormal walking patterns of nimodipine-fed *(solid bars)* and normally fed *(open bars)* senescent rats. Drug treatment started at the age of 24 months

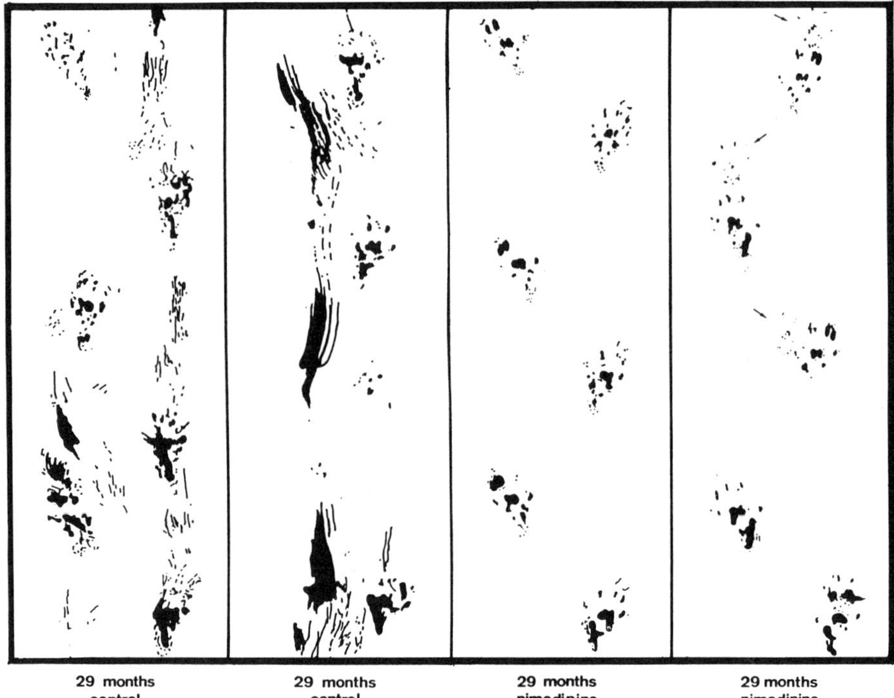

Fig. 7. Footprints of 29-month-old rats fed with normal food and prints of rats fed for 20 weeks with containing food nimodipine

These data show that long-term nimodipine treatment not only delays the onset of abnormal footprints, but also improves the age-related locomotion deficit. Results from electrophysiological and histological studies in the same animals strongly suggest that nimodipine inhibits neurodegenerative processes in the senescent rat (Gispen et al., this volume). This mechanism might explain part of the behavioural effects of nimodipine discussed in this paper.

Conclusions

Behavioural data obtained in old rats showed that the aging process in the rat is accompanied by a reduction or loss of different functions. Besides an impairment of learning and memory capacity, reduced social behaviour, decreased exploratory behaviour and impairment of sensorimotor functions and locomotion are characteristics of senescent rats. This variety of behavioural deficits and their progressive worsening in the course of aging mimics the multivariate symptoms of dementias in humans. Therefore the old rat might be a suitable animal model for the study of behavioural aspects of normal and pathological brain aging in humans and for the preclinical evaluation of geriatric drugs.

One of the proposed drugs for the treatment of dementias is the Ca^{2+} entry blocker nimodipine. Treatment of old rats with this drug resulted in a number of interesting behavioural changes. Exploratory behaviour of senescent rats was increased by nimodipine and learning and memory function as assessed in a water labyrinth was improved. Old rats treated with nimodipine preserved sensorimotor functions better than control rats (balance rod and climbing tests). Furthermore, the age-related walking impairment (footprint test) was significantly inhibited by long-term treatment with nimodipine.

These and other data provide a pharmacological basis for the use of nimodipine in age-related disorders of the nervous system. There is increasing evidence from animal studies (Landfield, this volume) that a dysregulation of Ca^{2+} homeostasis in the brain plays a role in the aging process of the brain, and it is very likely that the behavioural effects of nimodipine in old animals are the consequence of changes in Ca^{2+} currents in neurons.

References

Ader R, Weijnen JAWM, Moleman P (1972) Retention of a passive avoidance response as a function of the intensity and duration of electric shock. Psychon Sci Sect Anim Physiol 26: 125–128

Coper H, Jänicke B, Schulze G (1986) Biophysiological research on adaptivity across the life-span of animals. In: Baltes PD et al. (eds) Life-span development and behavior. Erlbaum, Hillsdale, pp 207–232

De Medicanelli L, Freed WJ, Wyatt RJ (1982) An index of the functional condition of rat sciatic nerve based on measurements made from walking trades. Exp Neurol 77: 634–643

Gage FH, Dunnett SB, Björklund A (1984) Spatial learning and motor deficits in aged rats. Neurobiol Aging 5: 43–48

Giurgea C, Mouravieff-Lesuisse F (1972) Effet facilitateur du piracetam sur un apprentissage repetitif chez le rat. J Pharmacol 3: 17–30

Hoffmeister F, Benz U, Heise A, Krause HP (1982) Behavioral effects of nimodipine in animals. Drug Res 32: 347–360

Le Vere TE, Brugler T, Sandin M, Gray-Silva S (1988) Recovery of function after brain damage. Behav Neural Biol (in press)

Schuurman T, Horváth E, Spencer DG Jr, Traber J (1986) Old rats: an animal model for senile dementia. In: Bès A et al. (ed) Senile dementias: early detection. John Libbey Eurotext, London, pp 624–630

Schuurman T, Klein H, Beneke M, Traber J (1987) Nimodipine and motor deficits in the aged rat. Neurosci Res Comm 1: 9–15

Transfer of Nimodipine and Another Calcium Antagonist Across the Blood-Brain Barrier and Their Regional Distribution In Vivo

W. van den Kerckhoff, and L. R. Drewes

Introduction

It is well kown that calcium currents across the cellular membranes are integrated in the regulatory process of many biological events. While there are complex regulatory systems supervising the equilibrium in the normal physiological state, these systems are strained to the point of ineffectiveness in many pathophysiological situations. In consequence, uncontrolled excessive influx of Ca^{2+} ions into the cells develops, causing a breakdown of the physiological extra-/intracellular concentration gradient: the cells are disregulated and lose their viability and biological potency [10, 25, 40]. The cumulative consequences of this development are diverse pathological reactions.

In recent years, several drugs have been developed to ameliorate those pathological events by diminishing the deleterious transfer of Ca^{2+} ions across the meembranes. These drugs, termed calcium antagonists or calcium entry blockers [17, 23], represent a direct causal therapeutic approach in different pathological disorders [15, 27, 33]. In chemical origin and in preferential efficacy they are heterogeneous.

One important group of those calcium antagonists belongs to the chemical class of the dihydropyridines (DHP). So far the most prominent derivative is nifedipine, well accepted as an effective cardioprotective as well as an antihypertensive drug [33]. Other potent derivatives of the same class have revealed different preferences. One, nimodipine, is characterized by its preferential cerebrovascular [28, 29, 41] and neuro- and psychopharmacological action [26, 39]. The mechanism of its cere-broparenchymal efficacy was explained by the documentation of binding sites for DHP in cerebral membranes in vitro [2, 6, 9, 24, 31, 32] and in vivo [36, 38]. These binding sites are not restricted to nimodipine but are also effective for other calcium antagonists, not only of the DHP type [16].

The question therefore arose of whether the preferential neuronal activity of nimodipine is due to a specific kinetic property that facilitates transfer across the blood-brain barrier (BBB), thus supporting the arrival of an adequate dose at the effector site.

To answer this question, the transfer kinetics across the BBB of nimodipine and, for comparison, nifedipine were studied. We also investigated the same parameters for sucrose, for the following reasons:
1. To test the techniques employed.
2. To compare the findings with published data to make sure that our methods produce reliable and comparable results.

Bergener, Reisberg (Eds.)
Diagnosis and Treatment
of Senile Dementia
© Springer-Verlag Berlin Heidelberg 1989

3. To confirm that the BBB was intact during the experiments.
4. To estimate the "trapped vascular volume".

The investigation was extended to encompass one further point: It is a relatively frequent, routine clinical procedure to estimate the concentration of a drug in the CSF, assuming that the results also represent its concentration in the cerebral parenchyma. It is often assessed from those results whether a drug has been administered in the effective concentration. In order to ascertain whether measurement of nimodipine or nifedipine in the CSF reliably reflects the concentration in the parenchyma, the transfer rates and distributions in the CSF were measured independently.

To extend the comparison between the characteristics of nimodipine and nifedipine, the regional cerebral distribution of both compounds was visualized by the histoautoradiographic technique.

Since it is known that physicochemical properties are limiting factors of the transfer potential across the BBB, we were interested in discovering whether those parameters might be behind the different transfer qualities of these compounds. For this reason the lipophilic characteristics of nimodipine and nifedipine were also evaluated.

Material and Methods

Remarks on the Method Employed

The transendothelial distribution of solutes depends upon a number of factors, including capillary blood flow and permeability [7, 8]. The general situation can be expressed in terms of "conservation of mass" [19]:

$$C_{\text{tis}}(T) = F_0 \int_0^T C_a(t)\, dt - F_0 \int_0^T C_v(t)\, dt \tag{1}$$

where $C_{\text{tis}}(T)$ is the concentration in tissue at time T, F represents the perfusion rate of the tissue, $\int_0^T C_a(t)\, dt$ is the concentration in the arterial blood during the recirculation time, and $\int_0^T C_v(t)\, dt$ represents the concentration in the venous blood during the recirculation time.

From the various techniques available to test different aspects of transfer across the BBB we have chosen "initial uptake rate analysis" after intravenous administration of the test substance. This technique was developed only recently and there are very few reports of its use to date [4, 18, 34]. It has several advantages; for instance, it allows model-independent analysis and provides a good means of quantifying transport across the BBB [for details see 1, 3–5, 12, 14, 19–22, 35]. In this technique the model of the BBB is a general one. It may be a single membrane or a complex system, because no specific time course of arterial concentration is assumed and no particular arrangement or number of compartments in the system is presupposed [11, 14, 35].

We performed the experiments using the "integral method with multiple time series." Basically, this method involves the determination of the amount of tracer present in the brain tissue at various times after an intravenous bolus injection of the radioactive substance. It is based on the relationship

$$C^*_{\text{tis}}(T) - C^*_{\text{vasc}}(T) = K_{\text{in}} \int_0^T C^*_a(t)\, dt \tag{2}$$

deduced from Eq. 1, where $C^*_{\text{tis}}(T)$ is the concentration of substance in the cerebral tissue at time T, $C^*_{\text{vasc}}(T)$ is the amount of substance trapped in the vascular space of the tissue sample, K_{in} is the "influx constant" or "initial transfer constant," which may also be called "clearance constant," and $_0\!\int^T C^*_a(t)\,dt$ is the integrated concentration-time curve until the time T [18, 20].

The most elegant and most informative way to interpret these results is to apply the "graphical analysis". It is published only from a few groups but a careful detailed deduction was published recently [35].

To prepare the results for the graphical analysis, the described general relationship (Eq. 2) is rearranged and both sites of the equation are divided by $C^*_a(T)$:

$$\frac{C^*_{\text{tis}}(T)}{C^*_a(T)} = K_{\text{in}}\; _0\!\int^T \cdot \frac{C^*_a(t)\,dt}{C^*_a(T)} + \frac{C^*_{\text{vasc}}(T)}{C^*_a(T)} \tag{3}$$

where the left equality denotes the "apparent volume of distribution" in milliliters per gram,

$$\frac{C^*_{\text{vasc}}(T)}{C^*_a(T)}$$

is the trapped vascular volume of the tissue in milliliters per gram, and

$$_0\!\int^T \frac{C^*_a(t)\,dt}{C^*_a(T)}$$

forms the "concentration-time integral", normalized for the concentration in the arterial blood at the end of the distribution time and expressed as a fictive time in minutes.

In the graphical analysis of this relation the expression

$$_0\!\int^T \frac{C^*_a(T)\,dt}{C^*_a(T)}$$

forms the abscissa, while

$$\frac{C^*_{\text{tis}}(T)}{C^*_a(T)}$$

is projected as the ordinate.

This analysis allows the determination of three parameters of interest:
1. K_{in}, the unidirectional influx or transfer constant that may also be called a clearance constant. It is derived from the initial straight slope of the resultant curve and expressed in milliliters per gram per minute.
2. The "apparent volume of distribution" (V; milliliters per gram) and its development during the experiment. It can be read from the ordinate.
3. Information on the compartmentalization of the BBB and the trapped vascular volume within the tested tissue. This can be derived from the ordinate intercept.

Test Substances and Materials

The radiolabeled test substances were tritiated nimodipine and nifedipine and [^{14}C]sucrose:
- [i-Pro-^{3}H]nimodipine (New England Nuclear)
  Specific activity: 150–160 Ci/mmol
  Radiochemical purity: 98% (repeatedly tested by thin layer radio-chromatography)
  Solution: ethanol
- [3-Methyl-^{3}H]nifedipine (New England Nuclear)
  Specific activity: 70–80 Ci/mmol
  Solution: ethanol
- [^{14}C(U)]sucrose (New England Nuclear)
  Specific activity: 0.6–1.5 Ci/mmol
  Solution: ethanol:water (9:1)

After each sampling from the stock solution the substances were stored under nitrogen gas at $-20°C$, and protected against light to avoid oxidation and radiolysis.

As tissue solubilizer, a mixture of soluene-350:n-butanol (1:1) was prepared. The samples were bleached with 30% H_2O_2 and neutralized with HCl (1 N). Unisolve 1 (Packard Instruments) served as scintillation cocktail.

Surgical Procedure

Male Wistar rats (Winkelmann) weighing 260–320 g were used. Under halothane anesthesia both femoral arteries and one femoral vein were catheterized. Following tracheotomy, the animals were injected with Curarin-Asta (2 mg/kg) for muscle relaxation and were artificially ventilated using a positive pressure respirator (Braun, Melsungen).

After preparation the animals were kept on 0.8% halothane and allowed to recover to a physiological steady state. This was confirmed by continuous measurement of blood pressure, heart rate, and temperature and intermittent measurement of acid-base status, Na^+ and K^+ concentrations in the blood (T 55, Eschweiler, Kiel), hematocrit (by centrifugation), and glucose concentration (glucose analyzer 23A, YSI, USA).

Transfer evaluation and preparation for assessment of regional distribution were started only when a steady state was achieved.

Experimental Procedure

Determination of Transfer Kinetics

Transfer measurements were initiated by starting the constant withdrawal of arterial blood – by means of a mechanical pump – to determine the "concentration-time integral". In parallel, the test solutes were administered by rapid (1 s) intravenous injection. These solutes were freshly prepared from the stock solutions: about 20 µCi [³H]nimodipine and 5 µCi [¹⁴C]sucrose were mixed. The volume was reduced with a light stream of nitrogen and then diluted with physiological saline to a total volume of 210 µl. [³H]Nifedipine was processed in the same way. With this procedure, the concentration of the solvent ethanol remained lower than 3% in the injected medium. The radioactivity of an aliquot was counted to normalize the injected material for the indicated activity.

At different intervals from 20 s to 600 s after injection of the tracers, the distribution was stopped either by decapitation of the animals or by sampling of CSF. In the use of decapitation, the brains were rapidly removed from the calvarium and pieces of the parietal cortex of both hemispheres (each about 70 mg) were sampled. In the case of CSF sampling, CSF was withdrawn using fine-tipped micropipettes after puncturing the cisterna magna: volumes of 20–50 µl were collected.

Parallel to the decapitation or CSF sampling, an arterial blood sample was withdrawn to determine the actual arterial concentration of the drug at the end of the circulation time. Cortical tissue or CSF, blood, and plasma were digested with 1.5 ml of the solubilizer (12 h), bleached with 0.5 ml 30% H_2O_2, and neutralized with HCl and the scintillation cocktail was added. Conventional liquid scintillation counting was performed to determine the radioactivity in the samples. The results were converted to dpm by means of standard quench corrections.

The data were prepared for graphical analysis as described above using a procedure integrated into a computer system. The graphs and statistical analyses were executed in the same PC system on the basis of the internally generated tables and calculations.

Visualization of Regional Distribution of Test Compound In Vivo

To avoid the danger of misleading interpretations owing to accidental distribution after bolus injection of the compounds, continuous infusion over a period of 3 min was performed using an infusion pump: 500 µl [³H]nimodipine or [³H]nifedipine, each diluted to a volume of 1 ml with NaCl, was infused. Thirty seconds before the end of the infusion the freezing of the heads was started by pouring liquid nitrogen onto the exposed calvarium. To maintain the cerebral supply of the not yet frozen tissue with blood and compound via the carotid arteries, a special procedure was developed that avoided direct contact between the nitrogen and the relevant circulation system.

After freezing for 5 min, the rats were decapitated. The brains were cut into 20 µm coronal sections at −10°C using a freezing microtome. The sections were mounted on glass slides and freeze-dried cautiously to avoid artifacts of tissue structure.

The sections were then exposed to a tritium-sensitive film for 3 weeks and developed using standard procedures.

The parallel processing meant that the resulting autoradiograms showing the regional cerebral distribution of [³H]nimodipine or [³H]nifedipine, were comparable.

Table. 1. General physiological variables of the animals before application of nifedipine or nimodipine

		Nifedipine	Nimodipine
pH		7.37 ± 0.02	7.40 ± 0.02
pO_2	[mmHg]	$107 \quad \pm 2$	$108 \quad \pm 4$
pCO_2	[mmHg]	38.7 ± 0.4	36.5 ± 0.8
Hct	[Vol%]	43.9 ± 0.6	46.3 ± 0.8
Na^+	[mmol/l]	$122 \quad \pm 5$	$128 \quad \pm 4.1$
K^+	[mmol/l]	4.2 ± 0.4	3.9 ± 0.2
Glucose	[mmol/l]	9.8 ± 0.3	9.1 ± 0.6
mBP	[mmHg]	$98 \quad \pm 4$	$102 \quad \pm 2$
Weight	[g]	$305 \quad \pm 6$	$300 \quad \pm 3$
Values are the mean $\pm$ SEM of		$n = 35$	$n = 80$

Results

Throughout the experiments the animals were in a respiratory steady state and under normal physiological conditions (Table 1). Also, hypermetabolism or stress could be excluded by the measurements of blood pressure and blood glucose concentration.

Transfer Kinetics from Blood to Brain and from Blood to CSF for [^{14}C]Sucrose, [^{3}H]Nimodipine and [^{3}H]Nifedipine

Hardly any [^{14}C]sucrose was transported across the BBB. The graphical analysis is shown in Fig. 1. The value for the initial transfer constant K_{in} amounted to only 0.0007

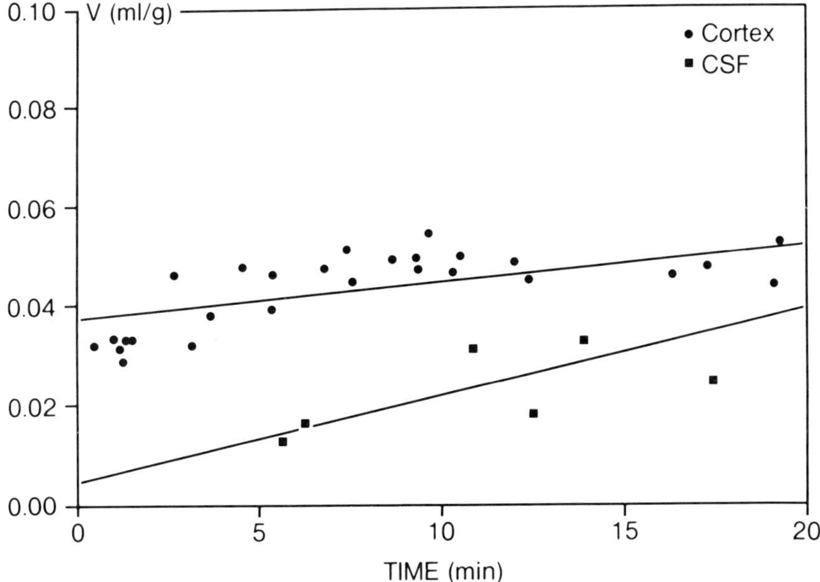

Fig. 1. Transfer kinetics of sucrose to cortex/CSF

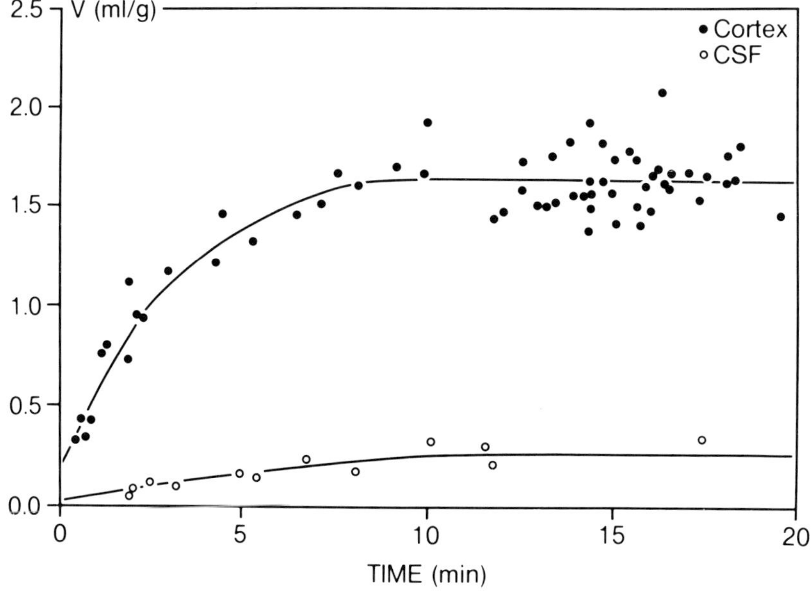

Fig. 2. Transfer kinetics of nimodipine to cortex/CSF

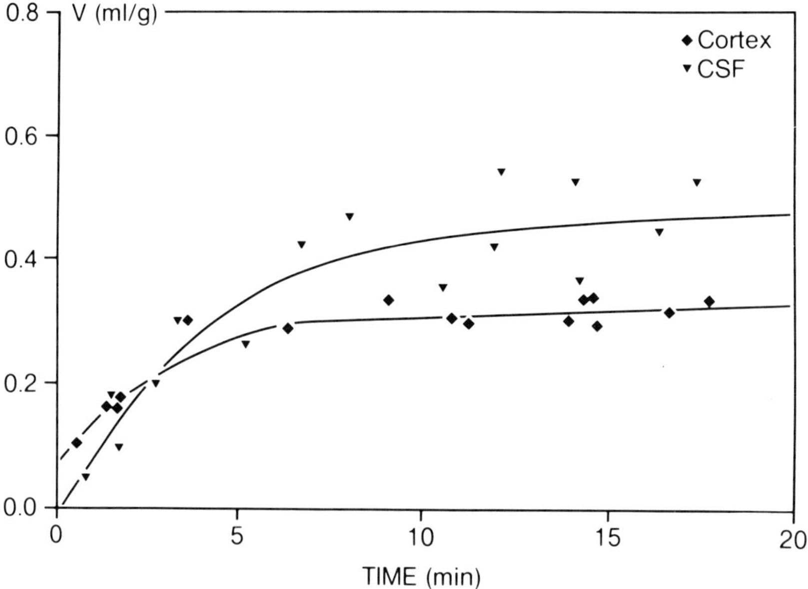

Fig. 3. Transfer kinetics of nifedipine to cortex/CSF

$\pm$ 0.0001 ml/g/min and the apparent distribution volume V increased very slowly but steadily.

Nimodipine (Fig. 2) is transported at a high rate across the BBB, as indicated by a value for K_{in} of 0.378 $\pm$ 0.054 ml/g/min. The value for V was 1.637 $\pm$ 0.121 ml/g. For the transfer of nimodipine from blood to CSF we found that K_{in} was 0.023 $\pm$ 0.006 ml/g/min while V was 0.252 $\pm$ 0.064 ml/g.

The BBB transport rates for nifedipine (Fig. 3) were distinctly lower: $K_{in} = 0.068 \pm$ 0.007 ml/g/min, $V = 0.292 \pm 0.016$ ml/g. Across the blood-CSF barrier, K_{in} was 0.088 $\pm$ 0.033 ml/g/min and V was 0.383 $\pm$ 0.089 ml/g.

Lipophilic Properties and Regional Distribution In Vivo of [³H]Nimodipine and [³H]Nifedipine in Rat Brains

Evaluation of the specific lipophilic properties of both compounds showed that nimodipine was distinctly more lipophilic than nifedipine (Table 2).

Table 2. Parameters of lipophilicity of nimodipine and nifedipine (expressed as R_m and log P values)

compound	R_m	log P
Nimodipine	+ 0.017	3.29
Nifedipine	− 0.144	2.35

As relevant examples of the regional distribution in vivo of both test compounds, two related sections from in the parietal region of the brains are presented (Fig. 4). The upper part of the figure represents the regional distribution of [³H]nimodipine in contrast to that of [³H]nifedipine. The different degree of blackening gives a relative measure of the corresponding concentration of the compounds in the respective structures.

The difference in the intensities of the two sections is obvious at first glance, implying a generally lower transfer of nifedipine. This impression is strengthened by the comparatively high intensity in the vascular system, exemplified by the sinus of the [³H]nifedipine-perfused brain (lower section). The generally low concentration of [³H]nifedipine is distributed relatively smoothly, even between grey and white matter. No specific affinity to circumscribed structures is indicated.

In comparison, [³H]nimodipine shows high concentrations in several structures of the brain and a remarkably low concentration in the sinus. This indicates a high extraction rate from the blood into the brain tissue. It is also obvious that the distribution of nimodipine is highly uneven, with only low activity in the white matter. High concentrations of nimodipine are located in the cortex, the dentate gyrus, and the hippocampus. Most of these structures are known to have high densities of specific binding sites.

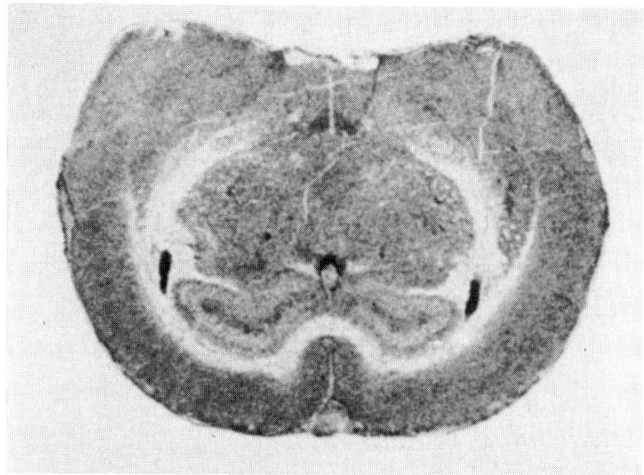

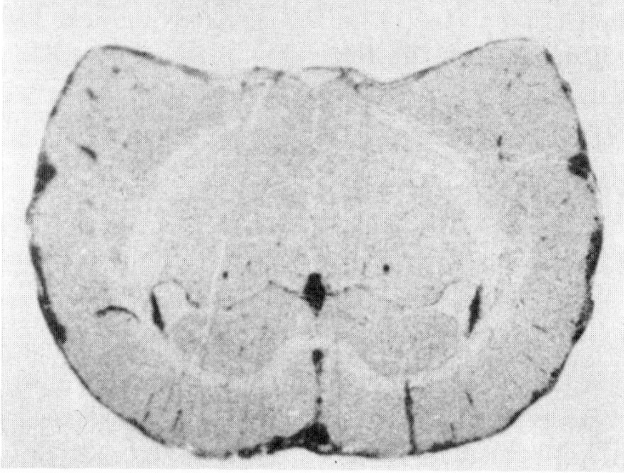

Fig. 4. Regional distribution of nimodipine (above) and nifedipine (below)

Discussion

As shown in Table 1, the animals were in physiological steady state. Thus, the differences determined in transfer or distribution potency really are related to the specific properties of the substances.

In these experiments the transfer of [^{14}C]sucrose is shown to be very low, in good agreement with the literature [21] (Table 3, 4). It is thus confirmed that sucrose is a vascular marker that cannot penetrate the blood brain barrier. The low transfer of [^{14}C]sucrose shows that the technique employed in these experiments was valid, that the extraparenchymal distribution volume for [^{14}C]sucrose was stable, and that the BBB remained intact during the experiments. In consequence, the results for nimodipine or nifedipine depend purely on the different kinetic properties of the two drugs.

In parallel with the measurements of the transfer of sucrose and of nimodipine in the same animals, it was striking that nimodipine passes the BBB to a great extent, as shown by the apparent distribution volume V and the initial transfer constant K_{in}. The

Table 3. Transfer constants and apparent distribution volumes in cortex and CSF for sucrose, nifedipine, and nimodipine

	Compound	$K_{in} \pm$ S.D. (ml $\times$ g^{-1} x min)	SIGN. LEV. P	$V_m \pm$ S.D. (ml/g)	SIGN. LEV. P	$V_i \pm$ S.D. (ml/g)	SIGN. LEV. P
parietal cortex	Sucrose	0.0007 ± 0.0001	< 0.001	∞	$-$	0.037 ± 0.002	< 0.001
	Nifedipine	0.068 ± 0.007	< 0.001	0.292 ± 0.016	< 0.001	0.065 ± 0.014	< 0.01
	Nimodipine	0.378 ± 0.054	< 0.001	1.637 ± 0.121	< 0.001	0.179 ± 0.087	< 0.05
CSF	Nifedipine	0.068 ± 0.007	< 0.001	0.383 ± 0.089	< 0.005	0.065 ± 0.014	< 0.01
	Nimodipine	0.023 ± 0.006	< 0.02	0.252 ± 0.064	< 0.01	0.026 ± 0.021	< 0.3

Table 4. Cerebral vascular permeability of various substances

Compound	K^* in (ml//100 mg $\times$ min)
Iodoantipyrine	83
Water	81
Flunitrazepam	67
Nimodipine	38
D-Glucose	15
Mannitol	0.24
Sucrose	0.075

transfer of nimodipine was also remarkably high in comparison to other reference substances whose transfer constants were determined using the same technique, (Table 4) D-glucose, for example, which is transferred by means of "facilitated diffusion," shows a K_{in} of only 0.15 ml/g/min, less than half that for nimodipine. The highest values for K_{in} were found for substances like iodoantipyrine and water, with about 0.8 ml/g/min. These substances are accepted as compounds which diffuse freely across the BBB and were chosen as tracers for the quantification of cerebral blood flow. Since the transfer constant for nimodipine amounts to about 50% of those for iodeantipyrine and water, it is concluded that nimodipine crosses the BBB eaadily with only slight limitation of diffusion.

The "apparent distribution" volume of nimodipine stabilized after about 180 s of circulation at the high level of about 1.6 ml/g. This indicates that the partitition coefficient of nimodipine between blood and brain is greater than 1 and suggests that a certain amount of nimodipine is in a bound rather than a free form, substantiating the observation of specific membrane binding sites in the brain.

Measurement of the transfer of drugs from blood to CSF has not been reported by others before, so no comparable results for other compounds are available from the literature. A few published experiments measured the transfer from CSF to brain parenchyma after the administration of drugs via the cisterna magna [37]. Our results clearly indicate a distinctly lower transfer to the CSF as well as a very low distribution volume. From the low apparent distribution volume it is concluded that nimodipine is distributed freely (unbound) in the CSF. The low degree of transfer into the CSF corroborates the results using histoautoradiographical techniques after continuous infusion of the tracer [30].

The transfer of nifedipine (Fig. 3) to the cortical parenchyma is less than one-fifth that of nimodipine. This indicates a remarkable limitation of diffusion across the BBB for nifedipine. The "apparent distribution volume" is also much smaller than that of nimodipine, so it can be concluded that there is little specific binding throughout the parenchyma or that the area of specific binding is very small. The latter can be excluded from the estimation of the regional distribution (Fig. 4).

The low "apparent distribution volume" of nifedipine is not a consequence of the low transfer rate across the BBB. This is clear from the plateau that was achieved within 2 min (Fig. 4). If there were a potentially large distribution volume that needed longer to reach equilibrium, the graph would show a steady slope, not a plateau. An example of such a slope is provided by flunitrazepam, with an "apparent distribution volume" of ∞ [19].

Interestingly, the transfer of nifedipine across the BBB (Fig. 3) is quite similar to that across the blood-CSF barrier. This suggests that for nifedipine the BBB is nearly equivalent to the blood-CSF barrier, in contrast to nimodipine.

These results may also be important for another reason: As mentioned in the Introduction, it is fairly routine to measure the concentration of a drug in the CSF in order to check the effective dosage or to test the "transfer to the brain." From the present data – showing a quite different transfer of the substances to the brain parenchyma than to the CSF – it is evident that the concentration of a drug in the CSF does not, a priori, allow any prediction as to its distribution or concentration in the brain parenchyma.

It is also clear from these experiments that nimodipine and nifedipine do not reach the CSF via the brain parenchyma. The graphical analysis shows that both radiolabeled compounds are found in the CSF immediately after intravenous administration – though in very low amounts. If they only reached the CSF via the brain parenchyma there would have been a delay especially since the samples were taken from the pooled CSF in the cisterna magna.

It is striking that the abilities of nifedipine and nimodipine to transfer across the BBB are so different since the two compounds are quite closely related in chemical structure.

It is well known that high lipophilia is a prerequisite for effective transfer across the BBB. By quantification of the lipophilic properties of the test compounds both techniques employed demonstrated, in very good agreement, that nimodipine is distinctly more lipophilic than nifedipine (Table 2). Comparing these results and the estimated transfer characteristics it seems clear that these different lipophilic properties are one reason for the differences in capacity for transfer across the BBB.

In conclusion, we found that our newly established technique is a valuable aid in quantifying several parameters of the blood-to-tissue transfer kinetics. It gives detailed information on the dynamic processes.

The most important result of these experiments (summarized in Fig. 5) is the impressive demonstration that nimodipine crosses the BBB easily, quickly, and to a

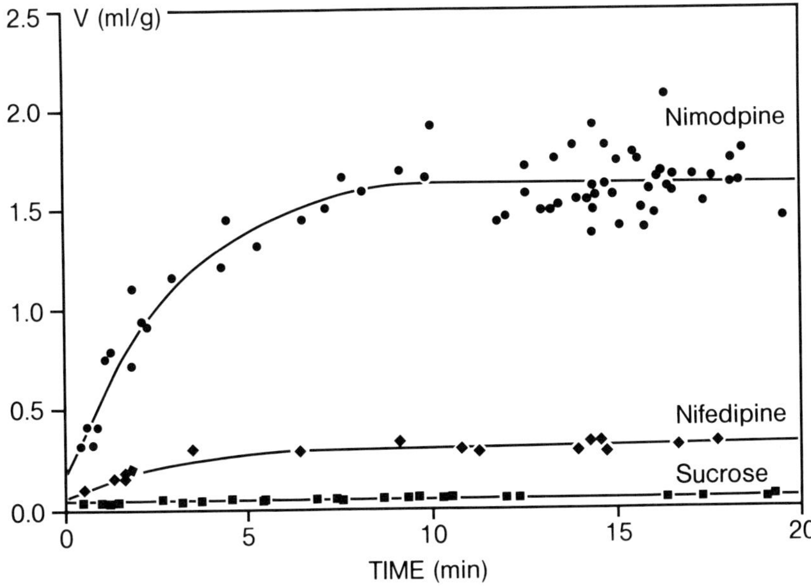

Fig. 5. Transfer kinetics of nimodipine, nifedipine, sucrose to cortex

considerable degree. The regional distribution corroborates these results, documenting a low, unspecific transfer of nifedipine and a contrasting high transfer of nimodipine with specific affinity to structures with noteworthy concentrations of binding sites. Since nifedipine shows a much lower transfer rate and is less effective in the brain parenchyma, it is possible that the pronounced transfer and the specific distribution of nimodipine are reasons for the preferential action of the latter compound against cerebral pathologic processes.

Summary

To quantify the transfer of nimodipine and nifedipine across the blood-brain and blood-CSF barrier the "integral method" with graphical analysis was employed in rats.

Nimodipine passes the blood-brain barrier quickly and to a considerable extent, this perhaps explaining its preferential effect in the central nervous system. However, the blood-brain barrier rather strongly resists the transfer of nifedipine into the cerebral parenchyma. The drugs do not reach the CSF via the brain parenchyma. The blood-CSF barrier is nearly equally resistant to the transfer of nimodipine and nifedipine.

The regional distribution of nimodipine, with high concentrations in specific brain structures, corroborates the kinetic data. The congruent findings with both techniques may explain the preferential potency of nimodipine against cerebral pathologic processes.

References

1. Banos G, Daniel PM, Moorhouse SR, Pratt OE (1973) The influx of amino acids into the brain of the rat in vivo: the essential compared with non-essential amino acids. Proc Roy Soc Lond B 183: 59–70
2. Bellemann P, Schade A, Towart R (1983) Dihydropyridine receptor in rat brain labelled with ^{3}H-nimodipine. Proc Natl Acad Sci USA 80: 2356–2360
3. Blasberg RG, Gazendam J, Patlak C, Fenstermacher J (1980) Quantitative autoradiographical studies of brain edema and comparison of multi-isotopes.1 In: Cervos-Navarro J, Ferszt R (eds) Brain edema. Proc Int Symp Berlin 1979. Raven, New York, pp 255–270 (Adv Neurol 28)
4. Blasberg RG, Fenstermacher JD, Patlak CS (1983) Transport of alpha-aminoisobutyric acid across the brain capillary and cellular membranes. J Cerebr Blood flow Metab 3: 8–32
5. Bradbury MWB, Kleeman CR (1967) Stability of the potassium content of cerebrospinal fluid and brain. Am J Physiol 213: 519–528
6. Cortes R, Supavilai P, Karobath M, Palacios JM (1983) The effects of lesions in the rat hippocampus suggest the association of calcium channel blocker binding sites with specific neuronal population. Neurosci Lett 42: 249–254
7. Crone C (1963) Permeability of capillaries in various organs as determined by use of indicator diffusion method. Acta Physiol Scand 58: 292–305
8. Crone C (1965) The permeability of brain capillaries to non-electrolytes. Acta Physiol Scand 64: 407–417
9. Ehlert FJ, Itoga E, Roeske WR, Yamamura HJ (1982) The interaction of ^{3}H-nimodipine with receptors for Ca-antagonists in the cerebral cortex and heart of rats. Biochem Biophys Res Commun 104: 937–943
10. Farber JL, Chien KR, Mittnacht S (1981) The pathogenesis of irreversible cell injury in ischemia. Am J Pathol 102: 271–281
11. Fenstermacher JD (1983) Drug transfer across the blood-brain barrier. In: Breimer DD, Speiser P (eds) Topics in pharmaceutical sciences. Elsevier Science, Amsterdam, pp 143–154
12. Fenstermacher JP, Rapoport SJ (1984) Blood Brain Barrier. In: Handbook of Physiology, Vol. 4, II Microcirculation Chap 21, p 969–1000
13. Fenstermacher JD, Patlak C, Blasberg R (1979) A new method of estimting plasma to tissue transfer contents. Fed Proc 38: 1138
14. Fenstermacher JD, Blasberg RG, Patlak CS (1981) Methods for quantifying the transport of drugs across brain barrier systems. Pharmacol Ther 14: 217–248
15. Ferry DR, Goll A, Rombusch M, Glossmann H (1985) The molecular pharmacology and structural features of calcium channels. Br J Clin Pharmacol 20: 233S–246S
16. Ferry DR, Goll A, Gadov C, Glossmann H (1984) (−) ^{3}H-Desmethyl-verapamil labelling of putative calcium channels in brain: autoradiographic distribution and allosteric coupling to 1,4-dihydropyridine and diltiazem binding sites. Naunyn Schmiedebergs Arch Pharmacol 327: 183–187
17. Fleckensten A (1983) History of calcium antagonists. Circ Res 52: 3–16
18. Gjedde A (1980) Rapid steady-state analysis of blood-brain glucose transfer in rat. Acta Physiol Scand 108: 331–339
19. Gjedde A, Rasmussen M (1980) Blood-brain glucose transport in the conscious rat: comparison of the intravenous and intracarotid injection methods. J Neurochem 35: 1382–1387
20. Gjedde A, Hansen AJ, Siemkowicz E (1980) Rapid simultaneous determination of regional blood flow and blood-brain glucose transfer in brain of rat. Acta Physiol Scand 108: 321–330
21. Gjedde A, Drewes LR, Christensen B (1983) Brain uptake of a "fluid microsphere": Comparison of Flunitrazepam, water and iodoantipyrine transfer across the blood-brain barrier. J Cerebr Blood Flow Metab 3 [Suppl 1]: S73–S74
22. Go KG, Pratt JJ (1975) The dependence of the blood to brain passage of radioactive sodium on blood pressure and temperature. Brain Res 93: 329–336
23. Godfraind T (1979) Alternative mechanism for the potentiation of the relaxation evoked by isoprenaline in aortae from young and aged rats. Eur J Pharmacol 53: 273–279
24. Gould RJ, Murphy KMM, Snyder SH (1982) ^{3}H-nitrendipine labelled calcium channels discriminate inorganic Ca agonists and antagonists. Proc Natl Acad Sci USA

25. Hass WK (1981) Beyond cerebral blood flow, metabolism and ischemic thresholds: an examination of the role of calcium in the initiation of cerebral infarction. In: Proceedings of 10th International Salzburg Conference on Cerebral Vascular Disease. Excerpta Medica, Amsterdam, pp 3–17
26. Hoffmeister F, Benz U, Heise A, Krause HP, Neuser V (1982) Behavioral effects of nimodipine in animals. Arzneimittelforsch/Drug) Res 32: 347–360
27. Katz AM, Hager WD, Messineo FC, Pappano AJ (1985) Cellular actions and pharmacology of the calcium channel blocking drugs. Am J Med 79 (4A): 2–10
28. Kazda S, Towart R (1982) Nimodipine: a new calcium antagonistic drug with a preferential cerebrovascular action. Acta Neurochir 63: 259–265
29. Kazda S, Garthoff B, Krause HP, Schloßmann K (1982) Cerebrovascular effects of the calcium antagonistic dihydropyridine derivative nimodipine in animal experiments. Arzneimittelforsch/Drug Res 32 (4): 331–338
30. van den Kerckhoff W, Steinke W (in preparation) The regional distribution of nimodipine, nifedipine and sucrose in vivo.
31. Lee HR, Roeske WR, Yamamara HJ (1984) High-affinity specific ^{3}H PN 200–110 binding to dihydropyridine receptors associated with calcium channels in rat cerebral cortex and heart. Life Sci 35: 721–732
32. Marangos PJ, Patel J, Miller C, Martino AM (1982) Specific calcium antagonist binding sites in brain. Life Sci 31: 1575–1585
33. Murphy KMM, Snyder SH (1982) Calcium antagonistic receptor binding sites labelled with ^{3}H-nitrendipine. Eur J Pharmacol 77: 201
34. Nayler WG, Grinwald P (1981) Calcium entry blockers and myocardial function. Fed Proc 40, 2855–2861
35. Ohno K, Pettigrew KD, Rapoport SJ (1978) Lower limits of cerebrovascular permeability to non-electrolytes in the conscious rat. Am J Physiol 235: H229–H307
36. Patlak CS, Fenstermacher JD (1975) Measurements of dog blood-brain transfer constants by ventriculocisternal perfusion. Am J Physiol 229: 877–884
37. Patlak CS, Blasberg RG, Fenstermacher JD (1983) Graphical evaluation of blood to brain transfer constants from multiple-time uptake data. J Cerebr Blood Flow Metab 3: 1–7
38. Quirion R (1983) Autoradiographic localization of a calcium channel antagonist, ^{3}H nitrendipine, binding site in rat brain. Neurosci Lett 36: 267–271
39. Scriabine A, Battye R, Hoffmeiste F, Kazda S, Towart R, Garthoff B, Schlüter G, Rämsch D, Scherling D (1985) Nimodipine. In: Scriabine A (ed) New drugs annual: cardiovascular drugs, vol 3. Raven, New York, pp 197–218
40. Shoemaker H, Lee HR, Roeske WR, Yamamura HJ (1983) In vivo identification of Ca antagonist binding sites using ^{3}H nitrendipine. Eur J Pharmacol 88: 275–276
41. Siesjö BK (1981) Cell damage in the brain: speculative synthesis. J Cerebr Blood Flow Metab 1: 155–185
42. Towart R, Wehinger E, Meyer H, Kazda S (1982) The effects of nimodipine, its optical isomers and metabolites on isolated vascular smooth muscles. Arzneimittelforsch/Drug Res 32 (4): 338–346

Tissue and Cellular Protective Effects of Nimodipine

R. L. Isaacson, J. M. Fahey, A. M. Danks, D. L. Maier, A. H. Mandel, and R. Van Buskirk

It is generally agreed that there is some point in the accumulation of intracellular calcium ions that, when exceeded, results in cellular dysfunction as well as the actual death of cells. Cells subject to this calcium-mediated trauma include nerve cells but other types of cells are also subject to this sort of damage. Prominent among such other types of cells are those of the heart, expecially those involved in the pacing of its functions, and the vasculature.

Calcium is a ubiquitous substance in the body that plays a vast number of different roles in cellular metabolism, the release of transmitters and other substances, and likely participates in many types of reactions that are beyond our imagination at the present time. One of the more interesting aspects of calcium metabolism is the large number of ways in which this ion can be bound and unbound in the cell after changes of the external and internal melieux.

One of the most intense lines of research being followed in our laboratory at the present time has to do with the role of calcium in cellular dysfunction and cell death caused in several different ways. In general, we are following the following hypotheses. Postischemic conditions and other toxic factors act to depolarize cell membranes and terminals. These conditions lead to the opening of some voltage-sensitive channels for longer than usual or more frequently in response to ongoing neuronal events. The depolarization of the terminals may lead to a greater release of transmitters than normal. Recently much attention has centered directly on the enhanced release of the excitatory amino acids. However, other transmitters may well be involved. In any case the increase in unbound intracellular calcium is thought to be an important cause of cellular disaster, although there is some disagreement as to just what aspect of the cellular response to this additional cytosolic calcium is most lethal. It is possible that calcium acts more or less directly on mitochondrial mechanisms but it is also likely that more complicated mechanisms are involved, such as the translocation of protein kinase C to neuronal membranes. The extra load of intracellular calcium is also likely to activate the production of additional amounts, and perhaps types, of enzymes that are problems for the cell.

Because it is now possible to reduce some of the influx of calcium into the neuron by the blocking of some of the calcium channels, we have undertaken to determine the extent to which the antagonism of the voltage-sensitive L channel (i.e., Miller 1987) can preserve cells in the face of hypoxic and toxic insults. Generally, we have concentrated our efforts on the effects provided by the drug nimodipine, although as a general principle we like to study, in parallel, the effects of equimolar doses of a

Bergener, Reisberg (Eds.)
Diagnosis and Treatment
of Senile Dementia
© Springer-Verlag Berlin Heidelberg 1989

calcium channel antagonist of a different drug family, i. e., verapamil. This drug is a phenylalkamine and not a dihydropyridine. Our view is that if similar qualitative effects are found with the two drugs, they are likely due to the calcium-related effects of the drugs and not to other changes in the biochemistry of the nervous system particular to a class of drugs.

Our approach to understanding the possible protection that can be provided nerve cells against insults differs from those of most other laboratories in two other ways. First, we try to establish situations where experiments testing the same or similar hypotheses can be undertaken in both cell cultures and in intact, or almost intact, animals. Second, we wish to establish a behavioral basis for determining whether or not our intervention with calcium ion entry produces effects on the behavioral disturbances usually produced by the insults. After all, it would be of little use to show substantial protection of cells from hypoxic insult and find that this protection, viewed histologically, was simply cosmetic and did not alter the behavioral effects of the trauma. Furthermore, coupling the behavioral and the histologic approaches tends to limit the possibility that a drug that can hasten the repair of one type of neural insult, such as the crush of a nerve tract (e. g., De Koning and Gispen 1987), also produces untoward behavioral disturbances in a different kind (e. g., Hannigan and Isaacson 1984).

In articles such as this, it is always a difficult matter to select which data to present. It is expecially true in our case where we have several dimensions of experiments from which to select. However, we have decided to first provide examples of how we are proceeding with the goals and methods of our studies using material that has not been presented elsewhere. We deviate from this plan only when we attempt to make some issues clearer. One other factor that influences what will be included here is that some of our recent results are a bit perplexing to us and may stir the creative minds of those who read them.

Historically we began our efforts by studying the protection nimodipine provides against hypoxia. Of course we were far from the first investigators to attempt such studies in an *in vivo* model. However, we have deviated from the usual approaches in two ways:

1. a different method of inducing an hypoxic state, and
2. a correlated study with *in vitro* intervention.

In our *in vivo* studies we did not try to occlude the blood supplies to the brains of our rats. This has been an effective tool in the hands of other investigators but we felt there would be advantages in finding a less intrusive way to induce the hypoxic state. We deprived rats of their normal oxygen supply to the brain by means of the induction of methemoglobinemia by the systemic (i. p.) administration of sodium nitrite 50 mg/kg (Isaacson and Fahey 1987). This produced major histologic changes in the brains of the animals 24 h afterwards. They were especially prominent in those areas shown by other methods to be most sensitive to short periods of ischemia (Wieloch 1985). Among these areas are both ends of the hippocampal formation, namely the CA1 and the dentate-hilar areas. The brains were perfused and fixed using a medium that has a small amount of formaldehyde and substantial amounts of methyl alcohol. They were paraffin embedded and sectioned before being stained with cresyl violet. We mention this because it now appears that the nature of the cellular deformation that is found

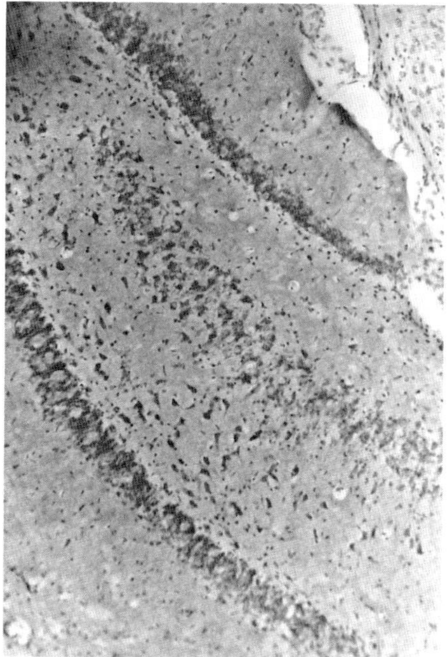

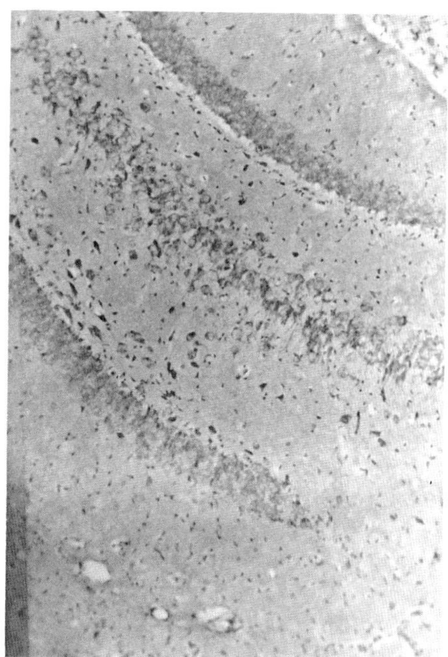

Fig. 1. Photomicrograph of ventral hippocampus, dorsal aspect, 24 h after sodium nitrite treatment. Nissl, × 100

Fig. 2. Photomicrograph of ventral hippocampus, dorsal aspect, 24 h after sodium nitrite treatment. In this rat nimodipine had been given as a "pretreatment" 2 h before the nitrite administration. Nissl, × 100

after nitrite exposure depends, in part, on the procedures used in perfusion and fixation. However, as expected the two poles of the hippocampus were affected. The signs of the effects were pyknosis of cells and processes along with an increase in "free space" caused by these retractions.

Figure 1 shows these effects, which can be found in the ventral as well as the dorsal aspects of the hippocampus. The reduction of cellular processes is especially prominent. If the animals are treated with 70 µg nimodipine in the PEG 400 vehicle 2 h before the nitrite is given, the histologic alterations are much less, as shown in Fig. 2. The amount of obvious cellular change is greatly reduced, although it is not entirely prevented. These results represent an independent confirmation that calcium channel antagonists do reduce hypoxic damage in cells.

However, it might be argued that the nimodipine acted to reduce the amount of methemoglobin in the nimodipine-pretreated animals. If this were the case, it would not be an example of cellular protection provided by the drug but rather a reduction in the amount of toxin formed. Therefore we assayed the levels of methemoglobin when the nitrite was given 2 or 24 h after i. p. injection of saline, nimodipine, or verapamil. The blood samples were taken 1 h after nitrite administration. The results are shown in Fig. 3. They show that the animals with no pretreatment before the nitrite had

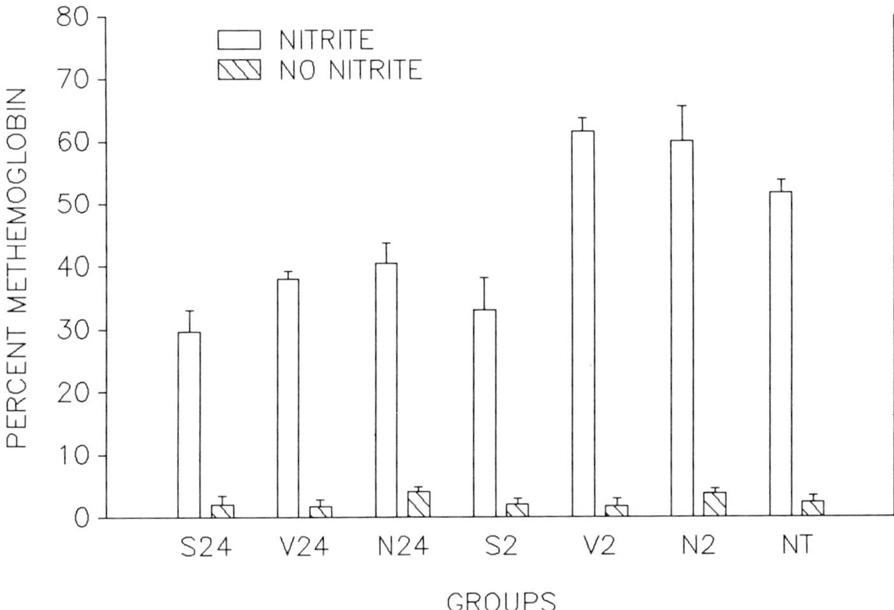

Fig. 3. Percentage of methemoglobin in blood after sodium nitrite treatment or saline vehicle (no nitrite) when saline *(S)*, verapamil *(V)*, or nimodipine *(N)* was given 24 h *(24)* or 2 h *(2)* before the nitrite. *NT* refers to a group that received no pretreatment before the nitrite administration

about 50% methemoglobin levels. An injection of labelled phosphate buffered saline (PBS) given 2 h before reduced that to about 30%, but this effect did not occur if one of the calcium channel blocking agents instead of saline was given 2 h before the nitrite. There was no significant difference among the groups treated 24 h before the nitrite.

Our hypothesis was that the handling and injection procedures induce a strong stress reaction in these animals and that some component of this stress response initiated enzymatic changes that either prevented the iron of the heme moiety from changing to the ferric state, or alternatively, returned it rapidly from the ferric to the ferrous state. We felt it likely that the antagonism of the calcium channels could result in a reduced amount of corticosterone being released in response to stress. Therefore, with the collaboration of Dr. Linda Dokas of the Medical College of Ohio, we assayed rat corticosterone levels 1 h after exposure to ether 1 min. All rats had been pretreated with saline, verapamil, or nimodipine 2 h before the exposure to ether. Two surprising results were obtained which were not in accord with our expectations. These are presented in Fig. 4.

The first was that a pretreatment with saline produces lower levels of corticosterone than normally found after ether stress. The usual levels found in animals given the same duration of ether stress, about 1 min, is over 200 ng/ml. There was a hint of long-lasting effects of the drug from our methemoglobin data and the present data confirm

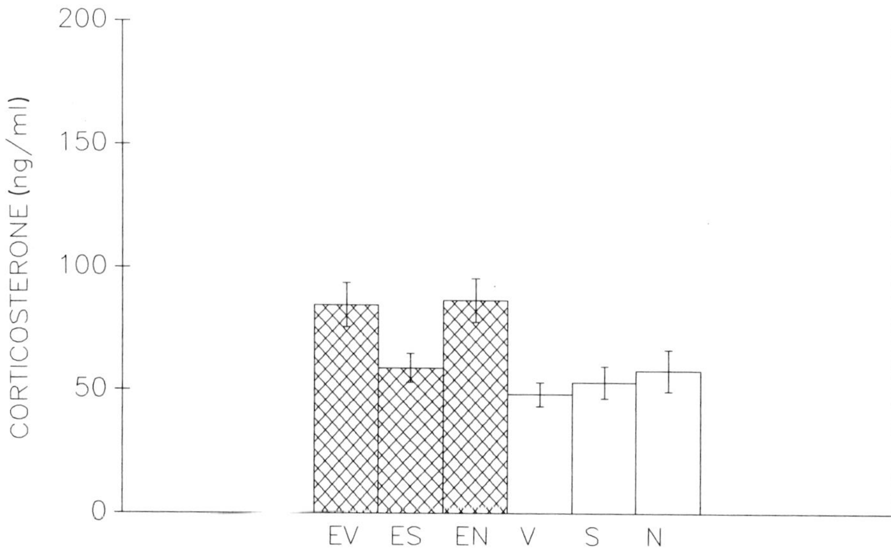

Fig. 4. Corticosterone levels obtained 1 h after ether stress (1 min; *shaded bars*) or no intervention *(open bars)*. Saline *(S)*, verapamil *(V)*, or nimodipine *(N)* was given 2 h before the ether stress, or 3 h before the blood sampling in the no-treatment groups. Ether stress groups: *EV*, verapamil pretreatment; *ES*, saline pretreatment; *EN*, nimodipine pretreatment. No-treatment groups: *V*, verapamil; *S*, saline; *N*, nimodipine

this. The second surprising result was that the injection of either of the calcium channel blockers raised, not lowered, measured corticosterone levels. The verapamil and nimodipine groups had significantly higher levels of corticosterone than the other groups. The drug did not restore the usual ether-induced stress response and the magnitude of the increase was not large, although significant. Therefore, it is likely that some other component of the stress response induced by the saline injection is responsible for the reduction in methemoglobin levels that we observed.

However, the results of the first *in vivo* studies of the induction of methemoglobinemia by sodium nitrite were encouraging and they justified the evaluation of nimodipine protection *in vitro*.

Led by Van Buskirk, we have developed an *in vitro*, three-dimensional matrix, vital dye system for assaying possible protective effects of different agents against various insults. Basically, cells of the pheochromocytoma cell line PC12 are seeded onto Millipore microporous membranes. Nerve growth factor (NFG) is added and most cells differentiate into neuron-like phenotypes. The cells are then incubated with rhodamine 123, a dye that does not affect the viability or the differentiation of the cells. The basic methods are outlined in Table 1. In our first study we created a hypoxic state by not supplying oxygen to the cells in culture for 48 h. We then counted the cells that still showed rhodamine fluorescence as it remained bound to mitochondrial membranes. Some cells were bathed in normal media, some in media with

Table 1. Protocol for the in vitro whole cell mitochondrial assay

Treat Milicell with matrix material
Add cells
Differentiate cells with NGF
Load mitochondria with rhodamine 123
Initiate treatment
Measure rhodamine outside Millicell (efflux)
Extract rhodamine with ethanol (extractable)
Quantify fluorescence with Fluroskan II

dimethysulfoxide (DMSO; the solvent for nimodipine), and others in baths that contained nimodipine disssolved in a minute amount of DMSO. Only a few appeared to retain viability. A summary of the effects of nimodipine based on cell counts is presented in Fig. 5. As can be seen at the extreme left, DMSO by itself is without effect. Nimodipine does increase the number of cells that retain viability, as indicated by their fluorescence, over the 48-h period. It does so in a curvilinear fashion, however, with the optimal levels being in the nanomolar range. Similar results can be shown as well by the measurement of rhodamine efflux is shown in Fig. 6. Here the least efflux of rhodamine indicates the smallest amount of cell destruction. Once again, the greatest protection occurs when the drug is given in the nanomolar range. This curvilinear protective effect seems to hold in studies using intact animals as well.

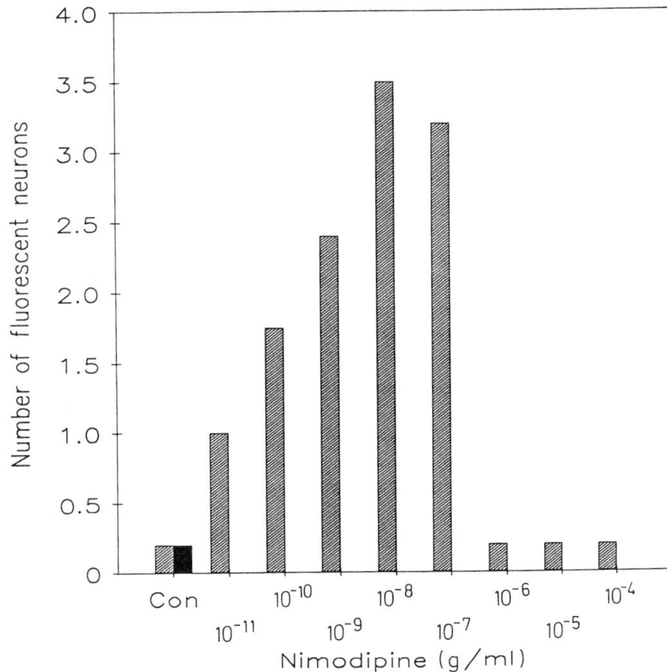

Fig. 5. The number of neurons showing rhodamine fluorescence under UV illumination after 48 h without osygen and with nimodipine added to the media at the doses indicated. *Con,* control; *filled bar,* water; *shaded bars,* DMSO vehicle

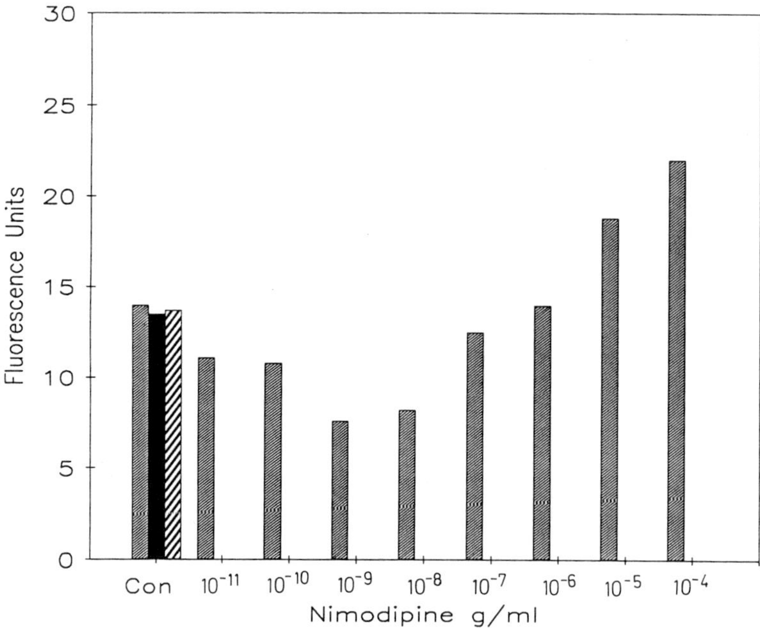

Fig. 6. The efflux of rhodamine after 48 h hypoxia from the cells in which the PC12 cells were placed on microporous membranes. Note that efflux is most reduced by doses of nimodipine in the nanomolar range 10^{-9} to 10^{-8} g/ml. *Con,* control; *filled bar,* water; *coarse shaded bar,* none; *fine shaded bars,* DMSO

This suggests that some negative findings reported in the literature may be due either to the timing of the drug administration relative to insult or to the amount of drug used.

While continuing with our attempts to study the strengths and weaknesses of our hypoxia model based on methemoglobinemia, we also investigated the question of whether the drug would also protect against other toxins. We began by investigating the effects of mercuric chloride. Figure 7 shows the toxicity of the mercury when measured by the efflux of rhodamine from the cells and by the amount remaining in the wells, i. e., the amount that is obtained when all remaining cell membranes are solubilized by the addition of 50% ethanol. The amount that remains in the tissue, the extractable rhodamine, is reduced in a more or less dose-dependent fashion while the efflux is most effected by the highest dose. This is shown in Fig. 8. The protection provided by nimodipine is measured by what remains.

A fundamental matter is to determine the extent of protection provided by nimodipine in the intact animals poisoned by mercury. At this point, we should mention we have used both mercuric chloride and methylmercury in these studies. The animals are injected with nimodipine 5.0 mg/kg 2 h before they are given mercuric chloride 1.5 mg/kg or methylmercury 10.0 mg/kg. The brains are processed using a standard intracardiac saline flush followed by 10% formaldehyde. They are sectioned while frozen and stained with cresyl violet.

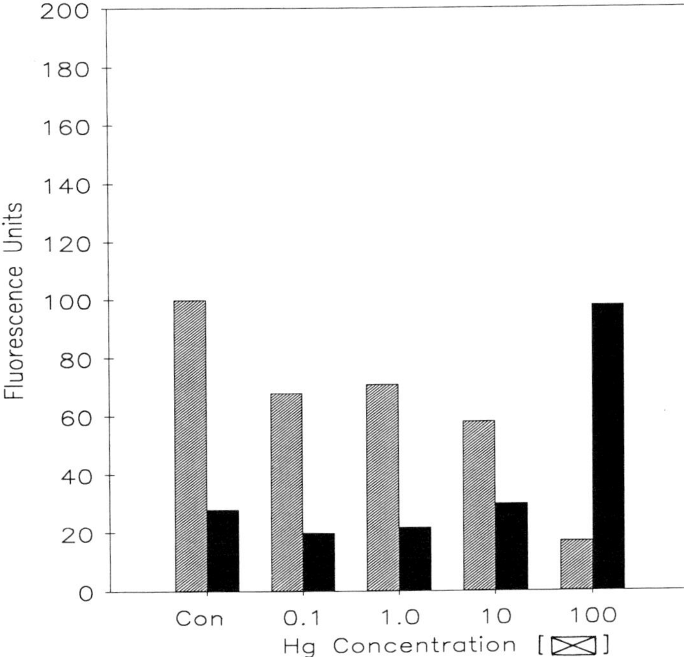

Fig. 7. The effect of mercuric chloride on PC12 cells in vitro as measured by efflux *(filled bars)* and amount *(shaded bars)* of rhodamine extracted by ethanol. *Con*, control

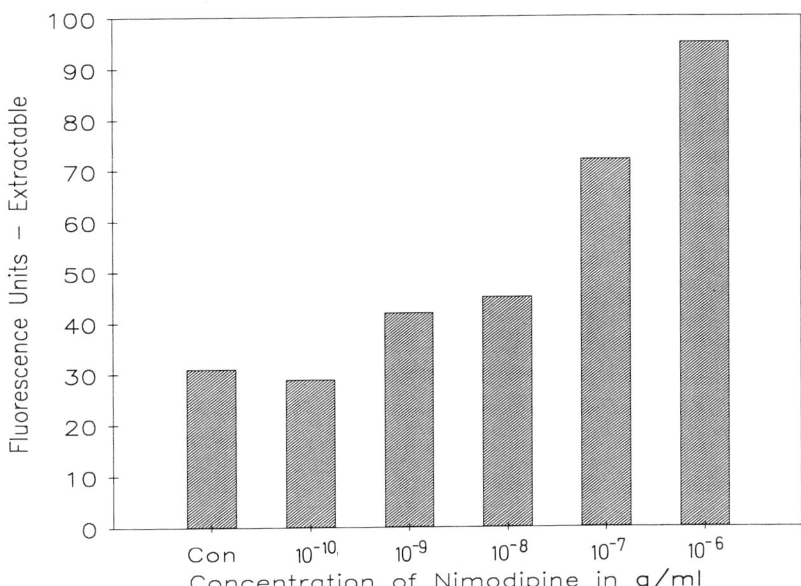

Fig. 8. Protection of PC12 cells against 10 μM mercuric chloride (2 h) by addition of nimodipine to the cell media 1 h before addition of mercuric chloride. *Con*, control

As far as we can determine, there is no difference between the two forms of mercury in producing the histologic abnormalities.

Since we have a large number of animals treated under various conditions, we must restrict our comments to some limited anatomical areas. On each of Figs. 9–11 the uppermost section will show the histological appearance of an animal that received a saline injection 2 h before sacrifice, perfusion, and further processing. The middle section will show the effect of the administration of the mercury, and the bottom portion will show a comparable section from an animal with nimodipine given 2 h before the mercury.

The effects of mercury toxicity produced by mercuric chloride or methylmercury were quite similar. The most frequent neurohistologic abnormality was chromatolysis. In many cases cells became as clear as glass marbles with small amounts of staining protein gathered either uniformly or clustered at the inner edge of the cell membrane. Cellular pyknosis was rare. In one or two of the 12 mercury-treated animals areas of pyknotic neurons replaced the chromatolytic cells found in the brains of the other animals.

Even in saline-treated animals, a few abnormal cells can be observed in the hilar region, but this is not unexpected, because it is possible that as many as 4% of the neurons in a normal, healthy animal may show histological anomalies. Mercury poisoning has a largely chromatolytic effect and partial compensation occurs in nimodipine-treated animals.

The dorsal subicular areas also show these changes, as shown in Figs. 9, 10. These are of the same general regions but at magnifications of 100 × and 250 ×, respectively.

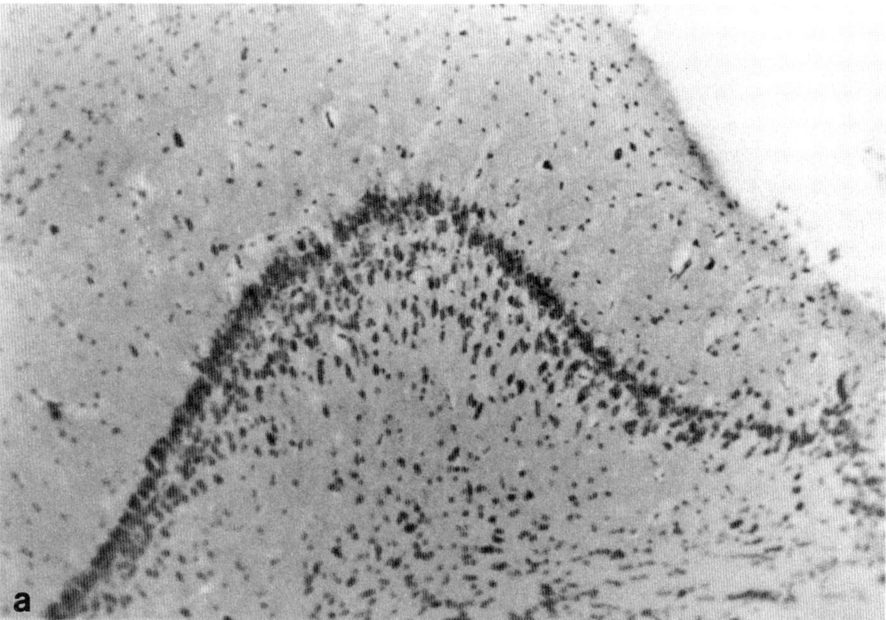

Fig. 9a–c. Photomicrographs of Nissl stained sections through the dorsal subicular regions. *Top, a* section from a saline-treated rat; *middle,* from a mercury-treated rat; *bottom,* from a rat pretreated with nimodipine before administration of the toxin. Nissl, × 100

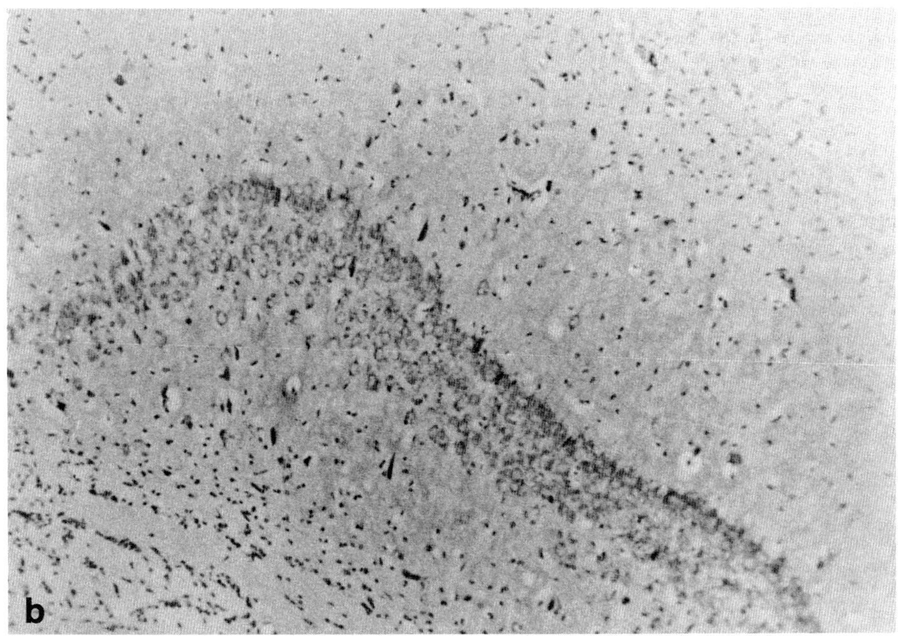

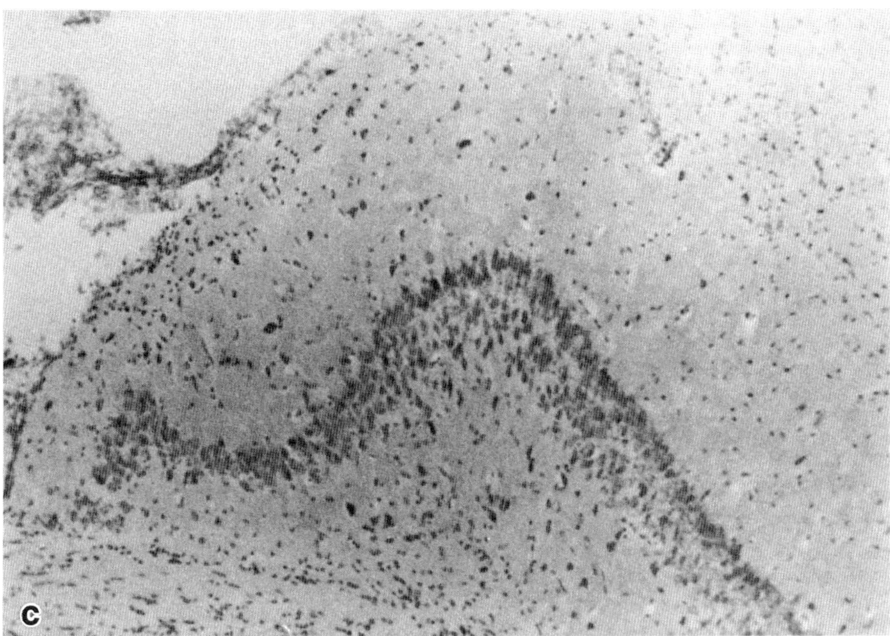

Fig. 9

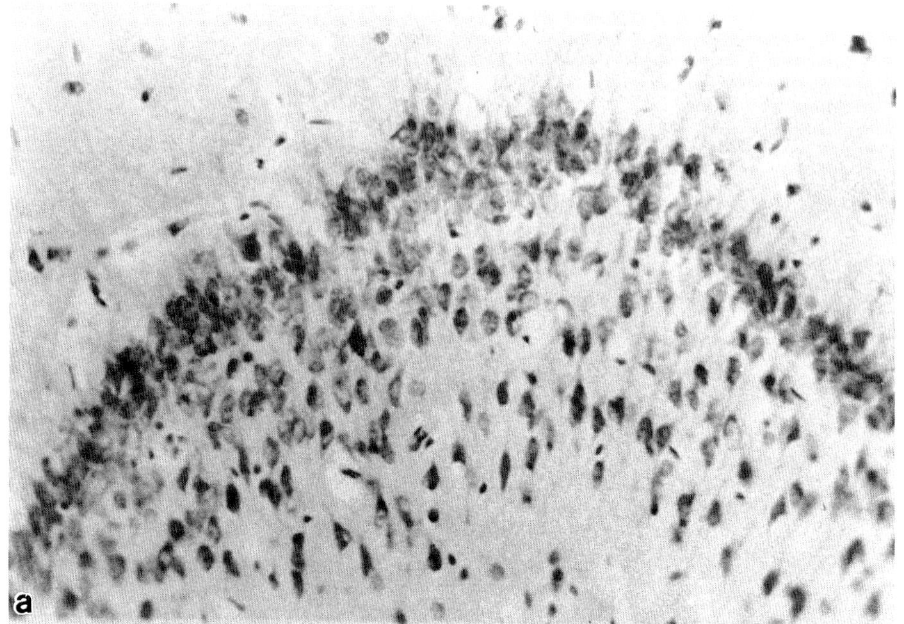

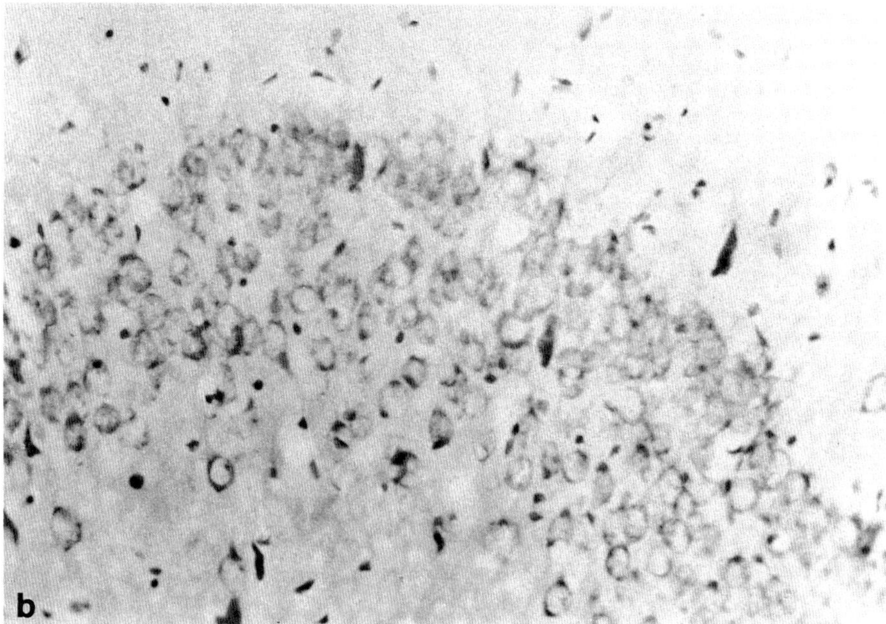

Fig. 10. Portions of the dorsal subiculum shown in Fig. 9 at a higher magnification. × 250

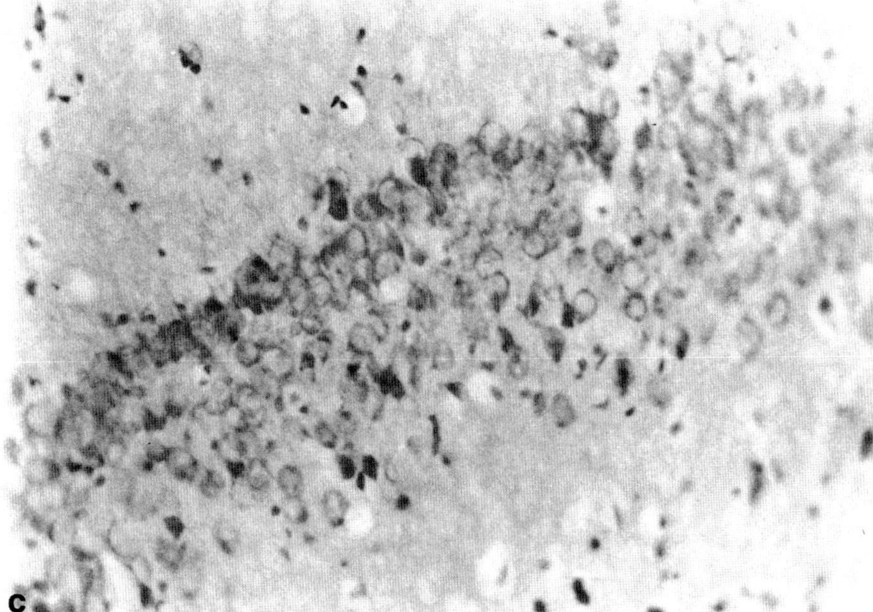

Fig. 10

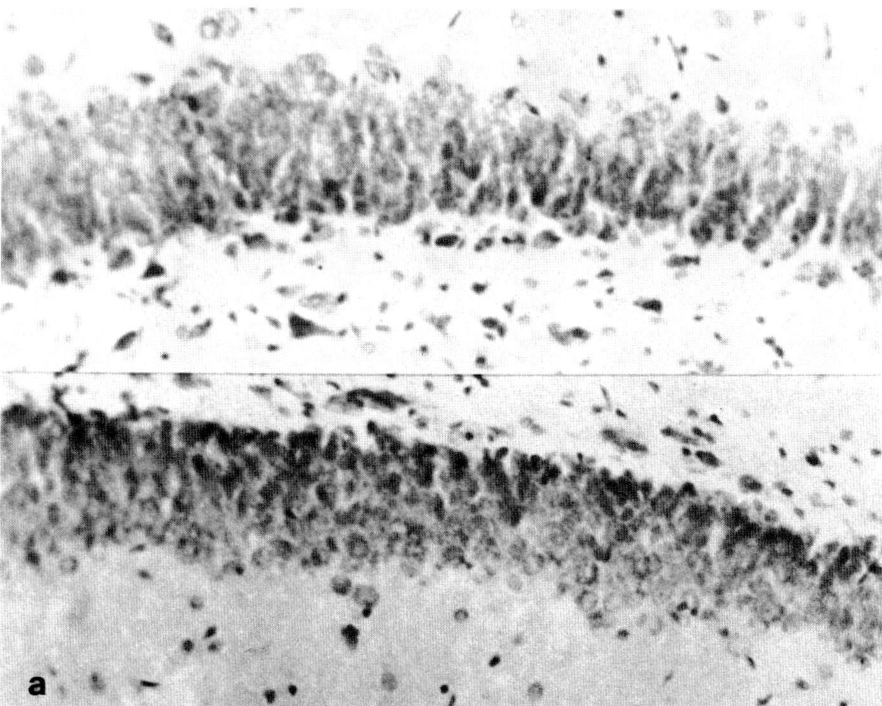

Fig. 11. Photomicrographs of dorsal and ventral blades of the dentate of rats treated as in Fig. 9. Nissl, × 100

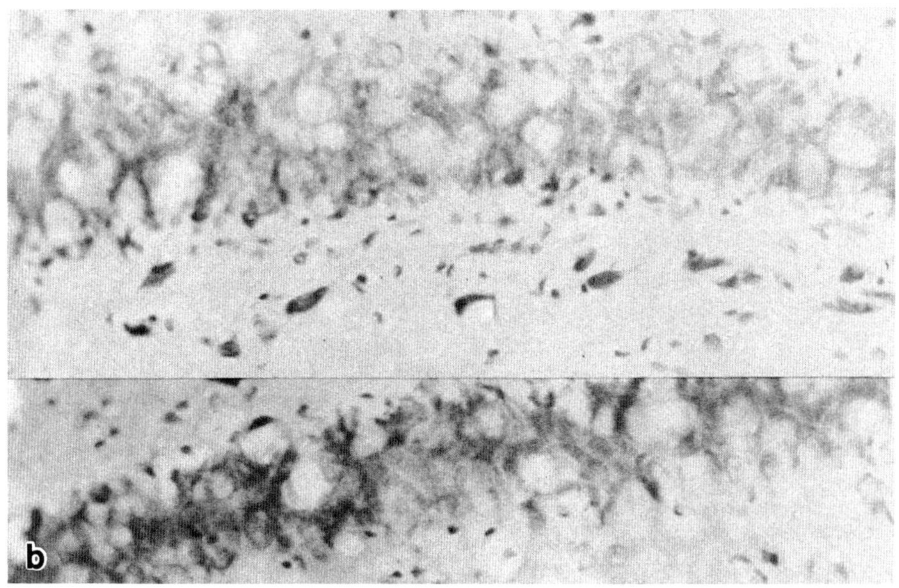

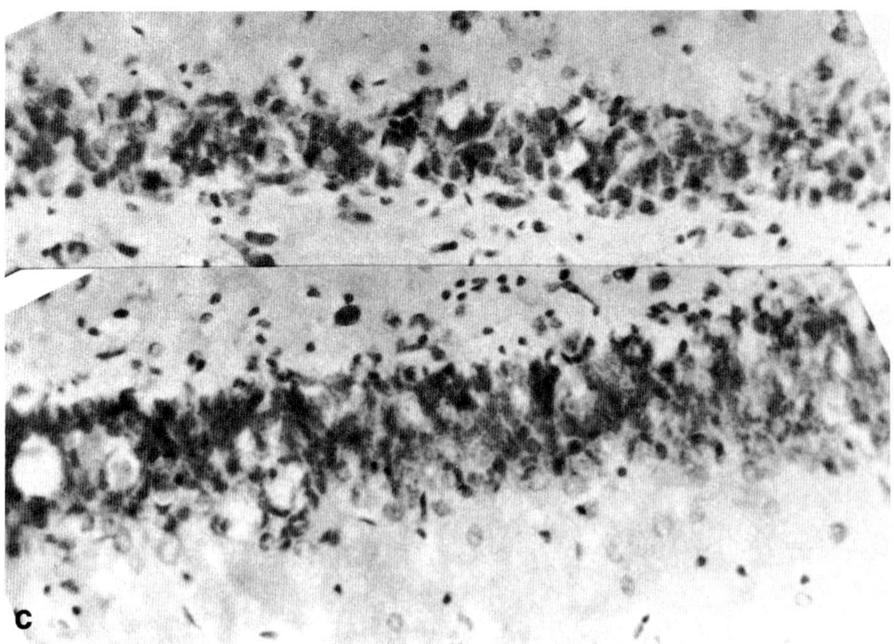

Fig. 11

The ventral subicular areas show similar changes. Although these results are so new that we haven't begun to quantify the effects, it does appear that some areas are offered better protection than others by nimodipine. A rough estimate of the ventral subicular areas indicates that about 65% of the cells show severe chromatolysis after mercury, but only about 25% after pretreatment with nimodipine. About 4 to 5% of the cells in the untreated animals appear abnormal. It may be that the nimodipine protection of hilar cells is so extensive as to limit dysfunction to 15% of the cells even though the percentage of cells in this area affected by mercury without pretreatment is also about 65%.

The best example of the protection offered by nimodipine against mercury toxicity may be seen in the blades of the dentate. Figure 11 is a montage that shows both dorsal and ventral blades of the dentate with most of the hilar area cut out. The chromatolysis of the blades produced by mercury is apparent in the middle portion of the figure. The protection provided by nimodipine is prominent, if not complete, as shown in the bottom section. All of our results indicate that pretreatment with relatively low doses of nimodipine does provide substantial protection against the destruction effects of mercury, although this protection is not absolute either in vivo or in vitro.

At the present time many questions remain to be answered, some of which are of substantial clinical and practical importance. These include the range of toxins against which nimodipine may offer protection, the effects of chronic administration of low doses of nimodipine on cellular protection (is the protection even greater?), and to what extend do these histological results correlate with behavioral disorders induced by the toxins? Nevertheless, a means of cellular protection against the high levels of environmental and industrial toxins that affect us in so many ways is a worthy goal.

References

De Koning P, Gispen WH (1987) Org 2766 improves functional and electrophysiological aspects of regenerating rat sciatic nerve. Peptides 8: 415–422

Exton JH (1988) Mechanisms of action of calcium-mobilizing agonists: some variations on a young theme. FASEB J 2: 2670–2676

Hannigan JH, Isaacson RL (1985) The effect of Org 2766 on the performance of sham, neocortical, and hippocampal-lesioned rats in a food search task. Pharmacol Biochem Behav 23: 1019–1027

Isaacson RL, Fahey JM (1987) Some anatomical and behavioral consequences of acute sodium nitrite administration. Neurosci Res Commum 1: 39–45

Miller RJ (1987) Multiple Calcium Channels and Neuronal Function. Science 235: 46–52

Wieloch T (1985) Neurochemical correlates to selective neuronal vulnerability. Prog Brain Res 63: 69–85

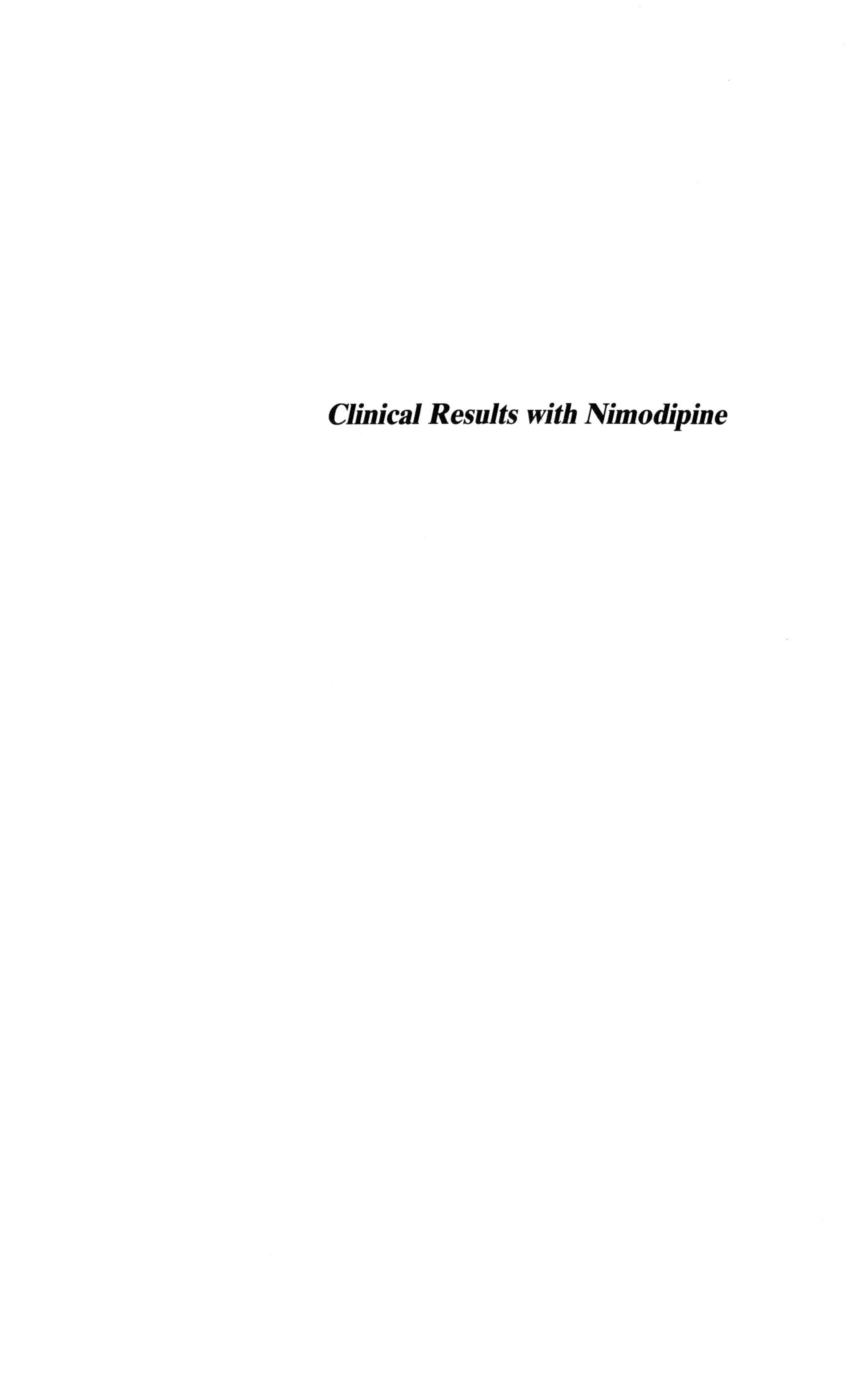

Clinical Results with Nimodipine

Therapeutic Efficacy of Nootropic Drugs –
A Discussion of Clinical Phase III Studies
with Nimodipine as a Model

S. Kanowski, P. Fischhof, R. Hiersemenzel, J. Röhmel, and U. Kern

Introduction

With regard to proving the clinical efficacy of nootropic substances there has been intense methodological discussion since 1975 (Kanowski 1975, 1986; Coper and Kanowski 1976, 1983; Kanowski and Hedde 1986; Comittee for Geriatric Diseases and Asthenias at BGA 1986). Both the selection of target parameters (outcome measures) and definition of diagnoses for inclusion are the subject of current debate, particularly given some of the differences in approach between research in the United States and that in Europe. In the United States, for instance, there has recently been a move to stop the use of traditional performance tests and symptom rating scales as therapeutic outcome measures and to adopt improvements within global clinical diagnostic rating scales instead, for example, a refinement to the Global Deterioration Scale (GDS; Reisberg 1982) as a target criterion (Gamzu 1987). It has been argued that an improvement from, say, GDS stage 4 (moderate impairment of cognitive function) to stage 3 (slight cognitive impairment) would certainly represent a change in elderly patients that is relevant to their daily lives.

With regard to the definition of inclusion diagnoses, there is a noticeable difference. From the European perspective, distinguishing in vivo between different forms of disease with different aetiopathologies poses problems for differential diagnosis and is the cause of heated discussion (Winblad 1987), whereas in the United States nootropic research is increasingly being equated with research into Alzheimer's disease (Gamzu 1987), and it is taken more or less for granted that this disease can be readily diagnosed.

This paper presents the results of a phase III study with a new calcium antagonist (calcium-entry blocker), nimodipine, which was conducted in 1985 and 1986 regarding the indication of impaired brain functions in the elderly, in accordance with the criteria determined by the B2 Preparatory Commission and published in 1986 (Committee for Geriatric Diseases and Asthenias at BGA 1986). This study reflects the current debate with regard to licensing in the Federal Republic of Germany for this indication. In addition, possible further developments to phase III models are considered, taking into account the current debate.

Bergener, Reisberg (Eds.)
Diagnosis and Treatment
of Senile Dementia
© Springer-Verlag Berlin Heidelberg 1989

Phase III Model to Prove Efficacy

Test Substance and Aims of Study

In its chemistry and pharmacology, nimodipine is related to the calcium antagonist nifedipine. Tests with pharmacological models suggest that nimodipine has a number of neuropsychopharmacological and cerebroprotective properties (Hoffmeister et al. 1982), confirming the view that its activity is not limited to disturbances of vascular origin. It seems able to influence symptoms of organic brain syndrome caused by metabolic disorders and may even have a positive effect regardless of aetiopathogenesis. The present study examines this hypothesis.

The aim of the phase III trial was therefore to investigate whether nimodipine effects a clinically relevant improvement in elderly patients with diffuse organic brain syndrome and a defined pattern of symptoms. The effects noted with nimodipine should prove to be reasonable indicators of its efficacy in the therapeutic sense.

Method

Study Design. The trial was randomised and double-blinded, with a controlled design using three parallel treatment groups (active, standard substance, placebo; each with 60 assessable cases expected) and involving in-patients at a psychiatric hospital (Klinik Baumgartner Höhe der Stadt Wien in Vienna). The 12-week treatment phase was preceded by a single-blind 4-week placebo run-in phase (test day 2); after 6 weeks treatment (test day 3) and after 12 weeks treatment (test day 4), the target and associated variables were measured. A treatment phase of 12 weeks was chosen because experience shows that an improvement in impaired cognitive functions becomes visible only after 2–3 months.

Patient Homogeneity. For controlling the homogeneity of the patients a set of inclusion and exclusion criteria were established. The chronic organic brain syndrome of diffuse type, from mild to moderate degree, was chosen as the target syndrome. This can be viewed as the core syndrome of any dementia process, independent of its special aetiology. Its main symptoms, as defined in the AGP (1982) system, are:
a) impairment of concentration,
b) impairment of memory,
c) impairment of perception,
d) impairment of thinking,
e) disturbed orientation, and
f) affective instability.

Aetiological homogeneity was not strived for because of the aetiological nonspecifity of the drug under study and because of uncertainty of clinical diagnosis, particularly in dementia of the Alzheimer type.

Male and female patients aged between 60 and 85 years with a clinical diagnosis of mild or moderate diffuse organic brain syndrome, according to the Lausanne grading (AGP, mental finding II), were included in the study. Cognitive status, particularly orientation, was documented with the aid of the Mental Status Questionnaire (MSQ;

Kahn et al. 1961). The clinical diagnosis was classified according to DSM III (American Psychiatric Association 1980). The Hachinski Ischemic Score (Hachinski 1975), which makes a differential diagnosis of primary degenerative and multi-infarct dementia, was added for descriptive purposes. The total score on the Clinical Assessment Geriatric Scale (SCAG; CIPS 1981) was used as a quantitative inclusion criterion. Patients were included whose total SCAG score was between 41 and 90, a range which covers mild to moderate organic brain syndrome, according to the results from reported random sampling. Psychopathological symptoms were noted on a symptoms check list. Memory impairment was an essential symptom. Patients then had to have at least three of the remaining eight symptoms: affective instability, low depressive emotional state, apathy, impaired concentration, insomnia, nocturnal agitation, anxiety and irritability.

Exclusion criteria were established to control for: transient organic psychoses, influence of multimorbidity, drug and alcohol abuse and long-term medication (Table 1). Note was also made of the following: previous and concomitant medication, case history, clinical examination findings including intensive monitoring of blood pressure, and heart rate.

Outcome Criteria. In order to monitor progress and assess target parameters for confirmatory statistical analysis, clinical symptoms were evaluated using the following target variables:

1. SCAG, a physician's rating scale using the total score on the scale, which reflects the extent of clinical symptoms and can be seen as a way of providing a systematised overall assessment.
2. The assessment scale for the behaviour of geriatric patients (BGP; CIPS 1981) a nurse's rating scale based on observations of the patient's behaviour in his or her natural environment (on the ward). It assesses affective and social behaviour,

Table 1. Exclusion criteria

- Transient organic psychoses (acute exogenous types of reaction)
- Stroke less than 6 months previously
- Patients with severe communication problems (sensorimotor aphasia); reading, writing and hearing difficulties
- Unstable hypertension
- Hypotension (blood pressure < 120/80)
- Poorly treatable risk factors (diabetes mellitus, gout)
- Renal or myocardial insufficiency, arrhythmias which may lead to secondary dementia
- Severe gastrointestinal disorders
- Patients with intercurrent diseases or moderately severe general illnesses which might interfere with the test result
- Existing alcohol or drug abuse
- Long-term consumption of the following substances which could not be withdrawn an appropriate length of time before the trial:
  - Psychotropic drugs
  - Nootropic drugs
  - Hypnotics (mild soporifics were allowed)
  - Calcium antagonists (calcium-entry blockers)
  - α-Methyldopa
  - Anti-arrhythmic drugs of the local anaesthetic type
  - β-blockers

---

interest and initiative, independence, and comprehension. Again, the total score was used.

3. The syndrome short test (SKT; Erzigkeit 1977), which records disturbances of attention and memory. The total score, used here, measures the degree of cognitive disturbance.
4. The trail-making test (ZVT-G; Oswald and Fleischmann 1986), which measures the speed of cognitive function in geriatric patients. In several pharmacopsychological trials it has proved a sensitive instrument for recording pharmacogenetic changes. The target parameter was the length of time taken to do the test, averaged from two test runs.

The Clinical Global Impression (CGI; CIPS 1981) and subscales of SCAG, BGP and SKT should be seen as accompanying, descriptive information. Tolerance of the substance was documented with the aid of a standardised scale for recording side effects (DOTES/TWIS; CIPS 1981).

The general working hypothesis was that nimodipine would induce an improvement of functioning on all of the four target variables listed above.

Medication and Dosage. Nimodipine was given in a daily dose of 90 mg (3×1 coated tablet). The standard substance used was co-dergocrine mesylate (Hydergine special, 4-mg active substance); the (active) placebo was Silecea tablets (strength D 6). The tablets were all encased in an identical outer coat and swallowed unchewed, making them indistinguishable from each other. The standard substance was taken in the morning, and a placebo tablet was taken at midday and in the evening, so that the dosage rhythm matched that of nimodipine.

Ethics. The patients were informed of the nature, significance and scope of the study and of the substances used, and they gave their verbal consent in the presence of a witness. The protocol was examined for its ethical justifiability and approved by an independent ethics committee.

Statistics. The nimodipine – placebo comparison (one-sided questioning) was planned as a confirmatory measure. The Hydergine group was added to enable comparisons to be drawn with a licensed substance, on a descriptive basis.

The four target variables (SCAG, BGP, SKT, ZVT-G) were subject to confirmatory data analysis. The Wilcoxon test served as a precise randomisation test. The assessment of statistical interference was made via dependent variables with gradual α-adjustment according to Bonferroni-Holm (Sonnemann 1981), firstly for the two scales of clinical symptoms (SCAG, BGP) and then for performance (SKT, ZVT-G). The resulting levels of significance per scale were then subject to another α-correction in order to give a total level of significance for the efficacy of nimodipine.

For group comparisons, the differences were noted between measurements of target variables before treatment (after the run-in phase, test day 2) versus after treatment (after 12 weeks treatment, test day 4). It was decided beforehand that only the result at the end of the treatment should be tested, because in the cognitive sphere marked improvements in performance and function can only be expected to appear after about 2–3 months treatment.

Sample Size and Description. A total of 202 patients were included in the trial. Five of these patients were excluded from the evaluation because they had received an additional nootropic drug (piracetam). The data on 197 patients (156 women, 40 men, one patient without gender identification) aged between 61 and 86 years (median of each group, between 77.5 and 79 years) were used for analysis. Only a small proportion of the patients (10%) had an educational status above that of school-leaving certificate. With regard to age, weight, height and inclusion diagnosis according to the AGP system, the χ^2 test showed no significant diffferences between the groups. In addition to compulsory memory impairment, the most common deficits were apathy and affective instability.

Drop-outs. A total of 19 patients left the trial prematurely: eight receiving nimodipine, eight on Hydergine and three on placebo. Three patients (two on nimodipine, one on Hydergine; aged 75, 82 and 85 years) died from acute cardiac decompensation against a background of severe cardiovascular and other pre-existing diseases. No connection with the test medication was established in any of these cases.

Side effects alone or combined with other factors led to eight drop-outs (three on nimodipine, three on Hydergine and two on placebo). The following side effects were given as reasons for withdrawal: nausea/vomiting in all three groups; dizziness and asthenia with nimodipine and Hydergine; with Hydergine only, hypotension, tendency to collapse and sensation of heat; with placebo only, rigor, sweating, pallor, difficulty in swallowing and epigastric pains. Lack of efficacy was given as a secondary reason for withdrawal of six patients (three on nimodipine and three on Hydergine) and as the principal reason for withdrawal of one patient (nimodipine). Other conditions accounting for drop-outs were intercurrent illness, transfer of the patient and withdrawal by the patient with no details of the reason.

Variations from the Original Protocol. As the trial was being conducted, it became clear from a practical point of view that the administration of concomitant vasoactive medication (particularly vasodilators in a peripheral indication) and, in a few isolated cases, psychotropic drugs (e.g. diazepam, bromazepam) could not always be avoided. In order to give equal consideration to therapeutic necessity and to the need for methodological purity, a deviation from the protocol was made, and two subgroups were formed for statistical analysis of the target variables: one group ($n = 144$) without and one group ($n = 53$) with unwanted concomitant medication. Results in these groups were used in addition to those in the overall group in order to clarify the question of whether such drugs had caused any additional effects.

Clinical Tolerability of Nimodipine

The accompanying symptoms, documented in DOTES/TWIS, which the investigator regarded as possibly connected with treatment are listed in Table 2; the number of instances mentioned per patient varied between one and 25 symptoms. Table 3 presents the percentage of patients complaining of the most commonly documented symptoms.

Table 2. Frequency of documented accompanying symptoms (DOTES/TWIS) with possible connection to treatment (number of times quoted)

Symptom	Nimodipine	Hydergine	Placebo
		Medication	
Stimulation/agitation	2		1
Depressive mental state	4		3
Increased motor activity	4		
Decreased motor activity		2	2
Insomnia	4	1	1
Sleepiness/somnolence/drowsiness		4	
Rigor			1
Dry mouth	1		1
Nasal breathing impaired			1
Constipation	1		1
Increased salivation	1		
Sweating		1	1
Nausea/vomiting	5	10	7
Diarrhoe	1		
Hypotension	17	26	8
Feeling of dizziness	21	28	6
Tachycardia	3	3	
Dermatological symptoms	1		1
Weight gain	6	1	3
Weight loss	2	1	3
Anorexia/loss of appetite	4	2	4
Headaches	6	1	2
Tendency to collapse		1	
Irritability			2
Precordial pain	1		
Eye pains			2
Unsteady gait/stumbling	3	3	
Tiredness/fatigue	1	2	2
Restlessness	1		
Fall in blood pressure	3	13	4
General malaise		1	
Breathlessness	2		
Heat sensation (extremities)	3	1	
Asthenia	1	2	1
Apathy/retiring behaviour		1	1
Pallor			1
Cold in extremities	2	2	
Mucosa – sensitive	1		
Hair loss			1
Difficulty in swallowing			1
Convulsions	1		
Gastric pains	1	1	2
Calf cramps		2	
Pressure around the heart		1	
Aggressiveness	2		
Spots in front of eyes		1	
Tinnitus	1		
Depression/dejection		1	

Table 3. Percentage of patients with adverse drug-related effects

Symptom	Nimodipine	Hydergine	Placebo
Dizziness	28%	36%	8%
Hypotension	19%	32%	10%
Fall in blood pressure	4%	14%	3%

Signs and symptoms indicative of a lowering effect upon blood pressure were recorded in both active groups, although descriptively these were less frequent with nimodipine than with Hydergine. These findings match the symptoms of the drop-out patients, who also complained largely of dizziness/asthenia and nausea/vomiting.

Median blood pressure measurements showed small and clinically insignificant decreases in systolic and diastolic levels for all three groups, and these were accompanied by a minimal rise in heart rate. Case histories revealed no relevant fall in blood pressure, even in patients with initially hypertensive blood pressure levels. There were isolated symptoms of central nervous stimulation (increased motor activity, insomnia, tachycardia and headaches) noted with nimodipine.

Therapeutic Efficacy of Nimodipine

For confirmatory analysis, the pre/post-treatment differences (baseline after the 4-week run-in phase versus test day 4 after 12-week double-blind treatment) was the object of group comparisons. This procedure reflects the way in which therapeutic efficacy is clinically assessed routinely ("What has changed?").

The extent of the patients' clinical symptoms, as shown on SCAG, improved in comparison with placebo ($p < 0.01$). From a descriptive point of view, Hydergine also proved superior to placebo ($p < 0.01$). Finally, nimodipine was significantly superior to Hydergine ($p < 0.01$). The superiority of nimodipine over placebo and the standard drug ($p < 0.01$) was found in both subgroups, for patients without concomitant vasoactive medication and those with (potentially misleading) concomitant medication (Fig. 1a).

The nurses' rating (BGP) also showed nimodipine to be superior to placebo ($p < 0.01$) and to Hydergine ($p < 0.05$). There was no significant difference between Hydergine and placebo in this respect. Taking together both of these target variables and after α-correction, it can be stated that the clinical symptoms improved with nimodipine ($p < 0.01$).

With regard to the psychological performance test (SKT), both active substances in the complete group and in the subgroup without concomitant medication proved significantly superior to placebo ($p < 0.01$); nimodipine was furthermore superior to Hydergine ($p < 0.01$; Fig. 1b).

The trail-making test (ZVT-G) also confirmed the working hypothesis that cognitive performance speed after treatment with nimodipine improves for the total group of patients and for both subgroups ($p < 0.01$).

For the total group and for the subgroup with additional vasoactive medication, the standard Hydergine was also found superior to placebo at the $p < 0.01$ level, and in the group without added vasoactive medication at the $p < 0.05$ level.

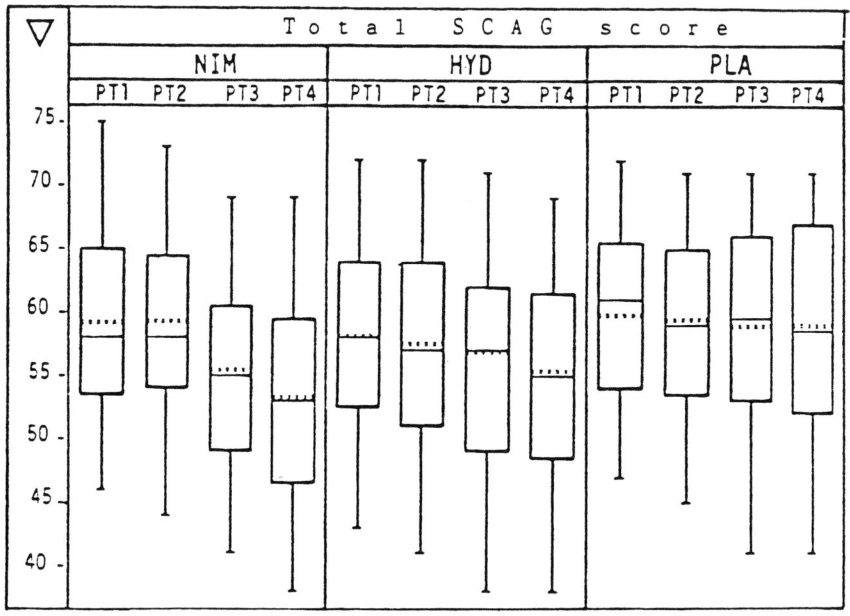

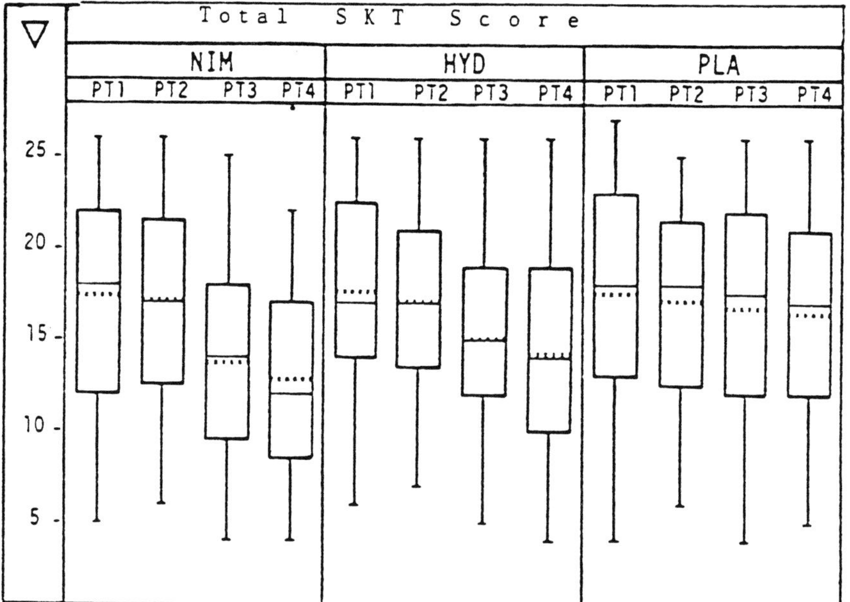

Fig. 1. Box-Whisker plots for the variables SCAG (**a**) and SKT (**b**). *Broken line in box* shows the mean, *solid line* the median. The box is limited by the 1st and 3rd quartiles (= 50% of the figures). *Columns above and below boxes* show the interquartile distances. The points and symbols are values within or outside defined quartile distances and are essentially freak values. The figure includes the measurements made at the start (*PT1*) and end (*PT2*) of the placebo washout (run-in) phase (pre-treatment), after 6 weeks treatment (*PT3*) and after 12 week's treatment (post-treatment; *PT4*). *NIM,* Nimodipine; *HYD,* Hydergine; *PLA,* placebo

After α-correction, a performance-enhancing effect of nimodipine ($p < 0.01$) could again be established.

Based on these multiple test procedures, the probability of error, when two levels are considered together, is less than 1%, i.e. with this level of significance it can be established that nimodipine not only improves clinical symptoms but also has a performance-enhancing effect.

The results found in the trial model were seen as clinically relevant, that is, to be important in the patients' daily lives. Treatment with nimodipine clearly improved impaired brain functions of in-patients with mild to moderate chronic organic brain syndrome with varying pathogenesis in a way that was observed by both the clinical investigators and the nursing staff, and that was evidenced in objective performance tests.

Exploratory data analysis on the question of whether vascular and primary degenerative dementia (separated using the Hachinski score) differed with regard to therapeutic outcome showed no difference.

Discussion: Is a Change of Model Needed?

The problems of demonstrating the clinical relevance of nootropic effects in phase III models is currently the subject of increasing critical debate (Zimmer et al. 1987). In the present trial necessary conditions were defined beforehand, and the effects detected in the phase III model were taken as a plausible indication of therapeutic efficacy, or clinical relevance (Herrmann and Kern 1987). In essence, the clinical relevance of effects measured in the study reported here is based on two conditions:
a) the effects detected point in the same direction and on several observation levels and derive from different data sources; and
b) the conditions for confirmatory data analysis are defined in advance.

The demands for clinically relevant outcome measures, such as an improvement by one or several degrees of severity on graduated rating scales (as described in the "Introduction"), go far beyond this. The underlying therapeutic demands are stricter than those associated with conventional phase III methods, although in the case of nootropic drugs these conventional methods still aim to detect more subtle effects. Whether one regards these rather limited effects as relevant is ultimately a matter of judgement and cannot easily be transformed into one of empirical indisputability. As, however, subjective suffering among elderly patients with impaired cerebral functions is certainly the norm, it is definitely worth considering whether to accept limited effects as relevant if the risks are minimal. The B2Committee (Committee for Geriatric Diseases and Asthenias at BGA 1986 p. 10) stressed that the overall somatic and psychoscial condition of the individual patient must be assessed when deciding on treatment. Such a decision cannot simply be substituted by general regulations; it also depends on the availability of alternative therapeutic strategies, which apparently do not exist yet.

It should be realised however, that a change of model in pharmacological research would bring with it a certain methodological dilemma. The move to criticise the appropriateness of established phase III models is usually associated with the development of new drugs. However, the manufacturers of pharmaceuticals that are already licensed are less interested, as a rule, in developing new test models. The dilemma, then, is: is it useful to change two crucial variables – the substance and the clinical model of evaluation – at the same time?

If no effect emerges, no conclusion on structural invariance can be drawn, i.e. it is impossible to decide whether the drug or the model were unsuitable. It would therefore be desirable to subject older substances in clinical trials to new model conditions in order to provide further information about the validity of altered models. Otherwise the comparative evaluation of old and new drugs will be rather difficult.

It should also be added that the changed clinical models demand a long process of construction. One sometimes has the impression in gerontopharmacological research that scales or tests created ad hoc or methods not fully tested for cross-cultural comparability are beginning to predominate, and that very little value is being placed on previous proof derived from classic test criteria. International communication is also being severely hampered by this development. This gives us a major point of departure for improving current test models.

A change of model is indicated in another respect, however: in the early 1980s the idea of supposedly uniform aetiology (e.g. based on the theory of cholinergic deficit in Alzheimer's disease) was abandoned, with good reason, in clinical trial models with nootropic drugs in favour of syndromal uniformity. In this respect organic brain syndrome was seen as a common pathogenic end stage regardless of its aetiology and was interpreted as the target syndrome of drug therapy (Kanowski and Coper 1982). This concept seems to be in accordance with the everyday clinical routine of physicians who are responsible for drug prescription.

The method of aetiologically oriented, differential diagnosis based on machine techniques (e.g. computed tomography, nuclear magnetic resonance, positron emission tomography) in order to achieve more precise patient homogeneity is to be recommeded only when a nootropic drug is reasonably linked with known specific aetiology, dependig on the biochemical or (neuro-)physiological working hypothesis. Hence on this level the old problem of responders/non-responders may be tackled afresh.

References

AGP. Arbeitsgemeinschaft für Gerontopsychiatrie. Ciompim L, Kanowski S (eds) (1982) Das AGP-System: Manual zur Dokumentation psychiatrischer Befunde bei Alterskranken. 2nd edn.

American Psychiatric Association (1980) Diagnostic and statistical manual of mental disorders, 3rd edn. DSM-III. American Psychiatrie Association, Washington DC

CIPS Collegium Internationale Psychiatriae Scalarum (ed) (1981) Internationale Skalen für Psychiatrie. Beltz, Weinheim

Coper H, Kanowski S (1976) Geriatrika: Theoretische Grundlagen, Erwartung, Prüfung, Kritik. Hippokrates 47: 303–319

Coper H, Kanowski S (1983) Nootropika: Grundlagen und Therapie. In: Langer G, Heimann H (eds) Psychopharmaka. Grundlagen und Therapie. Springer, Vienna New York, pp 409–430

Committee for Geriatric Diseases and Asthenias at BGA (1986) Impaired brain functions in old age. AMI-Heft 1, pp 1–264

Erzigkeit H (1977) Der Syndrom-Kurztest zur Erfassung von Aufmerksamkeits- und Gedächtnisstörungen. VLESS, Vaterstetten

Gamzu ER (1987) Drug development of cognition activators – clinical aspects (Abstract no 356 and Referat). The third congress of the International Psychogeriatric Association (sponsored by the IPA in cooperation with Northwestern University Medical School), Chicago, Ill. Aug 28–31

Hachinski VC et al. (1975) Cerebral blood flow in dementia. Arch Neurol 32: 632–637

Herrmann WM, Kern U (1987) Multizentrische klinische Prüfungen – Möglichkeiten und Probleme. In: Coper H et al. (eds) Hirnorganische Psychosyndrome im Alter. III. Springer, Berlin Heidelberg New York, pp 80–108

Hoffmeister F, Benz U, Heise A, Krause HP, Neuser V (1982) Behavioral effects of nimodipine in animals. Arzneimittelforschung/Drug Res 32: 347–360

Kahn RL, Pollack M, Goldfarb AI (1961) Factors related to individual differences in mental status of institutionalized aged. In: Hock PH, Zubin J (eds) Psychopathology of aging. Grune and Stratton, New York, pp 104–113

Kanowski S (1975) Methodenkritische Überlegungen zur Prüfung von Geriatrika. Z. Gerontol 5: 316–322

Kanowski S (1986) Möglichkeiten und Grenzen der Therapie mit Nootropika. Hospitalis 56: 400–409

Kanowski S (1987) Möglichkeiten eines modular aufgebauten Systems klinischer Prüfungen von Nootropika. In: Coper H et al. (eds) Hirnorganische Psychosyndrome im Alter. III. Springer, Berlin Heidelberg New York, pp 73–79

Kanowski S, Coper H (1982) Das hirnorganische Psychosyndrom als Ziel pharmakologischer Beeinflussung. In: Bente D, Coper H, Kanowski S (eds) Hirnorganische Psychosyndrome im Alter. II. Springer, Berlin Heidelberg New York, pp 3–19

Kanowski S, Hedde JP (1986) Arzneimittel für die Indikation hirnorganisch bedingter Leistungsstörungen (Nootropika). In: Dölle W, Müller-Oerlinghausen, Schwabe U (eds) Grundlagen der Arzneimitteltherapie. Bibliographisches Institut, Mannheim, pp 154–171

McKhann G, Drachman D, Folstein M, Katzmann R, Price D, Stadlan EM (1984) Clinical diagnosis of Alzheimer's disease: report of the NINCDS-ADRDA work group under the auspices of Department of Health and Human Services Task Force on Alzheimer's disease. Neurology 34: 939–944.

Oswald WD, Fleischmann UM (1986) Nürnberger-Alters-Inventar NAI. Published by author, Erlangen

Reisberg B et al. (1982) The Global Deterioration Scale (GDS): an instrument for the assessment in Primary Degenerative Dementia (PDD). Am J Psychiatry 139: 1136–1139

Sonnemann E (1984) Allgemeine Lösungen multipler Testprobleme EDV in Medizin u. Biologie. Internationale Biometrische Gesellschaft (ed) Vol 13, pp 120–128

Winblad B (1987) Alzheimer's disease – a Nordic perspective (Referat). The Third Congress of the International Psychogeriatric Association (sponsored by the IPA in cooperation with Northwestern University Medical School), Chicago, Ill. Aug 28–31

Therapeutic Results with Nimodipine in Primary Degenerative Dementia and Multi-Infarct Dementia

P. K. Fischhof, G. Wagner, L. Littschauer, E. Rüther,
M. Apecechea, R. Hiersemenzel, J. Röhmel, F. Hoffmeister,
and N. Schmage

Introduction

The diagnostic label of dementia is not justified in all elderly patients with cognitive decline. However, an organic factor of unknown aetiology can also be assumed in patients suffering from a milder decline. Therefore, the term "organic brain syndrome" is quite common, especially in German-speaking countries, to characterize these patients as a diagnostic category [6, 8]. This term covers a broad range of dementing and non-dementing processes with different aetiologies [14].

The characteristics of the dementia syndrome, of primary degenerative dementia (PDD) and of multi-infarct dementia (MID), as defined by DSM-III [10], have been widely accepted. The diagnostic criteria for dementia are based mainly on cognitive functions, but DSM-III does not explicitly refer to a cut-off score on a suitable psychometric scale. However, a Mini-Mental State [5] score of 23 or less has proven useful for supporting the diagnosis of dementia. Clear criteria together with differentiating scores are a substantial requirement for clinical trials with psychotropic drugs.

Nootropic drugs are a group of chemically diverse compounds which are expected to improve cognitive functions such as memory, learning, comprehension, thinking and ability to concentrate. It is assumed that nootropics influence the reduced functional state of still vital neurons, irrespective of their special mode of action.

Many clinical trials with nootropic drugs in the past have lacked precise diagnostic criteria for identifying the kind of disease or disorder that the patients were suffering from. This is the main reason that the results of these studies have not been accepted by scientists working in the dementia field. It has been argued that efficacy should be demonstrated in well-defined patient samples. Even if a drug has shown beneficial effects in patients from a mixed nonhomogeneous sample, the attempt should be made to investigate whether the therapeutic drug response depends on the underlying aetiology.

Kanowski et al. reported the results of a study in patients with organic brain syndrome [9]. Although the Hachinski score was assessed in this study for documentation purposes, no further differentiation of the diagnosis was made. As the results were favourable for both active drugs, a replication of this study with nimodipine against placebo including PDD and MID as separate entities seemed warranted. The aim of the present study was to confirm the efficacy in the whole patient sample composed of two different diagnostic dementia groups. Comparisons between PDD

Bergener, Reisberg (Eds.)
Diagnosis and Treatment
of Senile Dementia
© Springer-Verlag Berlin Heidelberg 1989

and MID should then clarify whether the therapeutic response of one group was superior to the other.

Methods

The trial was randomized, double-blind and placebo-controlled. The patients were stratified as diagnostic groups of PDD and MID. Each stratum was intended to include about 60 patients so that 30 patients under nimodipine and 30 patients under placebo could be compared. The two strata together were to include 120 patients. Inpatients from the Psychiatric Hospital of Vienna, Baumgartner Höhe, and from a nursing home in Wien-Lainz were involved, after giving their informed consent.

The 12-week double-blind treatment phase was preceded by a 4-week single-blind placebo wash-out phase. Ratings and testings took place at the start (test day 1) and at the end of the placebo wash-out phase (test day 2), then 6 (test day 3) and 12 weeks (test day 4) after the start of the double-blind treatment. Male and female patients aged between 50 and 85 with a clinical diagnosis of dementia were eligible for further testing and differentiation. Before inclusion into the study, the patients had to meet several criteria [3, 10, 11, 12, 16], as shown in Fig. 1. Patients with a Hachinski score [7] of 5 or 6 were excluded. A Hachinski score of 4 or less resulted in further procedures to confirm the diagnosis of PDD. If the score was 7 or higher, EEG and computed tomography (CT) scan had to be compatible with the diagnosis of MID for the inclusion into the study. After EEG and CT scan, a SKT [4] score of 9 or higher was mandatory.

The patients were excluded in the case of meeting any of the following criteria:
Brain Diseases
- Severe dementia with complete disorientation
- Disturbance of consciousness
- Dementia resulting from alcoholism or head trauma (including post-contusional residual state)
- Acute organic psychosis, e. g. delirium
- Suspicion of depressive pseudodementia
- Stroke less than 6 months previously
- Epilepsy
- Dementing processes following expanding lesions, Parkinson's disease, or other neurological diseases

Patients with Unstable Metabolic Conditions
- Congestive heart failure or decompensated or circulatory insufficiency
- Severe chronic pulmonary disease which may lead to cerebral hypoxia
- Non-compensated cardiac dysrhythmia
- Decompensated or insulin-dependent diabetes mellitus
- Thyroid disease
- Pernicious anaemia
- Severe dehydration

Diseases Which Prevent Adequate Psychometric Testing
- Serious communication problems (sensorimotor aphasia, apraxia)

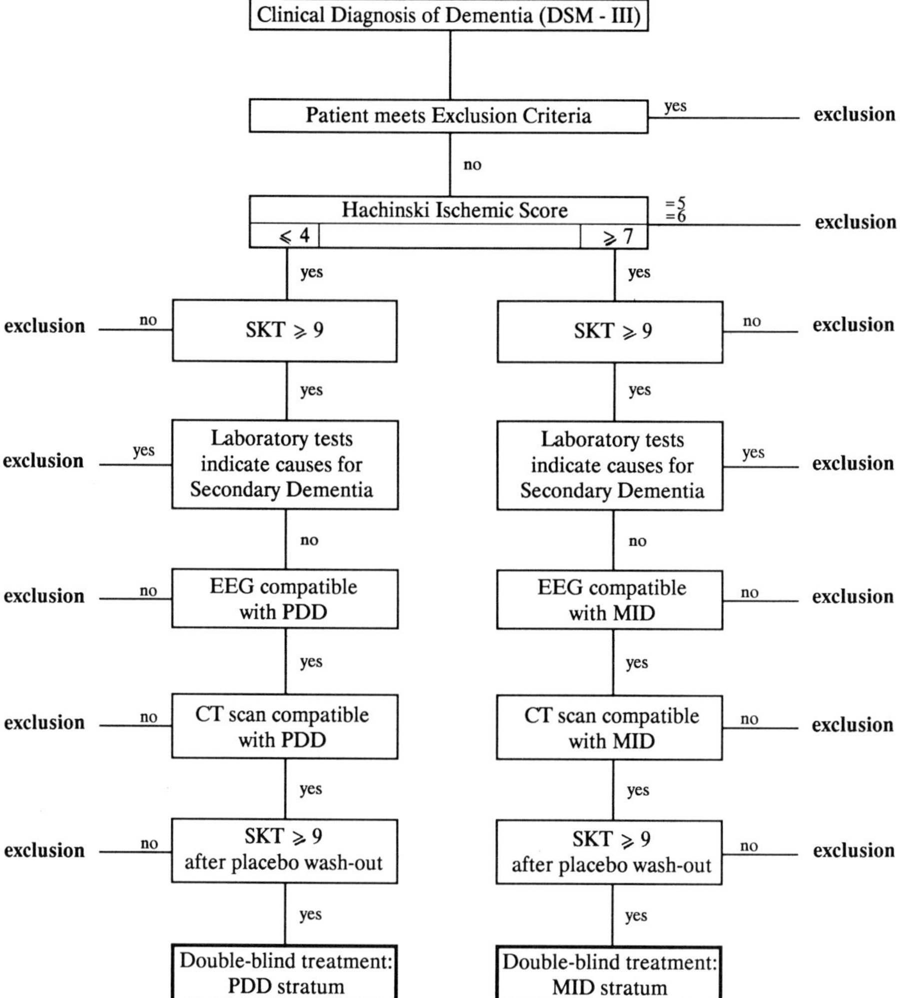

Fig. 1. Criteria for inclusion

– Inability to follow test instructions
– Non-compensated sensoric disturbances

Causes for Changed Pharmacokinetic Behaviour
– Severe gastrointestinal disorders
– Hepatic failure

Risks With Regard to Side Effects of the Drug
– Hypotension (systolic blood pressure < 105 mmHg)

Conditions Which Might Inferfere with the Psychometric Test Results
- Alcohol or drug abuse
- Concomitant treatment with other nootropics
- Concomitant treatment with other calcium antagonists
  (for methodological reasons)
- Concomitant treatment with cerebro-vasoactive compounds
- Irregular intake of other psychotropic drugs

At screening, the stage of the disease according to the Global Deterioration Scale (GDS [13]) and the Mini-Mental State score [5] were assessed for documentation and comparison purposes. The change of clinical symptoms during the course of the study was evalutated using the SCAG [2], and attention and memory functions were measured by the SKT [4]. The differences between end-point versus baseline assessments underwent confirmatory statistical analysis. Additionally, the Clinical Global Impressions (CGI [2]) was included as an overall clinical rating. The tolerability of nimodipine was recorded on the standardized scales DOTES and TWIS for side effects [1].

Nimodipine was given as a tablet of 30 mg. Placebo tablets looked identical. The dosage was one tablet three times daily.

The two target variables, SCAG total score and SKT total score, were subject to confirmatory statistical analysis using the one-sided Mann-Whitney U test. To test the working hypothesis that the score on the SCAG and the SKT in patients under nimodipine would have decreased at the end of treatment more strongly than in patients under placebo, two confirmatory tests were applied to the pre- and post-treatment differences of baseline (after placebo wash-out) versus 12-week assessments. The level of significance was set at $p < 0.05$, with an alpha-adjustment according to Bonferroni-Holm. Both target variables were then compared descriptively with regard to differences in therapeutic result between PDD and MID as separate strata. All other analyses including CGI or all measurements after 6 weeks of treatment must also be considered descriptive.

Results

A total of 228 patients aged between 50 and 85 years were screened for eligibility. In 31 cases the Hachinski score was 5 or 6, and these patients were not included. In 53 cases the CT scans were not compatible with the diagnosis of PDD or MID or were doubtful. Of 144 patients who entered the study after establishing the diagnosis, one patient dropped out during the placebo wash-out phase, and 13 dropped out during the double-blind treatment phase. The reasons for drop-out are shown in Table 1.

Of the 130 patients who completed the whole course of the study, 68 were diagnosed as having PDD and 62 as having MID. The age ranged between 61 and 83 in patients treated with nimodipine and between 67 and 84 in placebo patients. Initial values for height, sex ratio, Hachinski score, GDS stage and Mini-Mental State score were equally distributed in the two treatment groups. More women than men were included (nimodipine: 12 men, 49 women; placebo: 15 men, 54 women).

Table 1. Reasons for drop-out

| | Nimodipine | | Placebo | |
	PDD	MID	PDD	MID
Side effects	1	4	1	1
Deterioration of general condition	2	1	–	–
Discharge from hospital	2[a]	–	–	–
Non-compliance/withdrawal of consent	–	–	1	1
Total	5	5	2	2

[a] One patient was discharged from hospital during placebo wash-out

The measurements after the placebo wash-out period were considered baseline values for the efficacy variables SCAG and SKT. The corresponding comparison values for the confirmatory statistical analysis were assessed after the 12-week treatment phase. The measurements after 6 weeks were included for an exploratory analysis.

The mean SCAG total score for both strata, PDD and MID, decreased in patients under nimodipine from 71.6 to 65.9 and increased slightly under placebo from 70.9 to 71.0 after 12 weeks ($p < 0.001$; Fig. 2). The results were nearly the same when the

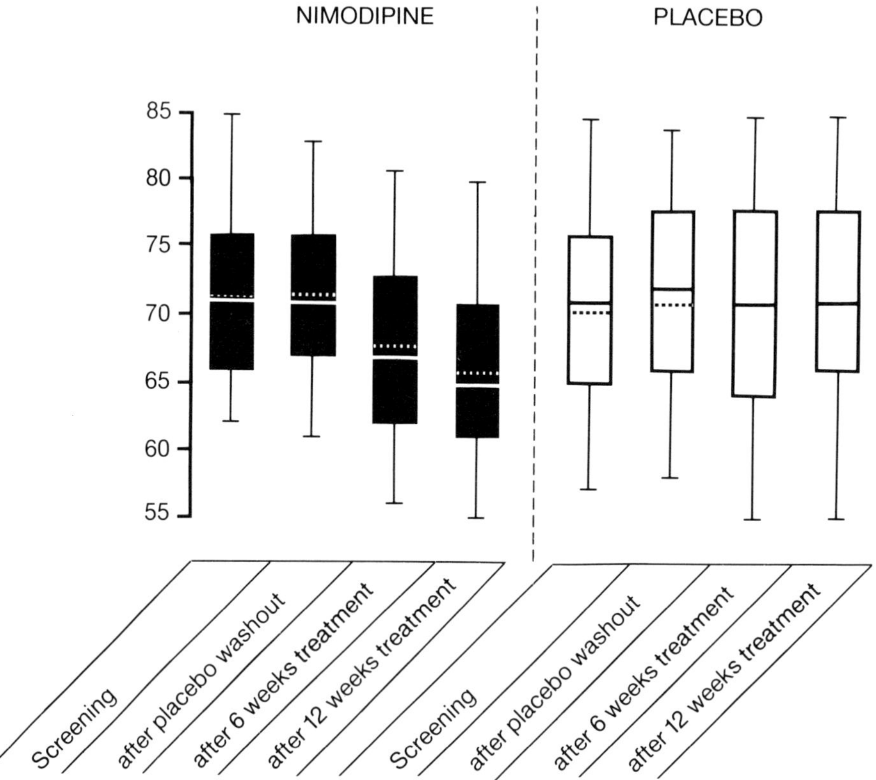

Fig. 2. SCAG total scores for those receiving nimodipine ($n = 61$) and those receiving placebo ($n = 69$)

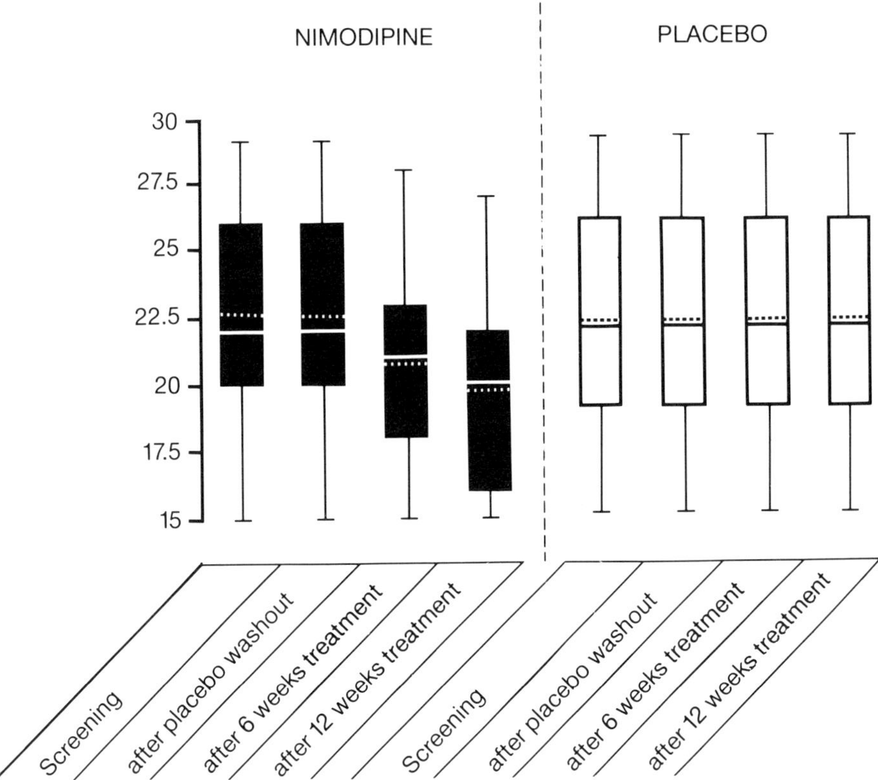

Fig. 3. Scores on SCAG factor "cognition" for those receiving nimodipine ($n = 61$) and those receiving placebo ($n = 69$)

PDD group was analysed separately. There was a decrease in the nimodipine group and a slight increase in the placebo group ($p < 0.001$). Also in the MID stratum similar changes could be observed. The only difference here was that under placebo there was a slight decrease ($p < 0.05$).

There was a decrease in the mean SCAG cognition score from 22.5 to 19.9 in nimodipine-treated patients in both strata and almost no change under placebo ($p < 0.001$; Fig. 3). The decrease in cognition score was also visible under nimodipine in the PDD stratum, and the changes under placebo were only marginal ($p < 0.01$). Again, similar changes could be seen in the MID stratum; the results, however, were not statistically significant.

The mean SKT total score decreased from 19.6 to 15.5 under nimodipine in PDD and MID together and decreased from 19.5 to 18.6 under placebo ($p < 0.001$; Fig. 4). Similar changes were noticeable when the PDD stratum was analysed separately. Here, the mean SKT total score decreased from 19.3 to 14.9 under nimodipine ($p < 0.001$). In the MID stratum the decrease in mean SKT total score was slightly less pronounced under nimodipine than in the PDD stratum; the score changed from 19.6 to 16.1 ($p < 0.05$).

356   P.K. Fischhof et al.

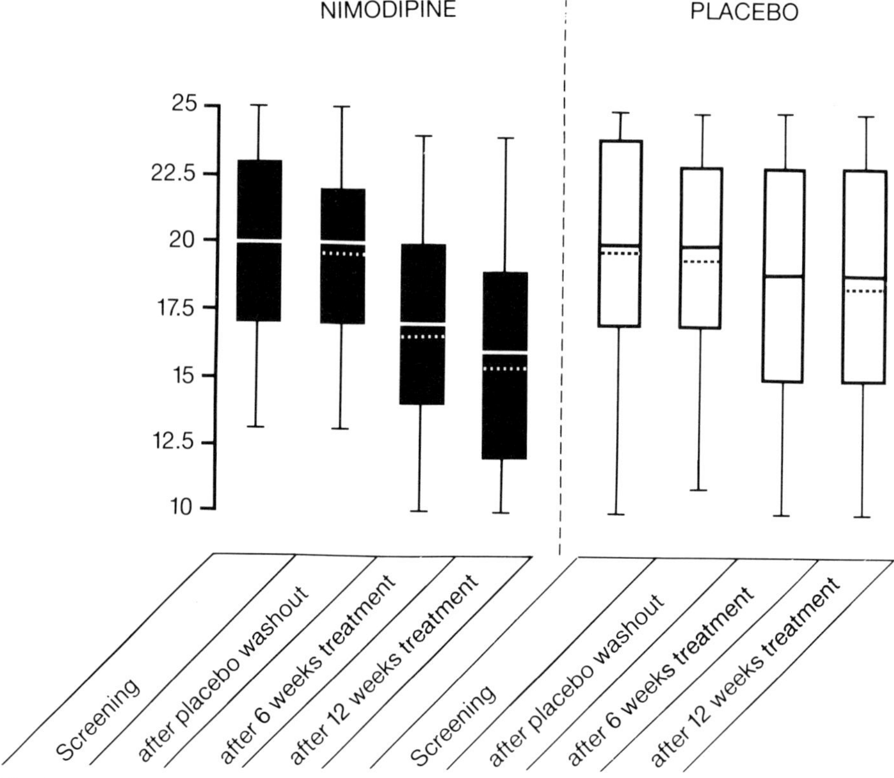

Fig. 4. SKT total scores for those receiving nimodipine ($n = 61$) and those receiving placebo ($n = 69$)

The CGI was also included in this study, but was defined as an exploratory variable in order to avoid problems of multiple testing and alpha-adjustments.

The global improvement rating (CGI) after 12 weeks is shown in Table 2 for both strata. There was a total improvement rate of 77% under nimodipine and 14% under placebo. In 59% of the placebo cases, there was no change. Minimally worse were 26% under placebo and only 5% under nimodipine ($p < 0.001$). Similar results were obtained when the PDD stratum was analysed separately. The improvement rate under nimodipine was 75% ($p < 0.001$). In the MID stratum, the total improvement rate under nimodipine was 78% ($p < 0.001$).

In view of the significance levels reached with the two target variables (SCAG total score, SKT total score) an alpha-adjustment is thus not necessary. It can be accepted that the nimodipine effects were superior to placebo.

Tolerability

In general, tolerability of the drug throughout the study was good. No major problems occured.

Table 2. Global improvement (CGI) after 12 weeks: PDD and MID together

Rating	Nimodipine		Placebo	
	n	*%*	*n*	*%*
Not assessed	0	0	0	0
Very much improved	7	11	1	1
Much improved	20	33	3	4
Minimally improved	20	33	6	9
No change	11	18	41	59
Minimally worse	3	5	18	26
Much worse	0	0	0	0
Very much worse	0	0	0	0
Total	61	100	69	100

As reduction of blood pressure is a known effect of dihydropyridine derivatives, blood pressure changes were analysed. Comparisons of baseline versus 12-week treatment values revealed that nimodipine lowered the mean systolic blood pressure by 11 mmHg in both strata taken together, whereas patients under placebo showed a mean reduction by 3.6 mmHg. The measurements at the end of the study ranged from 115 to 160 mmHg under nimodipine and from 120 to 170 mmHg under placebo. Mild to moderate drops in blood pressure as a side effect were noted in 12 cases under nimodipine and in 4 cases under placebo. This was a drop-out reason in one patient under nimodipine and in one under placebo. Dizziness was recorded in 14 nimodipine patients and in 8 placebo patients. This was a drop-out reason in three cases under nimodipine and in one under placebo. Other side-effects noted more often under nimodipine than placebo were nausea/vomiting, gastralgia, lack of appetite, headache and agitation.

Deterioration of general condition was a drop-out reason in three patients under nimodipine. As these patients suffered from multimorbidity (cardiovascular, pulmonary and gastric diseases, diabetes mellitus), the deterioration can be explained by the course of the primary diseases. A relation to the treatment with nimodipine seems rather unlikely.

Discussion

The results of this study show that nimodipine improves symptoms in patients with PDD and MID. Especially, the influence of nimodipine on cognitive functions was documented by the SKT and in the score of the SCAG factor "cognition". The global improvement rating of the CGI also showed nimodipine to be superior to placebo.

The progressive impairment of cognitive functions seems to be a good indicator of the functional stage of dementing processes. Definitions in the DSM-III are based on cognitive functions. Also the GDS characteristics of the individual stages refer to the extent of cognitive impairment. Improvement or stabilization of cognitive functions should therefore be meaningful for the patient. As the SKT measures attention and memory of the patient, and as the SCAG rating was performed by a clinical psychologist and the CGI rating assessed by a physician, efficacy of nimodipine was demonstrated by the patient's performance and by two independent raters with different methods.

The numeric change in the SCAG total score under nimodipine does not seem to be impressive at first sight. The decrease is in the range of one standard deviation. In former nimodipine studies higher numeric differences were reached. However, it is known that the SCAG does not offer precise anchor-points. Although Venn [15] published a manual for the SCAG with a rating guide, it has not been shown that this guide improved the rating situation. Individual raters may use a broad or narrow range when assessing the patient. In the case of this study the range of differences was narrow. But in patients treated with placebo there were almost no changes. As an experienced clinical psychologist performed the ratings under double-blind conditions, the results are obviously reliable. With respect to the results in the SKT and the CGI, the SCAG differences seem to be meaningful.

This study is one of the few with nootropic drugs in which a proper diagnostic differentiation was required. The criteria of DSM-III were adopted for the purposes of this study. For both diagnostic groups taken together, efficacy of nimodipine could be demonstrated by means of suitable instruments. The results were statistically significant. When analysed separately, nimodipine was effective in each of the two diagnostic strata. But it seems that the results in patients with PDD are slightly more favourable than in MID, based on the different levels of statistical significance. The SKT results in MID were significant at $p < 0.05$, whereas the PDD stratum reached $p < 0.01$. Furthermore, the SCAG factor "cognition" did not reach statistical significance in the MID stratum. These statistical differences in therapeutic response seem to have no clinical relevance. But the situation may be different in the case of larger samples.

The primary question as to whether there is a therapeutic effect of nimodipine in dementia irrespective of the underlying degenerative or vascular process can be answered affirmatively on the basis of these results. However, whether PDD patients respond better to nimodipine than do MID patients, cannot be answered definitely. Nevertheless, nimodipine is a promising drug in both PDD and MID.

References

1. CIPS – Collegium Internationale Psychiatria Scalarum (1981) (ed) Internationale Skalen für Psychiatrie, 2nd edn Beltz Test, Weinheim
2. CIPS – Collegium Internationale Psychiatriae Scalarum (eds) (1986) Internationale Skalen für Psychiatrie, 3rd edn Beltz Test, Weinheim
3. Eisdorfer C, Cohen D (1980) Diagnostic criteria for primary neuronal degeneration of the Alzheimner's type. J Fam Pract 11: 553–557
4. Erzigkeit H (1986) Der Syndrom-Kurztest zur Erfassung von Aufmerksamkeits- und Gedächtnis-störungen, 2nd edn. Vless, Vaterstetten
5. Folstein MF, Folstein SE, McHugh PR (1975) "Mini-Mental State". A practical method for grading the cognitive state of patients for the clinician. J Psychiat Res 12: 189–198
6. Gertz H-J, Kanowski S (1983) Die Therapie der senilen Demenz vom Alzheimer-Typ und der Multi-Infarkt-Demenz. Nervenarzt 54: 444–459
7. Hachinski VC et al. (1975) Cerebral blood flow in dementia. Arch Neurol 32: 632–637

8. Kanowski S, Coper H (1982) Das hirnorganische Psychosyndrom als Ziel pharmakologischer Beeinflussung. In: Bente D, Coper H, Kanowski S (eds) Hirnorganische Psychosyndrome im Alter. Springer, Berlin Heidelberg New York
9. Kanowski S, Fischhof P, Hiersemenzel R, Röhmel J, Kern U (1988) Wirksamkeitsnachweis von Nootropika am Beispiel von Nimodipin – ein Beitrag zur Entwicklung geeigneter klinischer Prüfmodelle. Z Gerontopsychol Psychiatrie 1: 35–44
10. Koehler K, Saß H (eds) (1984) Diagnostisches und statistisches Manual psychischer Störungen – DSM-III. Beltz, Weinheim
11. Ladurner G (1984) Die Klinik der vaskulären Demenz und ihre klinische Differentialdiagnose. In: Lechner H, Ladurner G, Ott E (eds) Klinik, Diagnostik und Therapie zerebraler Abbauprozesse. Perimed, Erlangen, pp 48–53
12. McKhann et al. (1984) Clinical diagnosis of Alzheimer's disease. Report of the NINCDS-ADRDA Work Group under the auspices of Health and Human Services Task Force on Alzheimer's disease. Neurology 34: 939–944
13. Reisberg B et al. (1982) The global deterioration scale for assessment of primary degenerative dementia. Am J Psychiatry 139: 1136–1139
14. Schmage N, Boehme K, Dycka J, Schmitz H (1989) Nimodipine for psychogeriatric use: methods, strategies and considerations based on experience with clinical trials. In: Bergener M, Reisberg B (eds) Diagnosis and treatment of senile dementia, p 374–381
15. Venn RD (1983) The Sandoz Clinical Assessment-Geriatric (SCAG) Scale – a general-purpose psychogeriatric rating scale. Gerontology 29: 185–198
16. Wagner O, Oesterreich K, Hoyer S (1985) Validity of the ischemic score in degenerative and vascular dementia and depression in old age. Arch Gerontol Geriatr 4: 333–345

Nimodipine Treatment Improves Cognitive Functions in Vascular Dementia

N. Tobares, A. Pedromingo, and J. Bigorra

Introduction

In recent years, the calcium antagonists in the group of dihydropyridine derivatives have been the subject of investigation for treatment of cerebrovascular disease [6]. Clinical and animal studies have provided promising results concerning the therapeutic value of dihydropyridines in cerebral ischaemia [3, 5, 7, 16]. Furthermore, it has been shown that in the brain, receptor binding sites for dihydropyridines are to be found in the blood vessels as well as in neural tissue [15]. Hence these compounds might act on the ischaemic tissue not only because of their potent dilator effect on the cerebral arterioles, but also by blocking the entry of calcium into neurons, an event which occurs after ischaemia. It is known that calcium-activated proteases and phospholipases produce cytotoxic free radicals and leukotrienes [13, 19]. In addition, dihydropyridines increase erythrocyte deformability [20].

The present study was undertaken to evaluate the effect of nimodipine, the most selective dihydropyridine derivative for cephalic blood vessels [4], on mental performance in senile vascular dementia.

Materials

All patients who participated in this study were living in a home for the elderly. Informed consent was obtained from the patients and/or from the relatives. The study was double-blind, placebo-controlled and randomized.

A group of 33 patients – 12 men and 21 women, aged 68–91 years (mean ± SD: 80.4 ± 4.6) – was treated with nimodipine (30 mg three times a day) for 24 weeks. The placebo group included 32 patients – 15 men and 17 women, aged 67–91 years (mean ± SD: 80.3 ± 5.4).

The diagnosis of dementia on the basis of DMS-III was made from the patient's history and/or from information given by close acquaintances and suggesting global mental impairment, as well as from physical and neurological examination. Vascular dementia was diagnosed on the basis of a Hachinski Ischaemic Score of more than 7 points [8]. Patients with coexisting depression as determined by the Brief Assessment Interview of Copeland et al. [2] and those with serious neurological or systemic diseases were excluded.

Bergener, Reisberg (Eds.)
Diagnosis and Treatment
of Senile Dementia
© Springer-Verlag Berlin Heidelberg 1989

Mental performance was evaluated by Pfeiffer's Short Portable Mental State Questionnaire [12], Wechsler's Digit Span Test [18], the Number Span Test of Bardizet and Camy [1], and the Sandoz Clinical Assessment–Geriatric Scale [17]. In addition, performance of daily living was assessed by the Crichton Behavioural Rating Scale as modified by Robinson [14], and the Performance Test of Activities of Daily Living published by Kuriansky et al. [11].

The tests were performed at baseline and after 4, 12 and 24 weeks of treatment.

The results are expressed as the mean ± SEM. The Mann-Whitney U test and analyses of variance and covariance with repeated measures (using BMDP2V) were used for statistical analysis of the data.

Results

As shown in Fig. 1, pretreatment severity of dementia, as determined by Pfeiffer's Short Portable Mental State Questionnaire, was comparable in the two groups of patients. The number of errors for the placebo group was 4.62 ± 0.15 and for the nimodipine group, the number of errors was 4.78 ± 0.16. According to Pfeiffer [12], for the nimodipine group, these scores are within the range of mild to moderate intellectual impairment. Analysis of covariance showed that the time–nimodipine treatment interaction led to a small but statistically significant improvement in the performance of this test ($p < 0.01$).

Evaluation of short-term memory for numbers was performed by the Digit Span Test [18] and by the Number Span Test [1]. Results for the Digit Span Test are shown in Fig. 2. The mean pretreatment score of the nimodipine group (8.96 ± 0.53) was higher than that of the placebo group (7.83 ± 0.62), although the difference did not attain statistical significance ($p = 0.083$). Analysis of the effect of nimodipine treatment as well as of the time–nimodipine treatment interaction showed a statistically significant improvement in the performance of this test ($p < 0.05$ and $p < 0.01$, respectively).

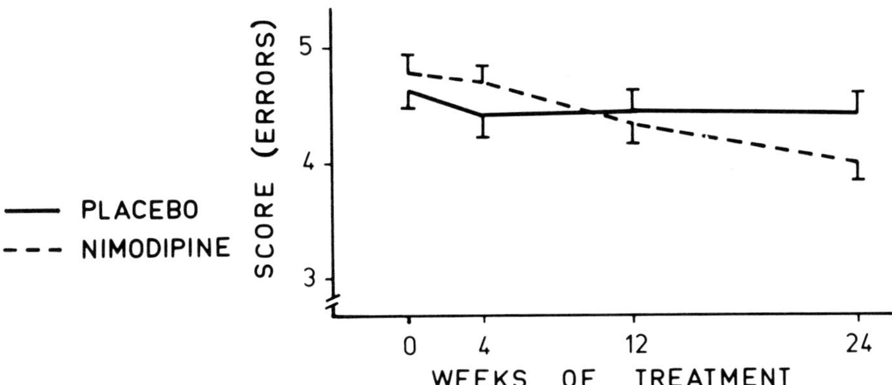

Fig. 1. Results from the Short Portable Mental Status Questionnaire in elderly patients suffering from cerebrovascular dementia treated with nimodipine ($n = 33$) or placebo ($n = 32$). Means ± SEM

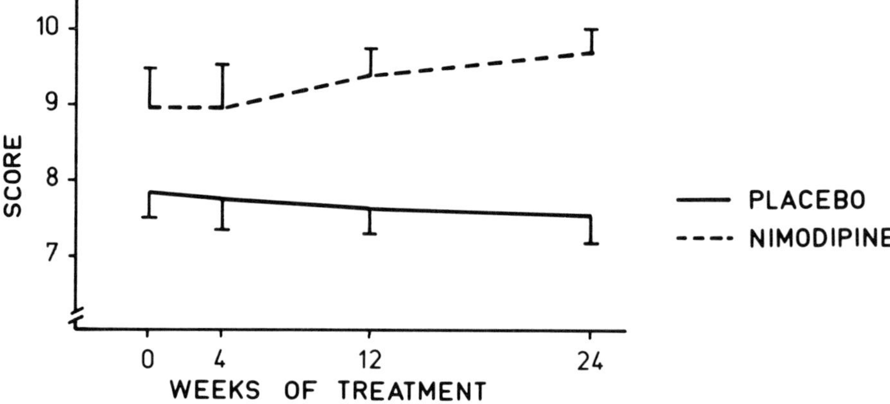

Fig. 2. Results from the Digit Span Test in elderly patients suffering from cerebrovascular dementia treated with nimodipine ($n = 33$) or placebo ($n =32$). Means ± SEM

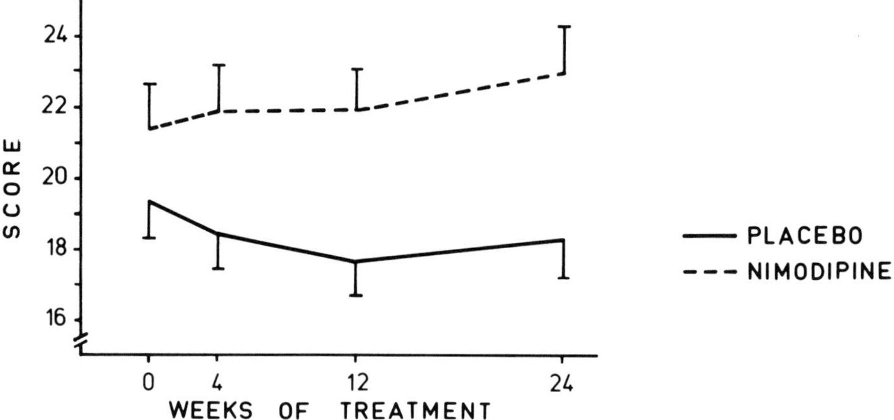

Fig. 3. Results from the Number Span Test in elderly patients suffering from cerebrovascular dementia treated with nimodipine ($n = 33$) or placebo ($n = 32$). Means ± SEM

The mean pretreatment score obtained for the Number Span Test (Fig. 3) was again higher in the nimodipine group (21.39 ± 1.23) than in the placebo group (19.32 ± 0.93), but this difference was not statistically significant ($p = 0.27$). While in the placebo group no changes were observed, after nimodipine treatment a higher score was obtained (23.03 ± 1.23; $p < 0.05$).

In the factor structure of the Sandoz Clinical Assessment-Geriatric Scale reported by Hamot et al. [9], the items mental alertness, confusion, impairment of recent memory and disorientation highly loaded on the factor named "cognitive dysfunction". A slight improvement in this factor in patients receiving nimodipine was statistically significant, both for the treatment factor and the time–treatment interaction ($p < 0.025$; Fig. 4).

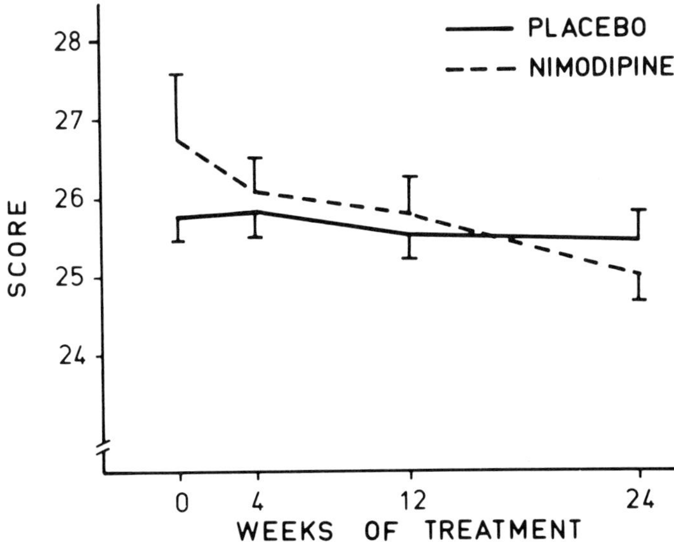

Fig. 4. Results from the Sandoz Clinical Assessment-Geriatric Scale in elderly patients suffering from cerebrovascular dementia treated with nimodipine ($n = 33$) or placebo ($n = 32$). Means ± SEM

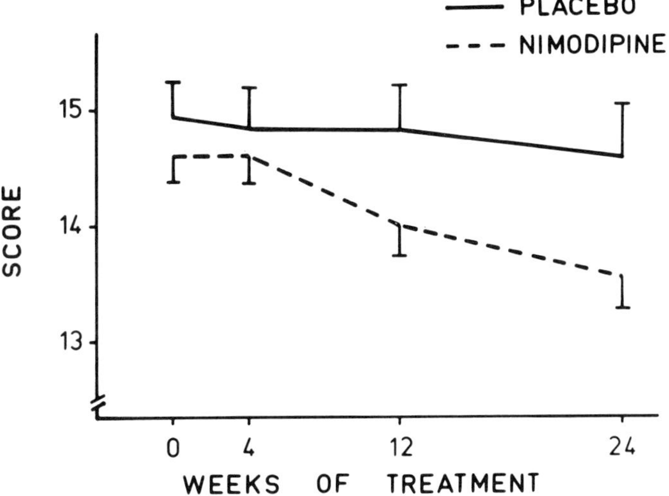

Fig. 5. Results from the Crichton Behavioural Rating Scale in elderly patients suffering from cerebrovascular dementia treated with nimodipine ($n = 33$) or placebo ($n = 32$). Means ± SEM

The patient's ability to perform everyday activities, assessed by the Crichton Geriatric Behavioural Rating Scale (Fig. 5), showed a statistically significant difference for the time–nimodipine treatment interaction ($p < 0.05$). However, when assessed by the Performance Test of Activities of Daily Living (Fig. 6), the effects under nimodipine did not differ from placebo treatment.

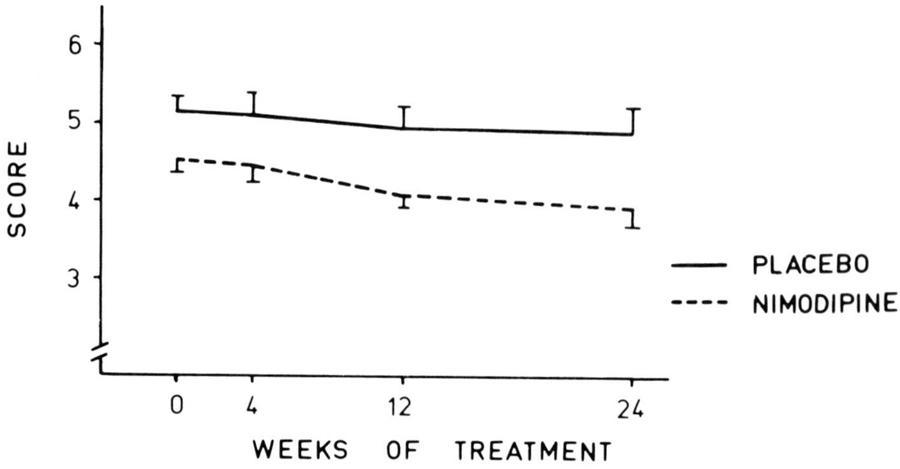

Fig. 6. Results from the Performance Activity of Daily Living Scale in elderly patients suffering from cerebrovascular dementia treated with nimodipine ($n = 33$) or placebo ($n = 32$). Means ± SEM

Finally, it should be mentioned that in all the above-mentioned tests, a statistically significant amelioration associated with the time factor was evidenced, possibly due to training effects.

Nimodipine was well tolerated, and no relevant side effects, including changes in blood pressure, were recorded.

Discussion

Our results show that in elderly patients suffering from mild to moderate cerebrovascular dementia, nimodipine treatment is associated with improvement of cognitive functions and activities of daily living. In all psychometric tests used in this study to assess cognitive function, patients receiving nimodipine showed improvement, whereas in some of these tests patients under placebo slightly deteriorated.

A variety of rating scales for the assessment of activities of daily living exist [10]. Of the two scales chosen for this study, the Crichton Geriatric Behavioural Rating Scale showed patients treated with nimodipine to perform better than patients under placebo, whereas the Performance Test of Activities of Daily Living Scale did not show any difference between the two treatment groups. These conflicting results may be explained by the assumption that the Activities of Daily Living Scale was not appropriate for the patient population included in this study. This scale asseses whether the patient performs each of the requested tasks without (task score = 0) or with help (task score = 1). Severe impairment of these functions is more likely to occur at later stages of dementia. In this study the initial total scores were rather low so that treatment effects may not have been reflected by this scale ("bottom effect").

In studies with psychotropic drugs it is always difficult to draw conclusions as to clinical relevance directly from results in psychometric tests. However, it is important to note that the improvement of cognitive functions under nimodipine was confirmed by all the tests used in this study. The impairment of cognitive functions is the first and essential sign of dementing processes. The further course is strongly associated with the progression of cognitive impairment. Therefore even slight improvement or stabilization of cognitive functions is a desirable therapeutic aim. Besides drug effects, training effects, both under nimodipine and placebo, must be taken into consideration. As improvement was also found to be statistically significantly associated with the time factor, such training effects must be discussed. Nevertheless, the results remain favourable for the patients treated with nimodipine. Since cognitive functions of the patients under placebo even deteriorated slightly, the clinical relevance of the results obtained with nimodipine is sufficiently demonstrated, even more, so as an accepted therapy for senile cerebrovascular dementia has so far not been established.

References

1. Bardizet J, Camy E (1968) Clinical and psychometric study of a patient with memory disturbance. Int J Neurol 7: 44–54
2. Copeland JRM, Kelleher MJ, Kellet JM, Gourlay AJ (1976) A semi-structured clinical interview for the assessment of diagnosis and mental state in the elderly: the geriatric mental state schedule. I. Development and reliability. Psychol Med 6: 443–449
3. Editorial (1985) Calcium channel blockers in the prophylactic treatment of vascular headache. Ann Intern Med 102: 395–397
4. Gelmers HJ (1983) Nimodipine, a new calcium antagonist in the prophylactic treatment of migraine. Headache 23: 106–109
5. Gelmers HJ, Gorter K, de Weerdt CJ, Weizer JHA (1986) Effect of nimodipine on clinical outcome in patients with acute ischemic strome (Abstract) Stroke 17: 145
6. Grotta JC (1987) Current medical and surgical therapy for cerebrovascular disease. N Engl J Med 317: 1506–1516
7. Grotta J, Spydell J, Pettigrew C, Ostrow P, Hunter D (1986) The effect of nicardipine on neuronal function following ischemia. Stroke 17: 213–219
8. Hachinski V (1978) Cerebral blood flow: differentiation of Alzheimer's disease from multi-infarct dementia. In: Katzman R, Terry RD, Bick KL (eds) Alzheimer's disease: senile dementia and related disorders. Raven, New York, pp 97–104
9. Hamot HB, Patin JR, Singer JM (1984) Factor structure of the Sandoz Clinical Assessment-Geriatric (SCAG) Scale. Psychopharmacol Bull 20: 142–150
10. Israel L, Kozarevic D, Sartorius N (1984) Source book of geriatric assessment, vols 1–2. Karger, Basel
11. Kuriansky J, Gurland BJ, Fleiss JL, Cowan PW (1976) The assessment of self care capacity in geriatric psychiatric patients by objective and subjective measures. J Clin Psychol 32: 95–102
12. Pfeiffer E (1975) Short Portable Mental Status Questionnaire. J Am Geriatr Soc 23: 433–441
13. Reichle ME (1983) The pathophysiology of brain ischemia. Ann Neurol 13: 2–10
14. Robinson RA (1961) Some problems of clinical trials in elderly people. Gerontol Clin 3: 247–253
15. Snyder SH, Reynolds IJ (1985) Calcium-antagonist drugs. Receptor interactions that clarify therapeutic effects. N Engl J Med 313: 995–1002
16. Steen PA, Newberg IA, Milde JH, Michenfelder JD (1983) Nimodipine improves cerebral blood flow and neurologic recovery after complete cerebral ischemia in the dog. J Cereb Blood Flow Metab 3: 38–43
17. Venn RD (1983) The Sandoz Clinical Assessment-Geriatric Scale. A general-purpose psychogeriatric rating scale. Gerontology 29: 185–198
18. Wechsler D (1945) A standardized memory scale for clinical use. J Psychol 19: 87–95
19. Wieloch T, Harris RJ, Siesjö BK (1982) Brain metabolism and ischemia: mechanism of cell damage and principles of protection. J Cereb Blood Flow Metab 2 (Suppl 1): 1: 55–59
20. Yamomoto M, Ohta T, Toda N (1983) Mechanisms of relxant action of nicardipine, a new Ca^{++}-antagonist, on isolated dog cerebral and mesenteric arteries. Stroke 14: 270–275

Nimodipine in the Treatment of Alzheimer's Disease*

B. Baumel, L. S. Eisner, M. Karukin, R. MacNamara, and H. Raphan

Introduction

Nimodipine is a calcium antagonist with a predilective action on the cerebral vessels. It has an effect on vascular tone of cerebral vessels and increases cerebral blood flow. It acts on small and large vessels. There is a dose-dependent effect in increasing the cerebral blood flow. At high dosages it can increase cerebral blood flow as much as 70%–100% compared to the baseline value of flow. Nimodipine prevents the cerebrovascular damage induced by transient ischemia, electroshock, anoxia or hypoxia. The electroshock-induced amnesia in the mouse and hypoxia-induced amnesia in the rat is prevented by nimodipine. The survivability of mice exposed to a hypoxic atmosphere is increased after prophylactic treatment with nimodipine [7].

The role of calcium in the etiology and pathophysiology of Alzheimer's disease is not known, although it is known that calcium and calmodulin control protein kinase in cell membranes [6]. The neurons from patients with Alzheimer's disease contain an excess amount of calcium. Calcium plays a role in ischemic cell death, and calcium-channel blockers prolong tolerance to ischemia in animal models [7]. The alteration of calcium flow in the cell membrane may be important in cellular function. Calcium accumulates in cells with neurofibrillar tangles. The clinical effect of nimodipine may be due to any of the many calcium cell functions.

In Alzheimer's disease there appear to be three populations of cells:
a) selective areas with neuronal cell loss and extensive reductions in levels of catecholamine acetyl-transferase (CAT) where cells virtually do not function;
b) cells that are marginally functioning with reduced levels of CAT and acetyl-cholinesterase; and
c) cells that are normal.

Clinical improvement should be apparent if marginally functioning cells are restored to health. Deterioration may be prevented by inhibiting degeneration in the normal population of cells [3].

The incidence of Alzheimer's disease is greatest in the older adult population. People over 80 years of age have a one in five incidence of dementia. This age group is the most rapidly increasing portion of our population [8]. Alzheimer's dementia is the

* The authors gratefully acknowledge the assistance of Miles Pharmaceuticals Inc. in preparation and support of this project; statistical services were provided by Miles and Abt Associates.

Bergener, Reisberg (Eds.)
Diagnosis and Treatment
of Senile Dementia
© Springer-Verlag Berlin Heidelberg 1989

most common type of dementia. This disorder is progressive over years and eventually causes complete dependence. Demented patients often require institutionalization because of behavioral problems [11]. Due to side effects of medications, there are limited means for control of their behavior. The progressive deterioration of a condition that frequently leads to institutionalization would justify treatment at any stage of the disease. Any improvement in the quality of life or any inhibition of deterioration would be a welcome benefit to the patient or to those caring for the Alzheimer's victim.

Safety studies have been conducted in both normal young and geriatric populations treated with nimodipine. No serious side effects have been found. Cardiovascular function has shown no differences from that in a placebo-treated group. Blood pressure and pulse rates do not significantly differ from placebo values. Even in severely stressed individuals suffering subarachnoid hemorrhage, nimodipine has been shown to be relatively safe [1].

Because of the protective nature of this drug on the central nervous system and the known effects of calcium on cellular function, a study was undertaken to evaluate the efficacy of nimodipine for the treatment or prevention of cognitive, behavioral, and affective impairments in Alzheimer's disease. This was done in a double-blind placebo-controlled randomized clinical trial. Standard psychometric and behavioral assessment scales were used as outcome measures.

Methods

This study was designed to assess the relative safety and efficacy of nimodipine to that of placebo. A total of 234 subjects were entered into the study, of whom 227 received either placebo or study drug. To demonstrate the effects of nimodipine, the evaluation of patients over a ten-visit, 14-week study was completed over a 2-year period. Data for this study was collected from nine sites in the United States.

This study was designed with essentially two phases: first, a 2-week single-blind placebo phase as a washout and screening period, followed by 12 weeks of double-blind, placebo-controlled randomization. The subjects were randomly assigned to one of three treatment groups. Patients received either 30 mg nimodipine three times a day, 60 mg nimodipine three times a day, or placebo.

Patients who entered this study were initially screened and tested against standardized criteria among all centers participating. Consent was obtained from all subjects, as well as from their caregivers. Initial evaluations included a medical history, physical and neurological examination, laboratory tests, scans, and psychological tests.

Participants included in the trial were over 45 years old, of either sex, and of any race. They all had to have a primary diagnosis of Alzheimer's disease according to the DSM-III criteria for primary degenerative dementia. Computed tomography scans could be normal or show evidence of atrophy only. In addition to diagnostic evaluations performed by each of the investigators, subjects were required to have a score of 4 or less in the Hachinski Ischemic Score, a score between 4 and 23 on the Folstein Mini-Mental State Exam, a score of less than 16 on the Hamilton Depression Scale, and a Reisberg Global Deterioration Scale of four 4, 5, or 6. In addition to standard serum chemistries, laboratory tests were screened for syphilis, thyroid disease, vitamin B_{12} deficiency, and folic acid deficiency.

Exclusion of subjects was based on the presence of unstable, serious illness or illness that would interfere with the evaluation of the study drug. Patients with unstable cardiac disease such as conduction defects, pathological bradycardia, angina, arrhythmias, or recent myocardial infarction were excluded from this trial. Patients with alcoholism, peptic ulcer disease, severe anemia, uncontrolled hypothyriodism, or target organ failure were also excluded. Other exclusions included CNS diseases and primary psychiatric diagnosis of anxiety or depressive disorders. Seizure disorder that preceded the dementia and head trauma with sequelae of cognitive defects were excluded. Vascular or metabolic dementias were excluded.

All subjects enrolled had medication administration supervised by a responsible party. Patients had to be able to swallow. This became important because of the testing of severely demented patients at the latter stages of the illness. They were not allowed to be on any other investigational drug study. Certain other medications were excluded from being administered concomitantly. These included other calcium antagonists, antihypertensives with CNS activity, cerebral vasodilators, metabolic enhancers, anxiolytics, phenothiazines, and antidepressants.

After subjects were found to meet the criteria for the study and appropriate consent was obtained, they began a 2-week single-blind placebo washout phase. At the end of this phase, the subjects returned for baseline safety and efficacy measures. Subjects then entered the double-blind phase of the study. Each subject was randomly assigned to one of the three treatment groups. After randomization patients were scheduled to return at interval visits for both safety and efficacy evaluations over the following 12 weeks. Visits 3, 4, 5, 7, and 9 were primarily for safety evaluations consisting of vital signs, blood tests, and assessment of any adverse experiences. Visits 6, 8, and 10 were primarily to assess efficacy as well as safety. Therefore patients would be seen at a total of ten visits over a 14-week period of time: one visit for screening, one visit for baseline, and eight treatment visits.

There were several instances in which subjects did not complete all scheduled visits. If a patient completed at least 10 weeks of therapy, and their end-of-study visit was not greater than 2 weeks from the last dose of study drug, the data from the end-of-study visit was used in both the efficacy and safety analysis. If the date of last dose was longer than 2 weeks from the end-of-study visit, or if the patient participated for less than 10 weeks, only the safety data were included from the final visit for the analysis of that subject's data.

Safety measurements, including the screening procedures at baseline, consisted of standard measures of physical health. Medical histories, physical examination, and laboratory tests were utilized as baseline data for subsequent evaluations of the same measures. The physical examination was repeated at the end-of-study visit. Vital signs, including blood pressure, pulse, and respiration, were recorded every 30 min for 1.5 h after an office dose of study medication. This set was performed at all visits through the 4th week of double-blind therapy. For the remainder of the follow-up visits, blood pressure was recorded 1 h after the office dose. An interval electroencephalogram and electrocardiogram were scheduled for visit 7, at the 6th week of double-blind treatment, and at the end-of-study visit.

Efficacy was defined to be an improvement in psychometric test scores, investigators' global opinions, as well as aspects of patient management. These parameters consisted of both subjective and objective data sets. Tests were administered in standardized order and where possible by the same tester. The efficacy measures were scheduled for baseline, weeks 4, 8, and 12 in the double-blind portion of the study. The Hamilton Depression Scale was repeated on the 6th week of therapy and again at the end-of-study visit. The Mini-Mental State Examination and Global Deterioration Scale were repeated only once, at the end-of-study visit.

Objective measures of efficacy included the Buschke Selective Reminding Test. The version for this study consisted of a ten-item, five-trial format. Additionally, the Word Fluency Subtest of Neurosurgery Center Comprehensive Examination for Aphasia was used. Other objective cognitive function tests included the Standardized Road Map Test, the First and Last Names Test, the Symbol Digit Modalities Test, and Tapping Speed Test.

Measures of efficacy included investigator evaluations and relative assessments of behavioral changes and levels of functioning. These scales included the Reisberg Brief Cognitive Rating Scale, Relative's Assessment of Global Symptomatology, and the Activities of Daily Living scale. Investigators' assessments also included Clinical Global Impressions and Clinical Global Impressions for Depression.

The set of efficacy variables in this study also included the following:
Mini-Mental State Examination
Hamilton Psychiatric Rating Scale for Depression
Activities of Daily Living: personal care
Activities of Daily Living: household care
Activities of Daily Living: work and money
Activities of Daily Living: social relationships
Activities of Daily Living: communication
Symbol Digit Written Score
Symbol Digit Oral Score
Word Fluency Test
Tapping Speed Test
Standardized Road Map Test
First and Last Names Test I–III
First and Last Names Test IV
Buschke long-term retrieval
Buschke short-term recall
Buschke long-term storage
Buschke list learning
Buschke random long-term retrieval
Brief Cognitive Rating Scale: concentration
Brief Cognitive Rating Scale: recent memory
Brief Cognitive Rating Scale: past memory
Brief Cognitive Rating Scale: orientation
Brief Cognitive Rating Scale: functioning and self-care
Clinical Global Impressions: severity of illness
Clinical Global Impressions: global improvement

Clinical Global Impressions: efficacy index
Clinical Global Impressions for Depression: severity of impairment
Clinical Global Impressions for Depression: global improvement
Relative's Assessment of Global Symptomatology: anxious score
Relative's Assessment of Global Symptomatology: disoriented score
Relative's Assessment of Global Symptomatology: speech score
Relative's Assessment of Global Symptomatology: excited score

The data collected for this study were generated from nine field investigators and pooled for statistical analysis. The combined data were tested for validity using Fisher's exact test for categorical data, rank tests for ordinal data the Student's t test for continuous data. Primary efficacy analysis was based on the comparison of nimodipine-treated patients at each dose level to that of the placebo group. The primary outcome measures were the Global Improvement Scales, improvement in psychometric tests and, behavioral management of the patient. These comparisons employed standard analysis of variance of outcome measures at each visit compared to baseline. Each treatment group was also evaluated with respect to demography, concurrent problems, and other medical characteristics.

A secondary statistical analysis of the efficacy parameters was employed to further elucidate possible subtleties using methods of covariance and reverse transformation (i.e., scores when necessary were transformed if appropriate to display greater improvement with higher values). These methods were then applied to the factor analysis of the Relative's Assessment of Global Symptomatology, in addition to the remaining efficacy measures.

Results

Study Groups and Demography

A total of 234 patients entered the study, with 227 continuing beyond the screening visit and receiving study medication; 221 patients were present at baseline and entered the double-blind portion of the study. There were 75 patients treated with 60 mg nimodipine, 70 patients treated with 30 mg nimodipine, and 76 patients given placebo. Efficacy analysis was performed on 195 subjects, all of whom had either a valid end-of-study visit or a valid week 8 visit.

No statistically significant differences were seen when the groups were compared with respect to sex, race, age, height, weight, occupation, education, past history of dementia and concurrent illnesses ($p \geq 0.10$).

In only one variable of 30 measures of efficacy tested at baseline (Standardized Road Map Test) were the three groups found to be statistically different ($p = 0.02$). These differences were taken into account in the final analyses by including a term in each analysis of covariance for the score at baseline.

Changes in Placebo Group

The placebo group on average had efficacy scores that increased over time (worsened). Of the 33 measures of efficacy on which changes could be measured, eight measures changed significantly ($p < 0.05$). Three of the measures were subsets of items in Activities of Daily Living: personal care, household care, and communication. Two of the measures were scores from the Buschke Selective Reminding Test: long-term retrieval and long-term storage. Two of the measures were from the Relative's Assessment of Global Symptomatology: anxious score and speech score. Increases in scores represent greater impairment, i.e., the placebo group got worse. This finding was important in that, should the drug be able to prevent further deterioration of dementia but not be able to lessen existing symptoms, this effect might only be detected if there were further deterioration in untreated (placebo) patients.

End point Analyses of Efficacy

Of the 33 measures of efficacy, in only one – Clinical Global Impressions for Depression: global improvement – was there a marginally significant main effect for drug ($p = 0.084$). A further test of the least-squares adjusted means revealed the 30-mg dose to be significantly better than placebo ($p = 0.029$) for this variable. There was no statistically significant main effect for drug (either in the 30-mg or the 60-mg group) for any of the other variables (at the $p = 0.10$ level). Using pairwise comparison of least-squares means, the 30-mg dose of nimodipine was significantly better than placebo for three of the Buschke measures: long-term retrieval ($p = 0.0553$), long-term storage ($p = 0.0475$), and list learning ($p = 0.0632$).

The degree of difference in pairwise comparisons of least-squares means for the 30-mg group with respect to these three Buschke variables exceeded the extent of further deterioration in the placebo group during this study. This suggests the possibility that the 30-mg dose of nimodipine prevented further deterioration. The 60-mg dose of nimodipine did not show a similar positive effect.

Since both memory and depression were affected in this study, it was suggested that nimodipine may be affecting memory by improving depression. To see whether this was indeed the case the Clinical Global Impression for Depression was examined in relation to Buschke scores in a covariate analysis. The Buschke scores in the depressed 30-mg patient group did not show greater efficacy for memory than in the nondepressed 30-mg patient group.

Safety Results

Treatment with nimodipine appears to be relatively safe. In the total sample of patients 23% had reports of adverse reactions. Eight patients experienced adverse reactions that were considered serious (three on placebo, one on 30 mg nimodipine, four on 60 mg nimodipine). The serious reactions were reported as urinary frequency, fecal impaction, rash, suspicion, agitation, flatulence, and nausea. One patient, with a history of hepatitis, experienced an asymptomatic elevation of liver enzymes. After discontinuing nimodipine (60-mg) the liver enzymes reverted to normal. There were no consistent laboratory results indicating organ toxicity due to nimodipine. No deaths were reported during the study.

Discussion

The findings obtained were, with slight variations, reported similarly throughout the nine study centers. The effectiveness of therapy was based upon improvement in managability as noted in relative's assessment (Relative's Assessment of Global Symptomatology, Activities of Daily Living), improvement on psychometric tests designed to measure changes in cognition, and a global assessment done by the investigator and the patient's family.

The Buschke memory measures of long-term retrieval, long-term storage, and list learning were significantly better than placebo in the 30-mg dose group. The magnitude of difference in the 30-mg group exceeded the magnitude of increase in impairment in the placebo group, i. e., the slight improvement exhibited by changes in these Buschke variables in the 30-mg group was statistically significant. The 60-mg group did not have a positive effect. The placebo group got worse. This suggests the possibility that the 30-mg dose of nimodipine had prevented further deterioration as measured by these three variables.

Effects on patient behavior were reported on a number of variables. For one variable, Clinical Global Impression for Depression: global improvement, the 30-mg dose was significantly better than placebo ($p = 0.029$). No significant effects for drug were found for the other variables.

Since the 30-mg dose had the only significant effect on memory, one wonders whether the drug might be treating depression rather than dementia. Depressed patients in the 30-mg group did not show efficacy when compared to patients in the same group that were not depressed. Therefore, the improvement of depression by nimodipine did not necessarily improve memory. This effect was not seen in the 60-mg group.

Treatment with nimodipine appears to be relatively safe. In the total sample of patients 23% had reports of adverse reactions. There were no consistent laboratory results indicating organ toxicity due to nimodipine. No deaths were reported during the study.

In a poster presented in 1987, we reported that 9 of 13 subjects with Alzheimer's disease showed either improvement or no deterioration in their condition during a 52-week period of open label treatment with nimodipine. In the minimally improved group, worsening difficulties were reported with subjects' behavior that was thought to be either a direct worsening effect on behavior by nimodipine or an indirect behavioral response to an improved cognitive or vigilant state. Severely impaired patients did not respond as well and generally deteriorated despite treatment [1].

Results of nimodipine therapy have been reported in a number of independent double-blind placebo-controlled studies in elderly patients with impaired brain function. These studies were carried out in Germany, Austria, and South America.

Generally these studies reported nimodipine to be superior to placebo as reflected in global assessment and/or psychometric test scores.

One double-blind, placebo-controlled study done in severe Alzheimer's patients showed a moderate improvement in many parameters, such as affect, behavior, and concentration. This effect was noted in a group treated with 60-mg nimodipine (T. Walsh, personal communication). These findings suggest that nimodipine may have a beneficial effect in Alzheimer's disease. This effect may be an ability of the drug to retard the inevitable progression of the disease. The drug may also reduce depression ratings for patients with depression more than for other patients. Future studies would need larger groups of subjects. Since rates of deterioration vary, less severely affected patients should be monitored over long periods of time.

References

1. Baumel B, Eisner L, MacNamara R, Karukin M, Raphan H (1987) Nimodipine in the treatment of primary degenerative dementia. Poster session, international symposium on calcium antagonists, New York Academy of Science, p 96
2. Becker JT, Huff F, Nebes R, Holland A, Boller F (1988) Neuropsychological function in Alzheimer's disease. Pattern of impairment and rates of progression. Arch Neurol March 263–268
3. Bowen DM (1984) Cellular aging: selective vulnerability of cholinergic neurones in human brain. Cell Aging Dev Biol 17: 42–59
4. Buschke H (1973) Selective reminding for analysis of memory and learning. J Verb Learn Verb Behav 12: 543–550
5. Folstein MF, Folstein SE, McHugh PR (1975) Mini-Mental State: a practical method for grading the cognitive state of patients for the clinican. J Psychiatr Res 12: 189–198
6. Frackowiak RSJ, Pozzilli C, Legg NJ, DuBoulay GH, Marshall J, Lenzi GL, Jones T (1981) Regional cerebral oxygen supply and utilization in dementia. Brain 194: 753–778
7. Harris RJ, Branston NM, Symon L, Bayhan M, Watson A (1982) The effects of calcium antagonist, nimodipine, upon physiological response of the cerebral vasculature and its possible influence upon focal cerebral ischemia. Stroke 13: 759–765
8. Katzman R (1976) The prevalence and malignancy of Alzheimer's disease. Arch Neurol 33: 217–218
9. Mabe H, Nagai H, Takagi T, Umemura S, Ohno M (1986) Effect of nimodipine on cerebral functional and metabolic recovery following ischemia in the rat brain. Stroke 17: 501–505
10. Petruk K, West M, Mohr G et al. (1988) Nimodipine treatment in poor grade aneurysm patients: results of a multi-center double blind placebo controlled trial. J Neurosurg 68: 505–517
11. Poeck K (1985) Pathophysiology of emotional disorders associated with brain damage. In: Vinken PJ, Bruyn GW (eds) Demyelinating diseases, no 3. Elsevier, Amsterdam, pp 343–346 (Handbook of clinical neurology, vol 47)
12. Reifler B, Larson E, Teri L, Poulsen M (1986) Dementia of the Alzheimer's type and depression. J Am Geriatr Soc 34(12): 855–859
13. Reisberg B, Ferris SH, De Leon MJ, Crook T (1982) The global deterioration scale for assessment of primary degenerative dementia. Am J Psychiatry 139: 1136–1139
14. Sjogren T, Sjogren H, Lingren AG (1952) Morbus Alzheimer's and morbus Pick. Acta Psychiatr Scand [Suppl] 82: 1–151

Nimodipine for Psychogeriatric Use:
Methods, Strategies, and Considerations Based on Experience with Clinical Trials

N. Schmage, K. Boehme, J. Dycka, and H. Schmitz

Introduction

The problem of diagnosis and questions of methodology in clinical psychogeriatric drug research have been discussed in several recent publications. A volume entitled *Assessment in Geriatric Psychopharmacology* was published in 1983, reviewing and discussing psychometric test instruments (Crook et al. 1983). A comprehensive source book for rating scales and psychometric tests was compiled by Israel et al. (1984). The assessment instruments reviewed are grouped into the three principal dimensions of physical, mental, and social functioning. Depending on the areas covered in one test, unidimensional, two-dimensional, and three-dimensional instruments were further differentiated. The authors emphasize that the physical, mental, and social aspects of health have to be considered as perspectives of functioning rather than as fields of independent activities since in reality they interact and are not separable.

In 1986, the Committee for Geriatric Diseases and Asthenias of the German Federal Health Office, which is in charge of drug regulation affairs, stated its position in a paper on drugs applied in the treatment of age-related or disease-related brain function disorders. It contains guidelines for evaluating the efficacy of drugs in patients with impaired brain functions in old age. The guidelines refer mainly to the organic brain syndrome. Suitable assessment methods are discussed.

More practical methodological aspects were discussed by Müller-Oerlinghausen et al. (1984) and by Kanowski and Hedde (1986) with special regard to the situation in the Federal Republic of Germany (FRG). Lehmann (1984) regards the physician's assessment of the global therapeutic result at the end of the study as a reliable method for detecting differences between treatment groups. He proposes to use global overall ratings as the main outcome measure.

According to the literature three principal categories of psychometric methods are used in psychogeriatric drug research: global overall ratings like the Clinical Global Impressions (CGI), specific rating scales as compiled in the *Source Book of Geriatric Assessment* by Israel et al. (1984), and performance tests which assess memory functions, attention, ability for calculation, for reproduction, for abstraction, and other functions. An interesting aspect is the requirement to include separate judgements on the same patient. Physician, psychologist, nursing staff, and relatives should independently evaluate the therapeutic outcome. It should preferably result in a high

Bergener, Reisberg (Eds.)
Diagnosis and Treatment
of Senile Dementia
© Springer-Verlag Berlin Heidelberg 1989

rate of agreement. A consensus of all raters would be significant to the assessment of therapy (Committee for Geriatric Diseases and Asthesias at BGA 1986).

A standard battery of tests for psychogeriatric patients has not been established yet. Due to different languages, it is difficult to develop test methods on an international basis. However, the attempt should be made whenever possible.

The Term "Organic Brain Syndrome"

Impairment of memory, of ability to concentrate, of thinking, of understanding, of orientation and of affectivity, as well as personality changes are characteristics of an organic brain syndrome (Gertz and Kanowski 1983; Kanowski and Coper 1982; Lauter 1986a, b). The presence of such symptoms in an elderly patient does not directly point to the underlying etiology, but requires differential diagnostic procedures.

After exclusion of other primary or secondary causes which can lead to an organic brain syndrome, a sample of patients can be identified who presumably suffer from underlying vascular or/and primary degeneration in the brain. The more severe forms meet the criteria of dementia, whereas the beginning forms may meet the diagnostic criteria of age-associated memory impairment (Crook et al. 1986). But there seems to be no generally accepted diagnostic label for patients whose symptoms are not severe enough for being classified as dementia. On the Global Deterioration Scale (GDS) these patients would be staged as 2 and 3 (Reisberg et al. 1982). The majority of these patients will not develop dementia (Reisberg et al. 1986).

Most epidemiological studies refer to patients who meet the criteria of dementia. It is not known whether degenerative and vascular processes have the same distribution in patients with organic brain syndrome as in patients with the diagnosis of dementia. Furthermore, computerized tomography (CT) scans are normally not a routine method of examination for these patients.

The term organic brain syndrome, as used here, covers demented and non-demented patients. A moderate organic brain syndrome is equivalent to mild dementia which is characterized by the presence of beginning disorientation.

Clinical Studies with Nimodipine

Nimodipine has been investigated in several open and double-blind studies in patients suffering from chronic organic brain syndrome. The following overview includes studies which were completed and reported by the beginning of 1988.

Nimodipine was superior to treatment with placebo in nine double-blind studies. Two double-blind studies showed no difference between the treatment groups. These 11 studies included 391 patients treated with nimodipine and 398 patients treated with placebo. The duration of treatment was between 8 and 16 weeks. In seven of the double-blind studies the patients received 3×30 mg nimodipine or placebo. The patients were treated partly during hospitalization and partly as outpatients. Each study was individually evaluated, whereby the treatment advantage of nimodipine could be shown to be statistically significant in nine studies. The data were then

Table 1. Battery of psychometric tests used to demonstrate efficacy

Method	Number of studies
Global Improvement Rating	11
Symptoms scale (ad hoc)	9
SCAG	6
Trail Making Test (ZVT-G)	7
BGP/NOSIE	3
Bf-S	2
SKT	2
Benton Test	2
Recall of numbers	4
Revision test	2
Reaction time and errors	1
Flicker fusion	1

SCAG, Sandoz Clinical Assessment Geriatric Scale; BGP Beurteilungsskala für geriatrische Patienten; NOSIE Nurses' Observation for Inpatient Evaluation; Bf-S Befindlichkeitsskala; SKT Syndrom-Kurztest

collected in a data pool. The separate studies involved a battery of various psychometric tests which were used to demonstrate efficacy (Table 1).

The global improvement rating, symptoms scale, Sandoz Clinical Assessment Geriatric Scale (SCAG), and Trail Making Test were the methods most frequently applied in the individual studies. The three principal categories of psychometric methods mentioned above (global overall result, symptoms rating scales, and performance tests) are represented with these measurements. The symptoms scale was developed as an ad hoc scale which was applied before the SCAG gained wider use in the FRG, but was also included in clinical drug trials in parallel to the SCAG in order to assess further symptoms.

As the individual data from these studies are stored in a clinical data pool, it seemed worthwile to reanalyze the global overall rating, SCAG, and Trail Making Test after combining the results of all 11 studies. As mentioned before, the physician's assessment of the global therapeutic result at the end of treatment is regarded as a reliable method for detecting differences between 2 treatment groups (Lehmann 1984) and was applied to all 11 studies.

The proportion of patients that do not respond or show deterioration is much larger in the placebo group than in the nimodipine group (Fig. 1).

The SCAG scale is a measure of the impairment of cognitive, affective, social, and somatic functions. It has been found to be a suitable instrument for supervizing the course of treatment (CIPS 1986, Committee for Geriatric Diseases and Asthenias at BGA 1986; Kanowski and Hedde 1986; Müller-Oerlinghausen et al. 1984). The SCAG scale was used in 6 of the 11 double-blind studies. The differences of the total score against baseline after 1, 2, and 3 months of treatment were compared. The reduction in the SCAG total scores after treatment is much more pronounced in the patients treated with nimodipine than in those treated with placebo. The effects under nimodipine increase with time (Fig. 2).

The Trail Making Test in the modified geriatric version has proven its value as a measure of performance. It is particularly suitable for gerontopsychiatric questions.

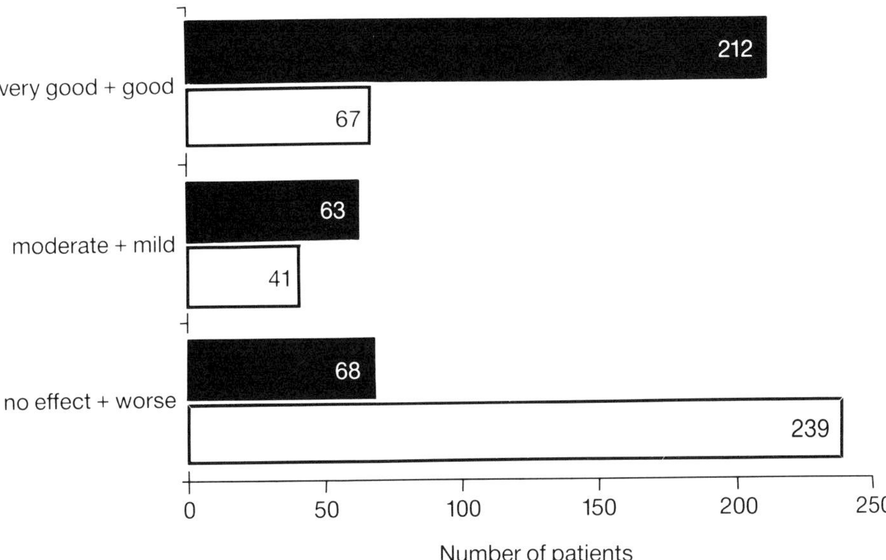

Fig. 1. Global therapeutic results after 2–4 months of treatment with nimodipine *(solid bars)* as compared with placebo *(open bars)*

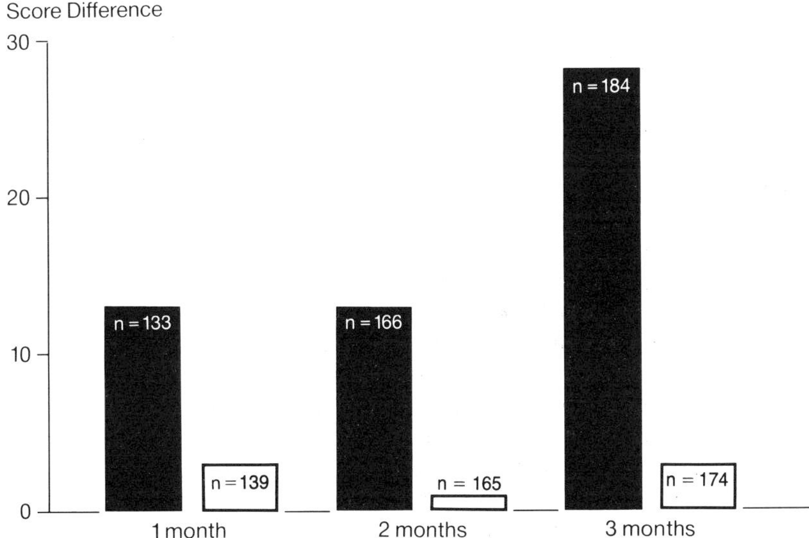

Fig. 2. SCAG scores against baseline (medians) after treatment with nimodipine *(solid bars)* as compared with placebo *(open bars)*

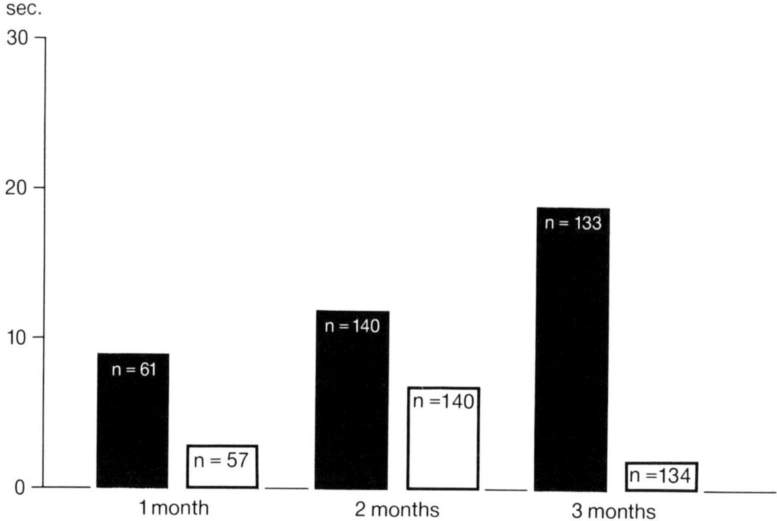

Fig. 3. Trail Making Test (ZVT-G Oswald) results against baseline (medians) after treatment with nimodipine *(solid bars)* as compared with placebo *(open bars)*

Plausible correlations between test performance, self-assessment, and assessment of personality were reported (Oswald et al. 1981). Differences in the performance against baseline after 1, 2, and 3 months of treatment were compared. The improvement in performance is much more pronounced under treatment with nimodipine than under treatment with placebo. Again, the effects under nimodipine increase with time (Fig. 3).

Such pool analyses of all studies can be conducted in order to condense data and to show trends like the time dependence of the drug effect. On the other hand, retrospective overviews are a valuable tool to generate further hypotheses or new aims.

Further analyses of single items of the SCAG and the symptoms scale revealed that impairment of memory and concentration improved more under nimodipine treatment than under placebo. As impairment of cognitive functions is a core characteristic of dementia, this finding should not be ignored. But instead of only using rating scales, the data pool results should be confirmed by a performance test. As the Syndrom-Kurztest (SKT) measures memory and attention, this test was chosen for the two studies reported by Kanowski et al. (1988) and by Fischhof et al. (1988).

The use of different assessment methods in psychogeriatric clinical trials makes it difficult to compare studies directly with each other. Therefore ways should be found to make the criteria and methods of clinical trials more transparent and comparable on an international basis. Applying the Mini-Mental State Examination (MMS; Folstein et al. 1975) and the GDS (Reisberg et al. 1982) to the study reported by Fischhof et al. (1988) was an attempt to approach this problem.

On the GDS these patients were staged between 3 and 6. As required by the inclusion criteria, the SKT total score was 9 or higher. The MMS scores did not exceed 23.

Table 2. Means, medians, and ranges of the MMS according to stage of GDS in the Fischhof et al. (1988) study

GDS	n	Mean	Median	Range
3	12	19.33 ± 2.35	20	15–22
4	48	18.17 ± 2.21	19	12–23
5	53	14.45 ± 2.71	14	10–21
6	31	11.00 ± 0.93	11	10–14

MMS, mini-mental state examination; GDS, global deterioration scale

Table 3. Means, medians, and ranges of the SKT according to stage of GDS in the Fischhof et al. (1988) study

GDS	n	Mean	Median	Range
3	12	15.25 ± 3.28	15	11–21
4	48	17.10 ± 2.92	17	10–22
5	53	20.75 ± 3.02	21	14–26
6	31	23.81 ± 1.58	24	18–26

SKT, Syndrom-Kurztest; GDS, global deterioration scale

Means, medians, and ranges of the MMS and SKT per stage on the GDS in the Fischhof et al., 1988 trial with the inclusion criteria described are shown on Tables 2 and 3. With increasing GDS stage, the MMS scores decrease, whereas the SKT scores increase. The Pearson correlation coefficient between MMS and SKT was -0.82.

Such investigations may assist in comparing the degree of agreement and range of coverage between different methods in psychogeriatric clinical research.

Tolerability

The clinical data pool is also a tool of drug safety surveillance. Therefore all data on adverse reactions from noncontrolled and from double-blind studies are collected, coded, and stored.

Nimodipine was, in general, well tolerated. Sensations of heat or warmth and reddening of the skin occurred more often under nimodipine than under placebo. In cases of elevated initial values, a blood pressure reduction due to nimodipine can be observed. Headache, gastrointestinal complaints, and nausea are more nonspecific and are also reported after placebo treatment.

Future Clinical Trials

Future clinical trials with nimodipine in psychogeriatric patients should be longer in duration (6 months or preferrably longer). Patients with less severe dementia may show some improvement. But also a stabilizing effect in comparison to placebo will be regarded as a therapeutic aim. Separate studies should include primary degenerative dementia and multi-infarct dementia.

Therapeutic Aims

Therapeutic aims should be expressed in terms of appropriate outcome criteria. Table 4 gives an overview on possible criteria. Treatment strategies in dementia should cover different areas and dimensions. Distinct functions, affectivity, and complex behavioral aspects have to be considered.

Table 4. Overview of possible outcome criteria

Clinical global impressions (CGI)
Cognitive functions
Affectivity
Orientation
Activities of daily living
Degree of independence (autonomy)
Social interaction
Quality of life and satisfaction

The more complex the outcome criterion is, like activities of daily living (ADL), the more difficult it is to develop suitable instruments which reflect the real situation. Such difficulties led to the development of a variety of rating scales for ADL. Israel et al. (1984) give many examples.

Drug therapy will not be the only factor responsible for therapeutic results. It should be discussed what a drug certainly is unable to do and what it may do.

Drug therapy cannot create a stimulating environment which is important for well being, activities of daily living, and social interactions. Also, behavioral training, physiotherapy, and personal contact to the patient cannot be replaced by administering a drug. The therapeutic setting has to be considered a cofactor in clinical drug trials. This fact will certainly influence the results of multi-center trials. The BGA Committee for Geriatric Diseases and Asthenias (1986) has also indicated that the therapeutic setting is an important contributing factor.

Drug therapy may be able to return certain potentials to the patient, like availability of or accessibility to cognitive functions. But the conversion of these potentials into more complex areas and dimensions of human life will also depend on the therapeutic setting. These conditions have to be considered when discussing questions of therapeutic relevance.

Conclusion

Nimodipine is a promising drug for elderly demented and nondemented patients. Several double-blind studies have shown that the drug may be effective for cognition deficits, performance, affectivity, and social integration. The conclusion can be drawn that the results from several behavioral experiments in animals are significant for predicting the clinical effects of nimodipine.

References

CIPS (1986) Internationale Skalen für Psychiatrie. Beltz Test, Weinheim

The Committee for Geriatric Diseases and Asthenias at BGA (1986) Impaired brain functions in old age. AMI-Heft 1/86, Institut für Arzneimittel des Bundesgesundheitsamtes, Berlin

Crook T, Bartus RT, Ferris SH, Whitehouse P, Cohen GD, Gershon S (1986) Age-associated memory impairment. Proposed diagnostic criteria and measures of clinical change – report of a National Institute of Mental Health work group. Dev Neuropsychol 2: 261–276

Crook T, Ferris S, Bartus R (eds) (1983) Assessment in geriatric psychopharmacology. Powley, New Canaan

Fischhof PK, Wagner G, Littschauer L, Apecechea M, Hiersemenzel R, Röhmel J, Rüther E, Hoffmeister F, Schmage N (1988) Therapeutic results with nimodipine in primary degenerative dementia and multi-infarct dementia. In: Bergener M, Reisberg B (eds) Diagnosis and treatment of senile dementia, pp 350–359

Folstein MF, Folstein SE, McHugh PR (1975) Mini-Mental State. A practical method for grading the cognitive state of patients for the clinician. J Psychiat Res 12: 189–198

Gertz H-J, Kanowski S (1983) Die Therapie der senilen Demenz vom Alzheimer-Typ und der Multi-Infarkt-Demenz. Nervenarzt 54: 444–459

Israel L, Kazerevic D, Sartorius N (eds) (1984) Source book of geriatric assessment. Karger, Basel

Kanowski S, Coper H (1982) Das hirnorganische Psychosyndrom als Ziel pharmakologischer Beeinflussung. In: Bente D, Coper H, Kanowski S (eds) Hirnorganische Psychosyndrome im Alter. Springer, Berlin Heidelberg New York

Kanowski S, Fischhof P, Hiersemenzel R, Röhmel J, Kern U (1988) Wirksamkeitsnachweis von Nootropika am Beispiel von Nimodipin – ein Beitrag zur Entwicklung geeigneter klinischer Prüfmodelle. Z Gerontopsycholpsychiatr 1: 35–44

Kanowski S, Hedde JP (1986) Arzneimittel für die Indikation „Hirnorganisch bedingte Leistungsstörungen". In: Dölle W, Müller-Oerlinghausen B, Schwabe U (eds) Grundlagen der Arzneimitteltherapie. Entwicklung, Beurteilung und Anwendung von Arzneimitteln. Bibliographisches Institut Mannheim, pp 154–171

Lauter H (1986a) Persönlichkeitsveränderung, organische. In: Müller C (ed) Lexikon der Psychiatrie. Springer, Berlin Heidelberg New York, pp 512–513

Lauter H (1986b) Psychosyndrom, organisches. In: Müller C (ed) Lexikon der Psychiatrie. Springer, Berlin Heidelberg New York, pp 567–568

Lehmann E (1984) Practical and valid approach to evaluate the efficacy of nootropic drugs by means of rating scales. Pharmacopsychiatry 17: 71–75

Müller-Oerlinghausen B et al. (1984) Psychopharmaka, Hypnotika und Nootropika. In: Kuemmerle H-P, Hitzenberger G, Spitzy KH (eds) Klinische Pharmakologie. Ecomed, München, pp 47–66 (III-2.1)

Oswald WD, Herrmann WM, Busch H (1981) Der Zahlen-Verbindungstest ZVT-G und Zusammenhänge mit Selbstbeurteilung, Alltagsaktivitäten und Persönlichkeitsmerkmalen bei N = 56 Probanden zwischen 63 und 84 Jahren. In: Oswald WD, Fleischmann UM (eds) Experimentelle Gerontopsychologie. Beltz, Weinheim, pp 90–104

Reisberg B et al. (1982) The global deterioration scale for assessment of primary degenerative dementia. Am J Psychiatry 139: 1136–1139

Reisberg B et al. (1986) Longitudinal course of normal aging and progressive dementia of the Alzheimer's type: a prospective study of 106 subjects over a 3.6 year mean interval. Prog Neuropsychopharmacol Biol Psychiatry 10: 571–578

Subject Index